Applied
Cardiovascular Physiology

Applied Cardiovascular Physiology

2nd Edition

G. R. KELMAN

M.D., Ph.D., M.R.C.P., D.I.C.
Until recently *Professor of Human Physiology*
University of Aberdeen

BUTTERWORTHS
London–Boston
Sydney–Wellington–Durban–Toronto

THE BUTTERWORTH GROUP

UK

Butterworth & Co (Publishers) Ltd
London: 88 Kingsway, WC2B 6AB

AUSTRALIA

Butterworths Pty Ltd
Sydney: 586 Pacific Highway,
Chatswood, NSW 2067
Also at Melbourne, Brisbane, Adelaide
and Perth

SOUTH AFRICA

Butterworth & Co (South Africa) (Pty) Ltd
Durban: 152–154 Gale Street

NEW ZEALAND

Butterworths of New Zealand Ltd
Wellington: 26–28 Waring Taylor Street, 1

CANADA

Butterworth & Co (Canada) Ltd
Toronto: 2265 Midland Avenue,
    Scarborough, Ontario, M1P 4S1

USA

Butterworths (Publishers) Inc
Boston: 19 Cummings Park,
    Woburn, Mass. 01801

First published 1971
Second edition 1977

ISBN 0 407 10881 5

© Butterworth & Co (Publishers) Ltd 1977

Library of Congress Cataloging in Publication Data

Kelman, George Richard.
    Applied cardiovascular physiology.

    Bibliography
    Includes index.
    1. Cardiovascular system.   I. Title.   [DNLM:
    1. Cardiovascular system—Physiology.   WG102 K29a]
    QP101.K4 1977   612'.1   76-48048
    ISBN 0-407-10881-5

Printed in Great Britain by
The Whitefriars Press Ltd, London and Tonbridge

Preface to Second Edition

When asked to prepare this second edition of *Applied Cardiovascular Physiology* I approached the task with a certain amount of trepidation because I was aware of the enormous amount of relevant new material which has appeared in the literature in the last five years. The task of distilling this vast amount of new information was a daunting one, and inevitably I have had to be selective in what I have chosen to include.

In preparing this edition I have tried to react to reviewers' comments on the first edition: the section on myocardial contractility has been completely rewritten; the section on the cardiovascular system during general anaesthesia has been much modified; and new material has been added where this seemed appropriate, including chapters on hypertension, and on the body's cardiovascular response to exercise.

In the first edition I complained about a lack of quantitative information about the human cardiovascular response to the stress of acute disease. To a large extent this situation still obtains: cardiovascular measurements on intact humans have not become any easier, nor has human variability become any less, and ethical committees are (quite rightly) scrutinizing human experiments more and more closely. But perhaps this lack of quantitative information is not as important as it once seemed, because our understanding of the pathophysiology of various disease processes has increased enormously in recent years; and we are now able to direct our therapy so as to aid a patient's recovery, while leaving it to the body's homeostatic mechanisms to deal with the quantitative details.

Of the new material in this edition the studies of Eger and his colleagues on the effects of various anaesthetic agents on the cardiovascular system of normal adults, and the studies of Prys-Roberts and his colleagues on myocardial contractility, and on anaesthesia in hypertensive patients are particularly worthy of comment. These important investigations have considerably helped our understanding of the response of the human cardiovascular system to the stress of general anaesthesia; they are reviewed here in full.

The style is little changed from the previous edition: as before I have tried to give a reference for most facts which are unexpected, or controversial, or just interesting; but I have not attempted to be comprehensive. A new feature which I hope will be helpful is the inclusion at the end of each chapter of a list of recommended further reading, consisting of selected review articles on the chapter's main topic(s).

In general all units have been converted into the SI system. But in the case of blood pressures and blood gas tensions I have resisted the temptation to adopt the foolishness of the kilopascal, taking the view that, since most blood pressures are still measured with mercury or saline manometers, the appropriate units are mm Hg or cm H_2O as appropriate, and not k Pa.

G. R. KELMAN

Preface to First Edition

This monograph on *Applied Cardiovascular Physiology* is intended to be a distillate of the vast literature available on this subject. It is aimed primarily at anaesthetists—both trainee and practising—but it is hoped that it may also prove valuable to physicians in other specialities, and to senior undergraduates studying physiology, particularly those preparing for a medical career.

The book was planned as a companion volume to Professor Nunn's *Applied Respiratory Physiology*. When I began to write it, however, it soon became apparent that my approach must be considerably less quantitative than John Nunn's. Respiratory physiology has developed until it is a fairly precise science; this is not, unfortunately, the case with cardiovascular physiology, where the approach is still often qualitative rather than quantitative.

We know that hyperventilation causes a reduction of cerebral blood flow, but we do not know the precise relationship between Pa_{CO_2} and cerebral perfusion in a given patient. We know that cardiac output is reduced in shock and that tissues are then deprived of blood as the body attempts to maintain perfusion of vital organs such as the heart and brain, but we do not know the blood flow through, say, the splanchnic circulation of a severely shocked patient, nor do we know at what level of tissue blood flow ischaemic damage is likely to occur.

The last two decades have seen the development of many exciting new techniques for the measurement of cardiac output and tissue blood flow, and for the estimation of parameters such as 'myocardial contractility'. Some of these techniques are suitable only for use in experimental animals, but some are applicable to intact man. I have discussed these latter techniques in considerable detail; indeed some would consider that I have devoted a disproportionately large amount of space to the techniques of measurement. I make no apology for this. I believe that only by making measurements on anaesthetized patients and on patients in intensive therapy units shall we improve our understanding of the physiological disturbances which occur in disease, and thereby reduce mortality in seriously ill patients. Accurate measurements can be made only by those who fully understand the techniques which they use.

Of the studies which are currently being made into the physiology of human anaesthesia the work of the Philadelphia School deserves special mention. Although some would question the ethics of anaesthetizing healthy subjects purely for experimental purposes, there is no doubt that these measurements are carefully and competently made, and that the results obtained are of inestimable value in the quantification of the response of the human cardiovascular system to general anaesthesia. As a result of these and similar studies it is likely that a future edition of this book, published in say 1980, will be considerably more quantitative in its approach than the present first edition, and will be closer in scientific style to Nunn's *Applied Respiratory Physiology*.

I predict that by 1980 quantitative information will be available about cardiac output and the perfusion of most, if not all, important organs under a variety of conditions both physiological and pathological. Such information must surely help the clinician to improve patient care, both in the surgical wards and operating theatres and in the intensive therapy unit. Clinical Physiology has come a long way in the past decade; I am sure, however, that what we have seen so far is just a beginning.

As regards references I have not attempted to be comprehensive. I have, however, tried to cite an authority for most statements which I have made where these appear to be controversial, unexpected or just interesting. I have tried also to include as many review articles as possible, because I believe that this is what most readers require.

I should like to acknowledge the help of my many colleagues, clinical and preclinical, who have given up their leisure time to read sections of my manuscript. I, of course, remain responsible for any errors that remain.

G. R. KELMAN

Contents

Chapter 1   Physical Principles

The cardiovascular system is responsible for the transport of nutrients, waste products and hormones round the body. It carries oxygen from the lungs to the tissues, and carbon dioxide in the opposite direction; it carries food materials from the gut to the tissues, and waste products from the tissues to excretory organs such as the liver and kidney. The circulatory system is concerned also with the transport of hormones from their production site to their target organ(s), and with the transport of heat from internal organs to the body surface, where it is dissipated by convection, conduction, evaporation and radiation.

An understanding of the factors which affect blood flow round the body and through its peripheral tissues must be based on at least an elementary knowledge of the physical laws governing the flow of liquids along tubes—on the science of hydrodynamics.

The rate at which a liquid flows down a tube depends on the pressure difference between the ends of the tube and the resistance to flow. If the tube has rigid walls, the liquid is Newtonian (*see* page 6), and the flow is streamline or laminar (*see* page 6), the flow rate is directly proportional to the pressure difference. This situation is analogous to the flow of electricity down a wire, when the current is directly proportional to the electrical potential difference between the ends of the wire, and inversely proportional to its electrical resistance. When the walls of the tube are not rigid, when the liquid is non-Newtonian, or when the flow is not streamline, the situation is more complex (*see* page 9).

PRESSURE

In physical terms pressure is defined as force per unit area. There is unfortunately no universally accepted unit in which this quantity is measured; the unit varies from science to science, and even within the same science, according to custom and tradition.

Units

In the non-medical sciences pressures are now usually measured in SI units, the SI unit for pressure being the $N\,m^{-2}$ (the pascal, Pa). In physiology and medicine, however, it is more customary to use the secondary units, mm Hg or cm H_2O (or cm saline). 1 mm Hg = 133.3 Pa = 0.013 k Pa, therefore a blood pressure of 120/80 mm Hg becomes approximately 16.0/10.6 k Pa. In keeping with normal clinical practice blood pressures in this book are given in mm Hg or cm H_2O, as appropriate.

Pressure of a column of liquid

The pressure exerted by a column of liquid of density ρ kg m^{-3} and of height h m is $g\rho h$ N m^{-2}, where g is the acceleration due to gravity (9.81 m s^{-2}).

This equation is derived as follows (*Figure 1.1*). Consider a column of liquid of area A m^2, density ρ kg m^{-3} and height h m. The mass of this column is ρhA kg; and the downward force (mass times acceleration) is therefore $g\rho hA$ newtons, that is, the force per unit area exerted by the column is $g\rho h$ N m^{-2}.

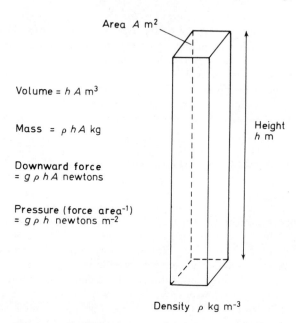

Area A m^2

Volume = $h\,A$ m^3

Mass = $\rho\,h\,A$ kg

Downward force
= $g\,\rho\,h\,A$ newtons

Pressure (force area^{-1})
= $g\,\rho\,h$ newtons m^{-2}

Height
h m

Density ρ kg m^{-3}

Figure 1.1.   *Pressure exerted by a vertical column of liquid. Pressure equals $g\rho h$ N m^{-2}*

The pressure exerted by a column of mercury 1 mm high is therefore equal to $9.81 \times 13\,600 \times 0.001 = 133.3$ N m^{-2}; the pressure exerted by a column of saline 1 cm high (density 1.04×10^3 kg m^{-3}) is $9.81 \times 1040 \times 0.01 = 101.9$ N m^{-2}.

Arterial blood pressure is usually measured by a mercury manometer, and is therefore expressed in the units, mm Hg; central venous pressure (*see* page 277) is usually measured by a saline manometer and is expressed in the units, cm saline. These two units are, of course, readily interconvertible; mm Hg may be converted to cm saline by multiplication by the factor $133.9/101.9 = 1.31$; cm saline may be converted into mm Hg by multiplication by the factor 0.76. The specific gravity of blood is approximately 1.06, therefore 1 mm Hg is roughly equal to 1.3 cm of blood ($1.31 \times 1.04/1.06$).

The torr

Some schools of physiology and anaesthesia prefer to measure pressures in torr (after Torricelli) rather than in mm Hg. A torr is defined as 1/760 of a standard atmosphere, which is itself defined as 1.013×10^5 N m^{-2}. For all practical purposes the torr is numerically identical to mm Hg, the difference being less than 2 parts in 10 million.

The advantage of the torr over the mm Hg is not at all clear, especially as in practice most manometers are calibrated against a column of mercury. Of course, under abnormal gravitational acceleration, mercury manometers are inaccurate, and, under conditions of zero *g*, unusable.

Physiological consequences of pressure differences due to gravity

The pressure difference which exists between the top and bottom of a column of liquid has important physiological implications.

Systemic blood pressure

The mean hydrostatic pressure at the aortic root is approximately 100 mm Hg; the vertical distance between the heart and the feet is some 130 cm. In the erect posture, therefore, the pressure in the *dorsalis pedis* artery exceeds that in the aorta by approximately 130 cm of blood or 100 mm Hg (*Figure 1.2*).

Similar considerations apply to the venous system, although here the situation is modified by the presence of valves which tend to break up the column of blood and prevent its full pressure being transmitted to the feet. This is particularly the case during exercise when the 'muscle pump' (*see* page 123)

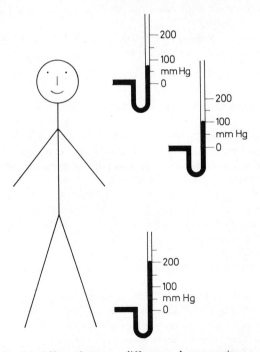

Figure 1.2. Effect of pressure differences due to gravity

propels blood centrally, and thus maintains a low peripheral venous pressure. If these valves become incompetent, the pressure in the vessels of the lower extremity may increase to such an extent that dependent oedema may form.

In the case of the cerebral circulation the situation is reversed. The arterial pressure transmitted to the brain is equal to the pressure in the aortic root minus the pressure of the column of blood lying between the aorta and the brain. In the erect posture this pressure is approximately 30 cm of blood, therefore cerebral arterial pressure is decreased by approximately 25 mm Hg. Similarly, on the venous side, the pressure in the jugular bulb is reduced below that in the right atrium.

Pulmonary circulation

The physiological consequences of gravitational pressure differences are greatest in the lungs. The mean pressure in the pulmonary artery is only about 17 mm Hg and, in the erect posture, this is comparable in magnitude to gravitational pressure differences between different regions of the lung. In the apices of the lungs the pulmonary arterial pressure is reduced to such an extent that it is below the pressure in the surrounding alveoli; the vessels therefore collapse (*see* page 163) and blood flow is greatly reduced. Lower down pulmonary blood flow occurs only during systole, when the pulmonary arterial pressure momentarily exceeds the surrounding alveolar pressure. But in the basal regions of the lung the pulmonary arterial pressure is increased by the effects of gravity, therefore the vessels are widely dilated, and a large proportion of the cardiac output flows through this region. The physiological consequences of the uneven distribution of pulmonary blood flow are discussed in detail by Nunn (1969); *see also* page 163.

In the supine or prone position the effects of gravity on the pulmonary circulation are reduced because the antero-posterior diameter of the thorax is less than its vertical height.

Variations of effective values of g

Under most conditions *g*, the acceleration due to gravity, is constant. In space exploration, however, this is not necessarily the case; and during aviation the body may be exposed to additional accelerations which may exaggerate the effects discussed in the previous paragraphs.

In a space capsule orbiting the earth the pull of the earth's gravity is counter-balanced by centrifugal force; the effective value of *g* is zero, and pressure differences due to gravitation effects are abolished. Conversely, in an aeroplane at the bottom of a loop, the centrifugal force acts in concord with the pull of the earth's gravity, and the effective value of *g* may be several times the normal. This may have dramatic physiological consequences because the pressure due to the column of blood between the heart and the brain may exceed the pressure generated by the heart. The cerebral blood vessels therefore collapse and the pilot suffers first 'black out' due to impaired retinal circulation, and then total loss of consciousness from cerebral ischaemia. A trained pilot is said to be able to retain consciousness when exposed to 4 *g* of footward acceleration (Whittingham, 1938).

Pressure measurement

It is necessary to take account of gravitational pressure differences when measuring arterial or venous blood pressure. If the measurement site is appreciably above or below the zero reference level, the pressure will be measured inaccurately, unless appropriate corrections are made. In the case of the arterial blood pressure, errors from this cause are small in relation to the actual pressure and are commonly ignored. When measuring venous pressure, however, where the actual pressure is relatively low, it is always necessary to take account of vertical distances between the zero reference level and the measuring manometer.

The usually chosen reference level is the right atrium. The position of this chamber may be determined with complete accuracy only by radiography, but it may be located for most purposes by assuming that it lies at the level of the sternal angle midway between the anterior and posterior thoracic walls (Winsor and Burch, 1945).

FLOW

Streamline versus turbulent flow

The flow of a liquid down a tube may be either streamline (laminar) or turbulent. With the former, the particles of liquid move parallel to the long axis of the tube; there is no component of motion across the tube (*Figure 1.3a*). In the case of turbulent flow, however, movement occurs both parallel and perpendicular to the long axis of the tube. Energy is wasted in causing this transverse motion which does not, of course, contribute to movement along the length of the tube (*Figure 1.3b*) therefore the resistance to flow is greater than

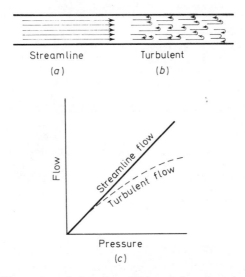

Streamline
(*a*)

Turbulent
(*b*)

Flow

Streamline flow

Turbulent flow

Pressure
(*c*)

Figure 1.3. Streamline versus turbulent flow. With turbulent flow the resistance to flow increases with the flow rate; with streamline flow the resistance is constant

under streamline conditions (*Figure 1.3c*). This effect is greatest at high flow rates when turbulence is most marked. Streamline flow may be treated mathematically more conveniently than turbulent flow.

Streamline flow

Under streamline conditions, the resistance to flow of a liquid along a tube depends on the geometry of the tube and the liquid's viscosity. The simplest case to treat is the flow of a liquid which has a viscosity independent of flow rate (a Newtonian liquid) along a rigid tube. Although neither of these conditions applies strictly to blood flow in the body, it is convenient to consider the simple case first before considering the more complicated case of the flow of a non-Newtonian liquid, such as blood, through a network of distensible vessels.

Parabolic velocity profile

With streamline flow the particles of liquid move parallel to the long axis of the tube but not all at the same velocity. The most peripherally situated layers move slowly; the liquid in the centre moves rapidly. The outermost layer, which lies in contact with the tube wall, is stationary. As a consequence the resistance to flow is little influenced by the condition, whether rough or not, of the tube's lining.

Mathematically, it may be shown that, if the force exerted by one layer of liquid on another layer moving relative to it is proportional to the velocity gradient at the junction between the layers, and the flow velocity at the tube wall is zero, then the velocity profile across the tube is parabolic (*Figure 1.4a*). A proof of this relationship is given in Appendix I.

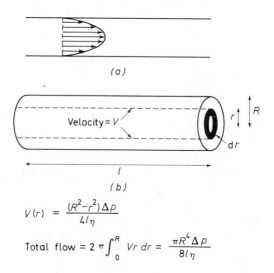

(a)

(b)

$$V(r) = \frac{(R^2 - r^2)\Delta p}{4l\eta}$$

$$\text{Total flow} = 2\pi \int_0^R Vr\, dr = \frac{\pi R^4 \Delta p}{8l\eta}$$

Figure 1.4. Streamline flow and the Hagen-Poiseuille relationship

The Hagen-Poisseuille Relationship

Given this parabolic relationship between flow velocity and distance from the tube centre, it is a simple matter to calculate the total flow along the tube per unit time.

Consider a thin annulus of liquid of radius r and thickness dr (*Figure 1.4b*) flowing along a tube of radius R and length l under the influence of a pressure difference ΔP. The velocity (V) of this layer of liquid is given (*see* Appendix I) by

$$V = (R^2 - r^2)\, \Delta P / 4l\eta$$

where η is the (constant) viscosity. This layer represents a volume flow per unit time of $V.2\pi r dr$. The total flow rate ($\dot{Q}$) may, therefore, be derived mathematically by simple integration as:

$$\dot{Q} = 2\pi \int_0^R Vr\, dr = 2\pi\Delta P \int_0^R \left(\frac{R^2 r - r^3}{4l\eta}\right) dr$$

$$= 2\pi\Delta P \left[\frac{2R^2 r^2 - r^4}{16l\eta}\right]_0^R$$

$$= \frac{\pi R^4 \Delta P}{8l\eta}$$

This is the familiar Hagen-Poisseuille formula.

It is perhaps useful to point out that, except for the dependence of flow on the fourth power of the radius, this formula is what would be expected from common sense considerations. It is reasonable to expect that, the wider the tube, the greater the flow, and conversely that, the longer the tube, or the more viscous the liquid, the less the flow caused by a given pressure difference. The factor $\pi/8$ is simply a proportionality constant, the π arising because the cross-section of the tube is circular.

Poisseuille's law only applies strictly when the length of the tube considerably exceeds its radius. The parabolic velocity profile is not fully developed for a distance along the tube equal to several times its radius. At the start of the tube, energy is expended in accelerating liquid from rest. More important, the law does not apply to the flow generated by a pulsatile pressure difference such as that which causes blood flow in the large arteries; in this case flow is not steady, therefore energy is expended in accelerating the blood, first in one direction, then in the opposite direction.

Pulsatile flow

Womersley (1955) showed that the flow of a Newtonian liquid through a rigid tube under the influence of a pulsatile pressure difference $A \cos wt$ could be expressed by the equation:

$$\dot{Q} = \frac{\pi R^4}{\eta} kA \cos(wt + \phi),$$

where $\dot{Q}$, R and η have the same significance as in the non-pulsatile case (*see* page 7).

ϕ is the phase angle between pressure and flow, and

k is a complex parameter whose value depends on the physical properties of the tube, the kinematic viscosity of the liquid (viscosity/density) and the frequency of oscillation.

The sigma effect

In very small vessels, erythrocyte diameter becomes comparable to vessel diameter. Under these circumstances it is no longer appropriate to speak of streamline flow; calculations based on the assumption that the blood velocity profile is parabolic across the vessel are incorrect, because the velocity now varies across the tube in a stepwise fashion rather than continuously. This phenomenon is sometimes called the 'sigma effect' since in the calculations considered on page 7 the integration ($\int$) must be replaced by a simple summation (Σ) because flow occurs as a finite and small number of cylinders moving parallel to the long axis of the vessel.

The sigma effect may account, in part, for the fact that the apparent viscosity of blood is reduced in small vessels (*see* page 11).

Transition between streamline and turbulent flow

If the mean velocity exceeds a certain critical value, flow ceases to be streamline and becomes turbulent. Turbulent flow is characterized by eddy formation (*Figure 1.3b*). These eddies represent a waste of energy, which is expended in accelerating liquid across the tube, therefore the pressure difference required to produce a given flow per unit time is greater than it would be if the flow were laminar.

Critical velocity and Reynold's number

The critical velocity (Vc) above which turbulent flow occurs is given by the formula:

$$Vc = \text{Re } \eta/\rho d,$$

where η is the viscosity,

ρ is the density of the liquid,

d is the diameter of the tube, and

Re a constant called Reynold's number.

Reynold's number is a so-called 'dimensionless number', that is its numerical value is independent of the system of units used for its calculation, provided of course that these units are compatible.

The above formula may also be written as $Vc = \text{Re } v/d$, where v, the kinematic viscosity, is the ratio of viscosity to density (η/ρ). (It is interesting that the kinematic viscosity of air at body temperature is approximately four times that of blood. Air flow in a bronchus may, therefore, be streamline at a velocity which is considerably above the critical velocity for blood in a vessel of comparable size.)

Under most circumstances, Reynold's number has a value in the region of 2000, although it varies somewhat with the conditions of measurement. When flow is pulsatile the critical velocity may be exceeded with a Reynold's number which is considerably less than 2000.

Is Reynold's number normally exceeded?

The linear blood flow velocity is normally greatest in the aorta. It falls rapidly as the total cross-sectional area of the vascular system increases down the arterial tree (*see Figure 3.6,* page 81). The critical velocity is therefore most likely to be exceeded in the aorta during ventricular systole. Is it? Assuming a value for Re of 2000, an aortic cross-sectional diameter of 2 cm, a blood density of 1000 kg m^{-3}, and a blood viscosity of 0.003 N s m^{-2} (a value fairly representative of the vast literature on this subject), it may be calculated that the critical velocity should be in the region of 0.3 m s^{-1}. If blood flow were steady, then, with a cardiac output of 5 l min^{-1} and an aortic cross-sectional area of 3 cm^2, the mean aortic flow velocity would be approximately 0.3 m s^{-1}, a value which is just about the critical velocity. However, aortic blood flow is pulsatile, not steady, therefore the peak velocity must exceed the critical velocity for a considerable proportion of the cardiac cycle. This is particularly likely to be so during exercise.

McDonald (1952) showed, by means of high-speed cinematography, that the blood flow in a rabbit's aorta was laminar during early systole, but became turbulent later in the cardiac cycle. Moreover, the turbulence, once developed, persisted well into diastole. McDonald (1960) concluded 'there is thus little doubt that there will always be marked turbulence in systole in the human aorta'; recent work has, however, cast doubt on this conclusion (*see* Recommmended Further Reading).

RESISTANCE TO FLOW

The resistance to blood flow through a given vessel equals the ratio of the driving pressure divided by the resulting flow. The situation is therefore analogous to the flow of electricity along a wire, in which case electrical resistance equals current divided by the electrical potential which causes it.

When flow is streamline, resistance is independent of the flow rate and depends only on blood viscosity and the physical dimensions of the blood vessel (resistance = $8l\eta/\pi R^4$ —*see* page 8). With turbulent flow, however, the resistance depends also on the flow rate; the higher the flow the higher is the resistance (*see Figure 1.3c,* page 5).

When considering flow through distensible vessels it is necessary also to take account of the fact that blood vessel diameter may be increased by an increase of transmural pressure, so that resistance to flow depends on the intravascular pressure as well as on the pressure difference between the ends of the tube (*see* page 12).

In general, changes of flow resistance are brought about by changes in vascular diameter, as considered in the next chapter. Because of the fourth-power relationship, a small change of vascular calibre can result in a large change in resistance to flow.

Blood viscosity

The subject of blood viscosity is complex. Not only is blood a non-Newtonian fluid, that is, it has a viscosity which varies with the velocity gradient or shear-rate, but, in addition, its apparent viscosity varies with the diameter of the tube along which flow is occurring. These peculiar properties arise from the fact that blood is a heterogenous system, composed of a suspension of relatively rigid particles, the erythrocytes, suspended in a colloidal solution, the plasma. Plasma itself behaves as an almost perfect Newtonian fluid with a viscosity somewhat greater (1.5 to 2 times) than that of pure water.

Units

In the older cgs system of units, viscosity is measured in poise (after Poisseuille). A liquid with a viscosity of 1 poise transmits a force of 1 dyne cm^{-2} when the velocity gradient is $1\,cm\,s^{-1}\,cm^{-1}$. By a fortunate accident the viscosity of water at $20.2^{\circ}C$ (room temperature in America if not in Britain!) is 0.010 000 poise.

In practice it is usually more convenient to express the viscosity of biological fluids in centipoise rather than in poise (1 centipoise = 0.01 poise). In SI units 1 centipoise equals $1 \times 10^{-1}\,N\,s\,m^{-2}$.

Effect of shear-rate

The variation of blood viscosity with shear-rate (*see* page 11) may be investigated by a cone-in-cone viscometer (Dintenfass, 1964). This consists of two concentric cones with a thin layer of blood between them. The outer cone rotates so that viscous drag tends to rotate the inner cone; and the viscosity is calculated from the transmitted force. Dintenfass (1963) has shown that, measured in this way, blood viscosity increases sharply at low shear-rates (*Figure 1.5b*); and this finding is thought to be due to red cell aggregation. At moderate to high shear-rates blood is some four or five times as viscous as water (Fahraeus and Lindquist, 1931).

Dintenfass has also made the observation (Dintenfass, Julian and Miller, 1966) that blood viscosity at very low shear-rates (0.01 to 0.1 s^{-1}) varies during the female menstrual cycle to a considerably greater extent than can be explained by any concomitant change of haematocrit ratio. The physiological significance of this interesting variation is at present uncertain; but it may conceivably be related to the well-recognized thrombogenic effects of the contraceptive 'Pill'.

Viscosity in vivo

Paradoxically blood *in vivo* behaves as if it were less viscous than it is *in vitro* (Djojosugito et al., 1970), and also much more as a Newtonian fluid. The reason for this experimental finding is complex, and not entirely clear; but it is thought to depend to a large extent on the fact that the apparent viscosity of blood decreases in small diameter vessels, probably as a result of axial streaming.

When a particulate suspension such as blood flows along a narrow tube the suspended particles tend to aggregate in the central stream, leaving a layer of relatively clear fluid peripherally. The viscosity of the peripheral fluid is less than that of the central stream, whereas it is at the periphery that the velocity gradient is greatest. As a result, the increased viscosity of the cell-rich fluid in the centre of the stream does not compensate fully for the relatively low viscosity of the peripheral layers; and the apparent overall viscosity is therefore reduced. The effect is especially marked in small vessels; it also increases with increasing flow rate, when axial streaming is accentuated.

The dependence of the apparent blood viscosity on vessel diameter may also be due partly to the 'sigma effect' (*see* page 8).

Plasma skimming.   The axial streaming of erythrocytes just mentioned may be of physiological importance outwith its effect on blood viscosity. In small vessels the peripheral layers of blood are relatively cell-free, therefore fluid which enters side branches leaving the main vessel at right angles tends to have a relatively low haematocrit ratio. This process is known as 'plasma skimming', and may account, in part, for the fact that the haematocrit ratio of blood from peripheral tissues is less than that from larger vessels (*see* page 272). Plasma skimming may also be concerned in the phenomenon of autoregulation (*see* page 92).

As would be expected, blood viscosity increases with the haematocrit ratio (Whittaker and Winton, 1933). The relationship is not, however, linear; the

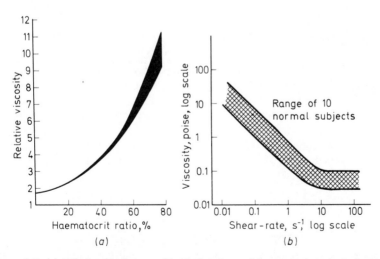

Figure 1.5. (a) Relationship between blood viscosity and haematocrit ratio (redrawn from Whittaker and Winton, 1933). (b) Relationship between blood viscosity and shear-rate (based on Dintenfass, 1963)

effect is more marked at high haematocrit ratios (*Figure 1.5*). As the ratio increases the relatively rigid erythrocytes become more closely packed together, with the result that the force needed to deform the blood rises steeply, as does its viscosity.

This dependence of viscosity on haematocrit ratio is important in anaemia and polycythaemia. The hypertension and tendency to intravascular thrombosis which may accompany the latter condition are due at least partly to increased blood viscosity.

The increase of blood viscosity at high haematocrit ratios (and the consequent increased resistance to flow) more than offsets the increased oxygen carrying-capacity of the blood. Conversely, the decreased oxygen carrying-capacity which characterizes anaemia more than offsets the decreased resistance to blood flow. It has been shown that in trauma the survival rate can be optimized by keeping the haematocrit ratio within reasonably normal limits (Crowell, Ford and Lewis, 1959; Greenbaum, 1969).

Vascular distensibility

Blood vessels are not rigid tubes; their diameter depends on the pressure difference between their lumen and their surroundings. The flow of a Newtonian liquid through a *rigid* tube is directly proportional to the pressure difference between the ends of the tube, but does *not* depend on the actual value of the intravascular pressure. It is of no consequence if the pressures at the two ends of the tube are 10 and 20 mm Hg or 110 and 120 mm Hg; the flow is identical in the two cases. With a distensible tube, however, the resistance to flow decreases when the transmural pressure difference is increased by an increase of intravascular pressure. This effect is seen particularly in the pulmonary circulation, where the increased intravascular pressures at the lung bases cause a decreased vascular resistance and a consequent overperfusion (*see* page 163). It is of some importance also in increasing blood flow to the legs in the upright posture.

Laplace's law

With a distensible tube the relationship between wall tension (*T*) and transmural pressure (*P*) is given by Laplace's law, $T = PR$, where *R* is the radius

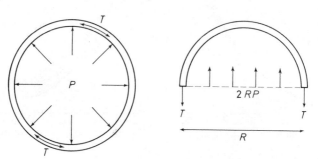

At equilibrium, $T = RP$

Figure 1.6. Derivation of Laplace relationship. Wall tension = RP

of the vessel. Tension is measured in the units, force per unit length, and is the force which would tend to distract the edges of a longitudinal slit in the vessel wall.

Laplace's law may be deduced as follows (*Figure 1.6*). Consider a cylindrical blood vessel of radius R and unit length. The transmural pressure (P) may be thought of as a force tending to split the cylinder into two halves. The force on the upper half is pressure times area, that is, $P \times 2R$; at equilibrium, this force is just balanced by the force ($2T$) due to wall tension. Laplace's relationship follows immediately.

Wall tensions

The probable wall tensions of some human blood vessels have been calculated by Burton (1972) from anatomical and physiological data (*Table 1.1*). The

Table 1.1   VASCULAR PRESSURES, SIZES AND WALL TENSIONS
(FIGURES FROM BURTON, 1972)

Type of vessel	*Mean pressure* (mm Hg)	*Radius* (cm)	*Wall tension* (N m^{-1})
Aorta	100	1.3	1.7×10^2
Other arteries	90	0.5	6.0×10^1
Arterioles	60	1.5×10^{-2} to 6.2×10^{-3}	1.2 to 5.0×10^{-1}
Capillaries	30	4×10^{-4}	1.6×10^{-2}
Venules	20	1×10^{-3}	2.6×10^{-2}
Veins	15	2×10^{-2}	4.0×10^{-1}
Vena Cava	10	1.6	2.1×10^1

tension varies enormously with vessel size from 170 N m^{-1} in the aorta to only 1.6×10^{-2} N m^{-1} in the capillaries. This decrease of tension is due mainly to the great decrease of vessel diameter between the aorta and the capillaries and, to a much lesser extent, to the accompanying decrease of intravascular pressure. The radius of the aorta is approximately 1.25 cm, that of the capillaries is several thousand times smaller; whereas the intravascular pressures are roughly in the ratio five to one. The transmural pressure in the veins is less than that in the capillaries; this reduction of pressure is, however, more than compensated for by the increase of vessel diameter, therefore the venous wall tension is considerably greater than that in the capillaries.

As would be expected, there is a marked correlation between the physical strength of a blood vessel wall and tension which it is required to withstand. The tension in the capillary walls is small, therefore their mechanical strength is correspondingly reduced, even though the transmural pressure is still fairly large (20 mm Hg). The veins are considerably stronger than the capillaries, despite the fact that venous pressure is only a few mmHg.

Relationship between vascular volume and intravascular pressure

The experimentally determined relationship between transmural pressure and the volume of a segment of blood vessel is non-linear (*Figure 1.7a*). With the aid of Laplace's law this curve may be manipulated to give the relationship between wall tension and vessel diameter (*Figure 1.7b*). The extra tension generated by a given degree of distension increases the more the vessel is distended; the more the vessel wall is stretched the greater is its resistance to further stretch. This is the opposite of what happens with, say, a piece of rubber when the degree of stretch caused by a given increase of extending force is nearly constant until the elastic limit is approached, at which point the material suddenly becomes very extensible, and if extended further, breaks.

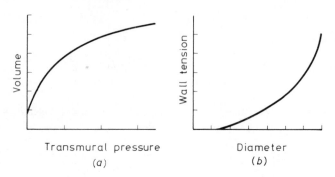

Figure 1.7. (a) Relationship between transmural pressure difference and the volume of a closed segment of blood vessel (diagrammatic). (b) Relationship between vessel diameter and wall tension (diagrammatic)

The non-linear relationship between stress and strain exhibited by the blood vessel wall is due to the special arrangement of its elastic and collagen fibres (Roach and Burton, 1957). Each of these materials alone shows a roughly constant modulus of elasticity (ratio of stress to strain), but the fibres are arranged in such a way that the unstretched lengths of the two components are different. The length of the elastic fibres is less than that of the relatively inextensible collagen fibres, therefore initial distension of the vessel is taken up by the extensible elastic tissue, whereas further distension is progressively resisted by the inextensible collagen. Young's modulus for elastin is approximately 3×10^3 N m^{-1}; that of collagen is in the region of 1×10^6 N m^{-1} (Burton, 1972). A simple analogy is to compare the blood vessel wall to a rubber hose, surrounded by a tough canvas sheath.

Graphical analysis of relationship between transmural pressure and vessel diameter

For a given blood vessel, Laplace's law predicts that, at any given transmural pressure, there is a linear relationship between wall tension and vessel diameter. This straight line may be superimposed on *Figure 1.7b* to intersect the experimentally determined relationship between diameter and tension (*Figure 1.8*). The relationship between wall tension and vessel diameter is, therefore, represented by two curves and, since for any individual blood vessel, there can be but a single diameter at a single wall tension, the actual values of these variables must be represented by the point at which the curves cross—point

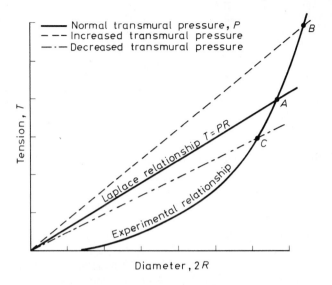

Figure 1.8. Relationship between blood vessel diameter and wall tension, superimposed on the Laplace relationship. Point A represents the equilibrium situation with a normal transmural pressure. Points B and C represent, respectively, the equilibrium situation with an increased or a decreased transmural pressure

A. (This is rather analogous to the way in which the relationship between cardiac output and right atrial pressure may be simultaneously represented by two curves (*see* Chapter 4).)

If transmural pressure is increased (dotted line in *Figure 1.8*), the system comes to a new equilibrium—point B—with a greater vessel diameter and a greater wall tension; a fall of transmural pressure takes the system to point C, with smaller vascular diameter and decreased wall tension.

Critical closing pressure

As would be expected from the previous section, it is found experimentally that the resistance to blood flow through a given vascular bed depends on the transmural pressure. At high pressures the resistance is low; as the pressure is decreased the resistance rises. In many cases, however, as the transmural pressure is decreased there comes a pressure at which flow ceases abruptly, that is, at which the vascular resistance becomes infinite. The pressure at which this phenomenon occurs is known as the 'critical closing pressure'.

Although there is considerable dispute about the precise nature of critical closure, Burton (1972) has suggested that there may be a simple physical explanation (*see* Appendix II). This simple explanation, however, assumes that the active tension which is generated by smooth muscle remains constant as the muscle shortens, and also that no tension is expended in deforming the vessel wall. Neither of these assumptions is, of course, strictly true; but nevertheless it seems that critical closure can in fact be demonstrated experimentally under some circumstances.

Vessels such as arterio-venous anastomoses possess very little elastic tissue; under these circumstances critical closure should occur with a very small active tension, that is, the vessel should be virtually either fully open or fully closed. This situation is ideal for by-pass channels such as arterio-venous shunts, but is less satisfactory in the case of most other vessels, where fine control of vascular diameter is necessary. This is provided by having an appropriate combination of elastic tissue and smooth muscle in the vessel wall, when vascular calibre can be finely adjusted by graded changes of smooth muscle tension.

VESSELS IN PARALLEL AND SERIES

The systemic circulation consists of a number of vascular networks connected in parallel between the arterial and venous sides of the circulation. Each vascular bed consists of a large number of separate vessels connected partly in parallel and partly in series. Although the complexity of the complete circulation, or indeed of any individual organ, is too great to permit an analysis of the ways in which the individual vessels are combined to form any given vascular bed, the way in which the total resistance to flow varies when vessels are connected in series or parallel must be briefly considered.

Vascular resistances in parallel

By analogy with Ohm's law, the resistance (R) of several vessels with individual resistances R_1, R_2, R_3, ... connected in parallel (*Figure 1.9a*) is given by $1/R = 1/R_1 + 1/R_2 + 1/R_3 + \ldots$

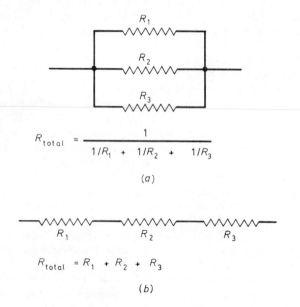

$$R_{total} = \frac{1}{1/R_1 + 1/R_2 + 1/R_3}$$

(a)

$$R_{total} = R_1 + R_2 + R_3$$

(b)

Figure 1.9. Resistances in parallel and in series

Vascular resistances in series

Similarly, the total resistance (R) of the same vascular resistances connected in series (*Figure 1.9b*) is $R = R_1 + R_2 + R_3 + \dots$

PHYSIOLOGICAL APPLICATIONS OF PHYSICAL PRINCIPLES

Vascular resistance

The vascular bed of an individual organ may be considered to consist of a succession of vessels of varying diameter interconnected in series. The total cross-sectional area of the bed increases from the arteries to the capillaries, and then decreases again towards the veins (*see* Chapter 3, page 81). Despite this marked increase of total cross-sectional area due to vascular branching, there is a considerable increase of total vascular resistance as vessel diameter decreases. This is a consequence of the marked dependence of resistance on vascular diameter predicted by the Hagen–Poisseuille relationship (*see* page 7).

The majority of flow resistance presented by any given vascular bed lies in the arterioles and precapillary sphincters (*see* page 79). The pressure drops which occur in the vascular network are, therefore, greatest in these vessels (*Figure 1.10*). The mean intravascular pressure decreases by only a few mm Hg in the large arteries, but has fallen to approximately 30 mm Hg at the arterial ends of the capillaries, and to approximately 12 mm Hg at their venous ends. Tissue blood flow is, therefore, readily regulated by changes in the calibre of these small vessels (*see* Chapter 3).*

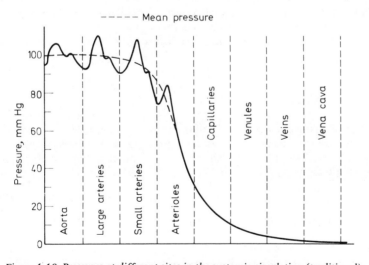

Figure 1.10. Pressures at different sites in the systemic circulation (traditional)

*When the peripheral vascular tree is widely dilated however, as in exercise, the pressure drop may be more evenly distributed between its different segments.

Resistance versus capacitance vessels

The arterioles are sometimes referred to as resistance vessels in contradistinction to the veins, the main function of which is storage of blood (capacitance vessels). The distinction between these two types of vessel is considered further in Chapter 3.

Total peripheral resistance (TPR)

The systemic vascular system comprises a number of vascular beds connected in parallel between the arterial and venous reservoirs (*Figure 1.11*). The total peripheral resistance (TPR) is, therefore, less than the resistance presented by any single organ. TPR is given approximately by the equation:

$$TPR = \text{mean arterial pressure/cardiac output}$$

and is, therefore, in the units, driving pressure/flow, for example mm Hg min l^{-1}.

With representative values for cardiac output ($5 \ l \ min^{-1}$), and mean arterial pressure (100 mm Hg) the total systemic peripheral resistance is approximately 20 mm Hg min l^{-1}. This value may be converted to the more fundamental (but considerably less convenient) units, N s m^{-5}, by multiplication by the factor 8000.* Under normal circumstances TPR is approximately equal to 160 000 N s m^{-5}, or 1600 dyne s cm^{-5} in the older units.

The peripheral resistance unit (PRU)

Vascular resistance may also be expressed in so-called peripheral resistance units (PRU). A resistance of one PRU permits a flow of 1 ml s^{-1} at a driving pressure of 1 mm Hg. With normal values of cardiac output and mean arterial pressure, TPR is approximately 1.2 PRU. Its value may, however, vary considerably under different pathophysiological conditions from about 0.25 to 4 PRU.

Pulmonary vascular resistance

In the pulmonary circulation the arterial pressure is approximately one-sixth to one-fifth of that in the systemic system, although the blood flow is the same; the calculated total resistance of the pulmonary circulation is therefore approximately 0.2 PRU or 30 000 N s m^{-5} (300 dyne s cm^{-1}).

Aortic input impedance

Under conditions of pulsatile flow it is not strictly correct to treat resistance to blood flow as just the ratio of the mean during pressure to the resulting flow.

---

*1 mm Hg = 133.2 N m^{-2} (*see* page 1), 1 l min^{-1} = 1/60 l s^{-1}, therefore a resistance of
1 mm Hg min l^{-1} = 133.3 × 60
= 8000 N $s^{-1} m^{-5}$

Under pulsatile conditions energy has to be expended in producing the pulsatile components of the flow; and under these circumstances it is more correct to speak about a hydraulic impedance, rather than just a simple resistance to flow (Bergel and Milner, 1965).

Such a hydraulic impedance describes the ratio of oscillatory pressure to oscillatory flow at a series of frequencies which are integral multiples (harmonics) of the fundamental heart frequency: it also takes account of phase

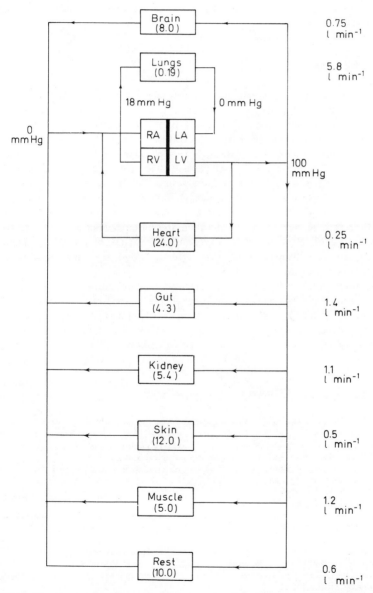

Figure 1.11. Flow, pressure and vascular resistance in various regions of the cardiovascular system. Figures in brackets are resistance in PRU (figures from Wade and Bishop, 1962)

differences between pressure and flow. The DC (or zero frequency) term of such an impedance is the same as the more usually measured total peripheral resistance, that is the ratio of the mean driving pressure/mean blood flow, as just considered.

A technique for determining the aortic input impedance in experimental animals has recently been described by Gersh and his colleagues (1972). Since it appears, however, that 90 per cent of the impedance to systemic blood flow is normally due to the DC component (that is to the ratio of mean driving pressure/mean flow) the advantages of this far-from-trivial calculation are disputable.

Tissue blood flow

The cardiac output is divided between the various tissues in inverse proportion to their individual vascular resistances (*Figure 1.11*). If the resistance of one tissue decreases there is a fall of total peripheral resistance, and therefore, if cardiac output remains constant, a decrease of arterial blood pressure (*see* page 213). If cardiac output is constant, however, a decrease of vascular resistance in one tissue must result in increased flow to that tissue and decreased flows to the remaining tissues. This decrease occurs despite the fact that vascular resistance in the deprived tissue remains constant; it is due to the fall of arterial pressure which occurs when total peripheral resistance decreases in the presence of a constant cardiac output. Usually, when the vascular resistance of one tissue is decreased, cardiac output is simultaneously increased, or there is compensatory vasoconstriction elsewhere, so that arterial blood pressure tends to remain constant (*see* page 213).

Although the concepts which determine the relationship between pressure and flow in individual vascular beds are theoretically straightforward, confusion often arises clinically, when it is sometimes difficult to define whether pressure or flow is the more important cardiovascular parameter under any given set of circumstances. This important topic is considered further in Chapter 9.

RECOMMENDED FURTHER READING

Anon (1975). 'Haemorheology, Blood-flow, and Venous Thrombosis.' *Lancet* ii, 113

Barra, J. P. (1969). 'Blood Rheology—General Review.' *Bibl. Haemat.* 33, 377

Bayliss, L. E. (1962). 'The Rheology of Blood.' In *Handbook of Physiology, Circulation*, Vol. 1, p. 137. Washington; American Physiological Society

Bond, A. G. and Parsons, R. S. (1970). 'Haemodilution and Plasma Proteins during Anaesthesia.' *Br. J. Anaesth.* 42, 1113

Charm, S. E. and Kurland, G. S. (1972). 'Blood Rheology.' In Bergel, D. H. *Cardiovascular Fluid Dynamics*, p. 158. London; Academic Press

Chien, S., Usami, S., Dellenback, R. J. and Gregerson, M. I. (1970). Shear-dependent Interaction of Plasma Proteins with Erythrocytes in Blood Rheology. *Am. J. Physiol.* 219, 143

Folkow, B. and Neil, E. (1971). *Circulation*, ch. 4. Oxford University Press

Haynes, R. H. (1961). 'The Rheology of Blood.' *Trans. Soc. Rheol.* 5, 85

Hershey, S. G. (1974). 'General Principles and Determinants of Circulatory Transport.' *Anesthesiology* 41, 116

Hill, D. W. (1972). *Physics Applied to Anaesthesia*, 2nd edn, chps 3 and 5. London; Butterworths

Magora, F. (1974). 'Blood Viscosity.' *Br. J. Anaesth.* **46,** 347

Wayland, H. (1967). 'Rheology and the Microcirculation.' *Gastroenterology* **52,** 342

Wells, R. E. (1964). 'Rheology of Blood in the Microvasculature.' *N. Engl. J. Med.* **70,** 832 and 889

Whitmore, R. J. (1968). *Rheology of the Circulation.* Oxford; Pergamon

Chapter 2   The Heart

The circulation of a viscous liquid such as blood through a series of vascular networks requires a source of energy to overcome frictional resistance. This energy is provided by the rhythmic contraction of the heart; it is the function of this organ to convert the chemical energy contained in complex food materials, such as glucose and fatty acids, into the mechanical energy which drives the blood round the circulatory system. Part of the energy imparted to the blood during ventricular systole is stored temporarily as potential (pressure) energy in the elastic reservoir ('Windkessel') formed by the aorta and other large elastic arteries (*see* page 73). This stored energy enables the pulsatile cardiac contraction to provide a tissue blood flow which is almost constant throughout the cardiac cycle.

The pumping action of the heart depends on the ability of its muscular fibres to shorten. Contraction of cardiac muscle is initiated by a wave of electrical depolarization which originates normally in the sino-atrial (S-A) node and then spreads centrifugally throughout the myocardium. This propagated wave of depolarization is known as an action potential, and its arrival at a given region of the myocardium causes the muscle there to contract to the best of its ability. In order to contract satisfactorily the myocardium needs an adequate supply of oxygen and nutrients and a satisfactory biochemical environment. An efficient cardiac pump needs a suitable geometrical arrangement of muscle fibres and a series of competent one-way valves, so that when the muscle fibres contract to compress the blood contained in the ventricles, this blood is expelled into the aorta and pulmonary arteries.

The normal cardiac output—the amount of blood which leaves the left ventricle each minute—is in the region of $5 \, l \, min^{-1}$ in a healthy adult male and somewhat less in an adult female. As explained in Chapter 4, however, cardiac output depends under normal circumstances more on the state of the peripheral circulation than on the efficiency of the cardiac pump.

Cardiac energy requirements

Since the mean aortic blood pressure is approximately 100 mm Hg, and the mean pulmonary artery pressure about 17 mm Hg, the amount of work done by the heart in expelling a stroke volume of 70 ml is approximately 1 joule.* (This calculation assumes that ventricular stroke work equals the product of stroke volume and mean arterial pressure; it therefore neglects the work done in

---

*1 mm Hg = 133.3 N m^{-2} (*see* page 1). Therefore left ventricular stroke work = 70 ml x 100 mm Hg = $70 \times 10^{-6} \times 100 \times 133.3$ N m = 0.93 N m. Total cardiac work therefore ≏ 1 N m = 1 joule. In the older units 1 joule ≏ 0.1 kp m.

imparting kinetic energy to the blood as it leaves the ventricle. When cardiac output is high, as during exercise, the velocity of blood flow is increased also; the kinetic component may then form an appreciable proportion of the total cardiac work, so that its neglect may no longer be justifiable.)

Since at rest the heart beats roughly 70 times a minute, its work rate is approximately 1 watt ($J\ s^{-1}$) compared with a total body energy expenditure at rest of perhaps 1500 Cal* 24 h^{-1}, that is, with a work rate of approximately 70 watts. Resting myocardial oxygen consumption is approximately 27 ml min^{-1} (Wade and Bishop, 1962), that is, 12 per cent of the total body oxygen consumption, whereas myocardial blood flow forms a much smaller proportion (4 per cent) of the total. Because of this disparity between blood flow and oxygen consumption, the oxygen content of coronary venous blood is considerably less than that from the rest of the body (*see* page 144).

CARDIAC MUSCLE

Functionally, the cardiac muscle may be divided into three relatively distinct masses—the atrial muscle, the ventricular muscle and the specialized muscular tissue which is concerned with generation of the cardiac action potential, and with its transmission throughout the myocardium. Although anatomically the ventricular muscle may be divided into several partially discrete bundles, from the physiological point of view these are so intertwined that they are best considered as a single entity.

The atrial and ventricular muscle masses are inserted into the fibrous framework of the heart, which also provides attachment for the one-way valves on which depends the functional efficiency of the cardiac pump. The atrial and ventricular muscles are separated anatomically and physiologically except where they are joined by the atrio-ventricular (A-V) bundle, which pierces the framework of the heart in the vicinity of the fibrous part of the interventricular septum.

The anatomy of the conducting system is considered in more detail on page 30.

Cardiac muscle compared with smooth and skeletal muscle

Cardiac muscle has properties which are, in many ways, intermediate between those of voluntary skeletal muscle and involuntary smooth muscle. Like skeletal muscle, cardiac muscle shows marked cross-striations under the microscope, but, like smooth muscle, it is not under voluntary control. Functionally, it resembles smooth muscle in undergoing spontaneous rhythmic contractions, in contracting as a single unit (a syncytium), and in the fact that both the frequency of contraction and the tension produced are influenced by hormones such as acetylcholine and noradrenaline. The rate of contraction of cardiac muscle is, however, closer to that of skeletal than to that of smooth muscle.

*1 Cal ≙ 4.1 kJ.

Histology (Naylor, 1963)

Although the myocardium is functionally a syncytium, its individual fibres are, in fact, histologically distinct; the cells are separated by a continuous membrane, the sarcolemma. If longitudinal sections of cardiac muscle are examined under the light microscope, the fibres are seen to be crossed in a stepwise fashion by dark bands called intercalated discs (*Figure 2.1a*). These are formed by the apposed membranes of adjacent cells with a small intervening space 100 to

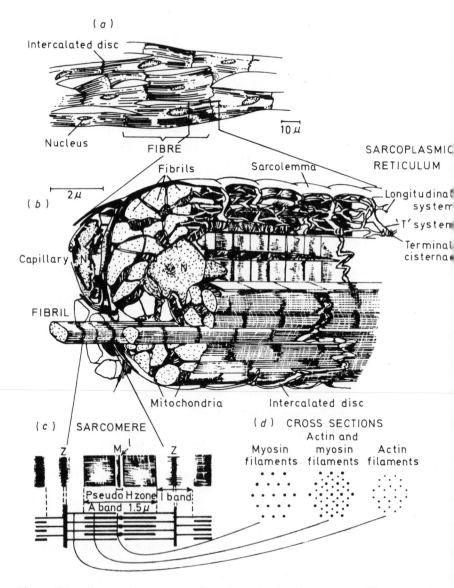

Figure 2.1. Microscopic structure of cardiac muscle (from Braunwald, Ross and Sonnenblick, 1967)

200 Å wide.* The myofibrils (*see* below) of adjacent fibres do not cross this space.

In places, the apposed membranes are fused across the disc at so-called tight junctions. It has been suggested that these junctions are regions of low electrical resistance, through which current can pass from one cell to another, thus permitting the muscle to contract as a single unit. Woodbury and Crill (1961), for example, found that the resistance of an intercalated disc was less than 5 ohm-cm compared with 2000 ohm-cm for normal myocardial membrane.

The sacroplasmic reticulum

The other striking histological feature of cardiac muscle is its sarcoplasmic reticulum (*Figure 2.1b*). This is involved in the complex coupling processes which link electrical depolarization of the cell membrane and mechanical contraction of the muscle proteins (*see* page 42). It consists of a network of anastomosing, membrane-lined intracellular channels running in close proximity both to the actual contractile units (the myofibrils) and to the cell surface.

The reticulum has two distinct components, the transverse and longitudinal tubules. In the region of the Z-lines (*see* page 50). the sarcolemma is invaginated into the interior of the cell; these invaginations are called transverse tubules (the 'T' system). The other component consists of a series of anastomosing longitudinal tubules running close to the myofibrils. Although the components are histologically separate, it is probable that the close proximity of the transverse system, filled with extracellular fluid, and the longitudinal system, filled with intracellular fluid, facilitates transmission of electrical excitation from the exterior of the cell to the immediate vicinity of the contractile apparatus.

The contractile proteins

The contractile proteins are regularly arranged in a way which gives the myocardial cell its typical striated appearance under the microscope. The basic contractile unit is the myofibril which is approximately 0.5 μm in diameter, and consists of interdigitating filaments of the proteins, actin and myosin. Under the electron microscope, the myofibril is seen to be crossed by a regular series of light and dark bands caused by the arrangement of the contractile proteins (*Figure 2.1c*).

In the centre of each light band (I-band) there is a thin, dark line—the Z-line. The region between two Z-lines is known as a sarcomere, and is shown diagrammatically in the lower half of *Figure 2.1c*. The dark A-Band, in the centre of the sarcomere, is formed by thick filaments of myosin; the I-band is composed of thinner filaments of actin, attached on either side of the Z-line. The interdigitation of the actin and myosin filaments is shown diagrammatically in transverse section in *Figure 2.1d*.

The actin and myosin filaments are linked by chemical bonds, the nature of which is uncertain. According to the sliding filament hypothesis of muscular contraction (Huxley and Hanson, 1954), activation of the contractile proteins

*1 A = 1 x 10^{-10} m

produces forces which cause the thick and thin filaments to slide past one another, thus decreasing the inter-Z distance, and shortening the muscle (*see also* page 50).

Cardiac muscle cells contain more mitochondria than do the cells of skeletal muscle. This finding is probably related to the fact that cardiac muscle is required to produce energy almost continuously, whereas skeletal muscle is inactive for much of the time. Also in keeping with its high metabolic rate is the large number of capillaries found in cardiac muscle—almost one per fibre.

Polarization of the myocardial cell membrane

As is the case with other tissues, the interior of myocardial cells is electrically negative with respect to the surrounding extracellular fluid. If a microelectrode is slowly advanced into the myocardium, the electrical potential at its tip suddenly decreases by approximately 80 mV as the cell membrane is penetrated. Provided the electrode tip is sufficiently small (less than 1 μm), however, the cell continues to function normally, and it is possible to study changes of transmembrane potential in response to electrical stimulation, or to changes of extracellular environment.

Intra- and extracellular ionic concentrations

The transmembrane electrical potential difference depends on differences of ionic composition between the intracellular and extracellular fluids, and on the differential permeability of the cell membrane to various ions. The observed concentration differences depend on the activity of a sodium–potassium 'pump', *see*, for example, Marsden (1970). This pump actively extrudes sodium ions from the cell and moves potassium ions in the opposite direction; both of these ionic movements occur against gradients of electrochemical potential and therefore require the expenditure of metabolically-produced energy.

The precise concentrations of potassium, sodium and chloride ions in mammalian cardiac muscle cells are not known, but they probably do not differ greatly from the values which have been determined in cardiac muscle fibres of lower animals (*Table 2.1*). The intracellular concentration of potassium is

Table 2.1   INTRACELLULAR AND EXTRACELLULAR CONCENTRATIONS OF Na$^+$, K$^+$ AND Cl$^-$ AND MEMBRANE EQUILIBRIUM POTENTIAL PREDICTED BY NERNST EQUATION (FIGURES FROM WOODBURY, 1962)

	Intracellular fluid (mmol l^{-1})	*Extracellular fluid* (mmol l^{-1})	ΔE (mV) *predicted by Nernst equation*
Sodium (Na$^+$)	18	110	46
Potassium (K$^+$)	90	2.5	−90
Chloride (Cl$^-$)	15	112.5	−50

Experimentally-determined   transmembrane   potential   averaged   over   one   cardiac cycle $\simeq$ 50 mV considerably greater than its extracellular concentration: the opposite is the case with sodium, which is concentrated extracellularly. Intracellularly, potassium ions are electrically balanced by phosophate and large organic anions such as protein; in the extracellular fluid sodium is balanced mainly by chloride and bicarbonate.

The intracellular potassium concentration is some 30 times greater than its extracellular concentration; and since the membrane is relatively permeable to potassium there is a marked tendency for potassium ions to diffuse down the concentration gradient into the extracellular fluid, leaving the interior of the cell negatively charged. This intracellular negativity tends to prevent further movement of potassium out of the cell so that an equilibrium is established in which the forces which are tending to extrude potassium ions from the cell are just balanced by the electrical potential difference which is tending to hold potassium ions intracellularly. (This is not to say, of course, that no exchange of potassium occurs across the membrane at equilibrium; radioactive isotope studies have shown that there is a constant movement of ions both into and out of the cell. The net transfer rate is, however, zero: the equilibrium is dynamic, not static.)

In contrast to the situation with potassium, the cell membrane appears to be relatively impermeable to sodium ions. The intra-extracellular sodium ratio therefore has very little effect on the resting membrane potential.

The Nernst equation

It may be shown (Woodbury, 1965) that the chemical force tending to cause diffusion of a substance out of a cell equals $RT \ln c_i/c_o$, where

R is the gas constant,

T is the absolute temperature, and

c_i and c_o are, respectively, the concentrations inside and outside the cell.

(ln means logarithm to the base e—natural or Naperian logarithm.)

The electrical force tending to keep an ion inside the cell is $zF\Delta E$, where

z is the valency (number of charges) of the ion,

F is Faraday's constant, and

ΔE is the electrical potential difference across the membrane.

At equilibrium, in the absence of active transport, these two forces must be equal, that is:

$$zF\Delta E = RT \ln c_i/c_o,$$

or

$$\Delta E = \frac{RT}{zF} \ln c_i/c_o.$$

At 37°C the value of RT/zF for a univalent cation is such that the previous equation may be rewritten as:

$$\Delta E = 60 \log c_i/c_o,$$

where ΔE is measured in mV and log means logarithm to the base 10. This is the Nernst equation (*Figure 2.2*).

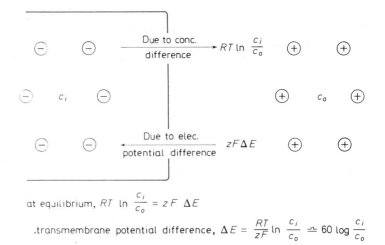

at equilibrium, $RT \ln \dfrac{c_i}{c_o} = zF \, \Delta E$

.transmembrane potential difference, $\Delta E = \dfrac{RT}{zF} \ln \dfrac{c_i}{c_o} \simeq 60 \log \dfrac{c_i}{c_o}$

Figure 2.2. Derivation of Nernst equation (for explanation see text)

If the electrical potential difference across the membrane is zero ($\Delta E = 0$), it follows that, at equilibrium, log c_i/c_o must also be zero, that is, $c_i = c_o$. (The logarithm of 1 to any base is zero). Similarly, if the substance under consideration is uncharged ($z = 0$), it follows that log c_i/c_o must again be equal to zero, that is, c_i must equal c_o, whatever the potential difference across the membrane. Both of these conditions agree with what would be predicted by common sense.

Active transport compared with passive distribution

The Nernst equation may be used to determine whether an ion is distributed across a membrane purely in accordance with physico-chemical principles, or whether some 'active' process is involved. If the ion is distributed purely passively, the value of ΔE predicted by the Nernst equation agrees with the experimentally-determined transmembrane potential difference. If active transport is involved, however, there is a discrepancy between the two values.

During diastole the transmembrane potential of ventricular muscle is approximately 70 mV. However, as described later, the membrane undergoes rhythmic depolarization and the mean transmembrane potential, averaged over one cardiac cycle, is approximately 50 mV.

The potential differences which would be required to explain the experimentally-determined distributions of potassium, sodium and chloride ions across the myocardial cell membrane are given in the third column of *Table 2.1*. The equilibrium potential for chloride (−50 mV) is similar to the actual membrane potential; chloride ions are therefore thought to be distributed across the membrane entirely passively.

In the case of potassium ions, however, the calculated potential difference is approximately 40 mV greater than the experimentally-determined value, and this implies that potassium ions are actively transported into the cell. With sodium ions the transmembrane potential is actually in the opposite direction to that predicted by the Nernst equation; that is, concentration gradient *and* the transmembrane potential difference both act in a direction to cause sodium ions to enter the cell. Since the membrane is permeable to sodium, although much less so than to potassium, it is clear that there must be some mechanism by which sodium ions are actively extruded from the cell. It has been calculated that at least 20 per cent of the cell's resting metabolism is expended in maintaining ionic concentration differences across the cell membrane (Keynes and Maisel, 1954).

The sodium pump

The precise mode of action of the sodium pump (or more correctly, the sodium–potassium pump) is unknown. One suggestion (*Figure 2.3*) is that sodium ions combine with a (hypothetical) carrier molecule at the inside of the membrane to form a sodium-carrier complex. This complex then diffuses to the outside of the membrane and there dissociates into sodium ions and uncombined carrier molecules. The carrier is then able to combine with potassium ions, and this potassium-carrier complex diffuses to the interior of the cell, where it again dissociates into uncombined ions and carrier molecules. Under this hypothesis the active transport of sodium and potassium is accomplished by simple diffusion because, in each case, the ion-carrier complex moves across the cell membrane down a concentration gradient. If this process is to be cyclic, however, at least one of the chemical reactions involved must be endergonic, that is, it must be supplied with metabolically-produced energy.

Although it is likely that the transport of potassium is linked in some way to

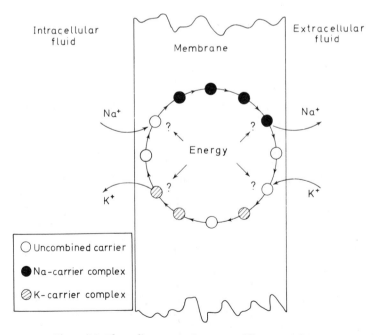

Figure 2.3. The sodium–potassium pump (diagrammatic)

that of sodium, there is not necessarily the one-to-one relationship implied in the previous paragraph. The carrier theory allows carrier molecules to diffuse across the membrane without necessarily being combined with potassium. This is represented diagrammatically in *Figure 2.3*, where some carrier molecules return combined with potassium, and some return in the uncombined state. The ratio which is currently favoured is two potassium ions to three sodium ions.

Membrane depolarization

As explained in the previous section, the membrane of myocardial cells is polarized during diastole with a transmembrane potential difference of approximately 70 mV. This potential varies rhythmically throughout the cardiac cycle, and it is these changes of membrane potential which are responsible for the initiation of myocardial contraction (*see* page 43).

When the heart is beating normally in sinus rhythm, each contraction is initiated by spontaneous depolarization of the sino-atrial (S-A) node, which causes an action potential to spread throughout the remainder of the myocardium (*see* below). In the normal mammalian heart the ability of myocardial cells to depolarize spontaneously is limited to the S-A and atrio-ventricular (A-V) nodes and to the upper part of the bundle of His. The rhythmicity (rate of spontaneous depolarization) of the S-A node normally exceeds that of the A-V node, therefore the normal cardiac pacemaker is the S-A node. The wave of depolarization initiated here reaches the A-V node and depolarizes it before it can become spontaneously depolarized.

ANATOMY OF THE CONDUCTING SYSTEM

The impulse-generating and conducting system of the heart comprises the S-A node, the A-V node, the atrio-ventricular bundle (of His) and the ventricular Purkinje tissue.

The S-A node lies in the wall of the right atrium near the opening of the superior vena cava. It is composed of cells which are rather smaller than those of the remaining myocardium. The A-V node lies in the interatrial septum near the opening of the coronary sinus. Inferiorly, it is continuous with the atrio-ventricular bundle which pierces the fibrous tissue separating the atrial and ventricular muscle masses, and then divides into right and left branches. These pass down on either side of the interventricular septum towards the apex of the heart. The A-V bundle is liable to damage during open-heart surgery.

The final ramifications of the conducting system form a network running over the endocardial surfaces of both ventricles. These fibres are larger than the normal ventricular fibres; they contain much glycogen and relatively few myofibrils, and are modified to conduct electrical impulses rather than to undergo physical contraction. Their conduction velocity is some six times (1.5 to 2.5 m s^{-1}) that of the remainder of the myocardium.

CARDIAC ELECTRICAL ACTIVITY

Depolarization of the pacemaker

If a microelectrode is inserted into the interior of a cell in the S-A node, the intracellular potential at the start of diastole is approximately 70 mV negative with respect to the extracellular fluid. This potential difference does not, however, remain constant as it would in, for example, a skeletal muscle cell, but declines slowly towards zero (*Figure 2.4*). When it reaches a threshold value of approximately 50 mV negative the rate of decrease accelerates enormously and the potential inside the cell falls rapidly to zero, and then overshoots to become some 20 mV positive.

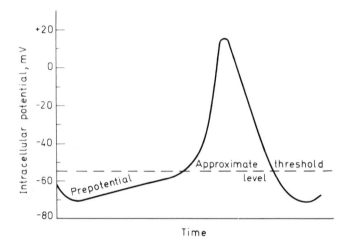

Figure 2.4. Variation with time of transmembrane potential of typical pacemaker cell (redrawn from Hoffman and Cranefield, 1960)

This spontaneous decrease of diastolic potential is called the prepotential or pacemaker potential and is characteristic of the cells of the S-A and A-V nodes. It appears to be due to the fact that, in these situations, the cell membrane is relatively permeable to sodium ions (Trautwein and Kasselbaum, 1961); therefore this ion is able to diffuse into the cell faster than it can be extruded by the sodium pump. The slope of the prepotential region is greater in the S-A than in the A-V node, thus accounting for the greater inherent rhythmicity of the former structure.

The cause of the rapid reversal of transmembrane potential which occurs when the membrane is depolarized to its threshold value is probably the same as in other excitable tissues. Depolarization causes an increase of sodium permeability which causes further depolarization; a postive-feedback process develops and sodium ions enter the cell at a rate which completely swamps the activity of the sodium pump. The transmembrane potential therefore quickly falls until it is approximately equal to the sodium equilibrium potential.

The level of the threshold for this positive-feedback process is relatively constant. The rate of impulse generation by the pacemaker cells is determined mainly by the rate of change of the prepotential, and by the extent to which the membrane is polarized at the start of diastole. Sympathetic stimulation increases the rate of spontaneous depolarization and therefore, by allowing the trans-membrane potential to reach threshold sooner, causes an increase of heart rate; stimulation of the vagus decreases the slope of the prepotential, thus slowing the heart. Excessive parasympathetic stimulation may cause the heart to come to a standstill with the cells of the S-A node in a stable, hyperpolarized state.

Electrical transmission through the heart

Atrial depolarization

The depolarization process spreads from the S-A node throughout the atrial muscle with a velocity of rather less than 1 m s^{-1}. Spread from cell to cell is electrical; depolarization of one cell lowers the membrane potential of adjacent cells which become depolarized in turn. Although there is no histological evidence of specialized conducting tissue in the atria, there is some evidence that the depolarization process may spread preferentially along certain channels (Paes de Carvalho, de Mello and Hoffman, 1959).

Transmission between atria and ventricles

Transmission of the cardiac action potential from the S-A node to the vicinity of the A-V node takes about 40 ms (0.04 s). The impulse is then delayed in the proximal part of the A-V node where the velocity of conduction is very slow, perhaps 0.2 mm s^{-1} (Hoffman et al., 1963). Therefore ventricular depolarization does not start until some 150 ms after depolarization of the S-A node. This delay improves the pumping efficiency of the heart because it allows time for atrial contraction to force an additional amount of blood into the relaxed ventricles before closure of the A-V valves prevents further filling.

The muscle fibres which link the atrial muscle to the A-V node are known as junctional fibres. These specialized cells have a conduction velocity of only about 0.05 m s^{-1}; the cells of the A-V node itself conduct at about 0.1 m s^{-1}. These rates are both considerably less than the conduction velocity of the remaining atrial muscle and of the A-V bundle and Purkinje tissue.

The A-V node may contain more than one conducting pathway; and although these normally conduct simultaneously they may not always do so, and may then be responsible for 're-entrant' dysrhythmias (Wallace and Daggett, 1964).

Ventricular depolarization

The cardiac action potential passes from the A-V node to the main mass of ventricular muscle via the atrio-ventricular bundle, its R and L branches and the Purkinje fibres. Because of the high conduction velocity of these tissues, depolarization spreads rapidly over the endocardial surfaces of both ventricles. It then spreads at a much slower rate (0.3 m s^{-1}) towards the epicardial surface of the heart. A perpendicular cut in the ventricular muscle does not affect conduction between adjacent areas of myocardium provided the Purkinje tissue is not damaged (Lewis and Rothschild, 1915).

The first part of the ventricular muscle to be depolarized is the interventricular septum. Purkinje tissue is more plentiful on its left-hand side, therefore this area is initially more extensively depolarized than the right side. The wave of depolarization then spreads rapidly over the endocardial surfaces of both ventricles, and then outwards towards their epicardial surfaces.

The wall of the right ventricle is thinner than that of the left, therefore the right ventricle is completely depolarized at a time when the left ventricle is still partially polarized. As seen later (*see* page 39) the partial myocardial depolarization is responsible for the QRS complex of the electrocardiogram. The last parts of the ventricular muscle to be depolarized are the posterior wall of the left ventricle and the basal part of the interventricular septum, which is poorly supplied with Purkinje tissue. Ventricular depolarization is complete in just over 200 ms.

Shape of the cardiac action potential

In most excitable tissues the reversal of membrane potential which occurs at the start of the action potential is followed by a rapid repolarization of the membrane (*Figure 2.5a*). This is due to decrease of the membrane's permeability to sodium ions, accompanied by increase in its permeability to potassium. Potassium therefore diffuses out of the cell, thus restoring the transmembrane potential to its normal resting value.

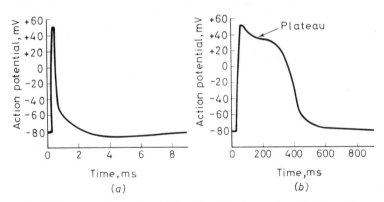

Figure 2.5. *Shape of action potential in (a) skeletal muscle and (b) cardiac muscle (semi-diagrammatic). Note different time-scales*

The cardiac action potential

In cardiac muscle, however, the time course of events is very different. The initial depolarization is followed by a period of approximately 200 ms, during which the transmembrane potential remains close to the sodium equilibrium potential (*Figure 2.5b*); at the end of this period the membrane gradually repolarizes. The precise explanation of this plateau in terms of ionic permeabilities is uncertain; various hypotheses are reviewed by Brady and Woodbury (1960).

During the plateau of the action potential the ventricle is completely inexcitable, and unable to respond to external stimuli; this is very necessary if the heart is to pump efficiently under all conditions. If it were not so, the random stimulation of the ventricle which accompanies atrial fibrillation would cause continuous ventricular contraction and cessation of effective cardiac action.

The duration of the plateau depends, to some extent, on heart rate. At very high rates the action potential is shortened so that an increase of heart rate is accompanied by a decrease of systolic duration. This decrease is not, however, as marked as the accompanying decrease of diastolic duration (*see* page 63).

The QRS complex of the electrocardiogram is due to the (rapid) spread of the depolarization process through the ventricular muscle mass.

Ventricular repolarization

The T wave of the electrocardiogram is due to ventricular repolarization. Since this deflection is in the same direction as the R wave it appears that, contrary to what might be expected, repolarization occurs in the *opposite* sequence to depolarization; the last part of the myocardium to become depolarized is the first to be repolarized. The reason for this anomaly is not clear. It appears, however, that the pathway taken by ventricular repolarization is influenced by factors other than simple cell-to-cell electrical conduction. As was first suggested by Lewis and Rothschild (1915), ventricular repolarization is influenced by pressure gradients in the myocardium and, as a result, it starts in the regions where the pressure is least, that is, just under the pericardium. This is, of course, the last area to be depolarized.

Repolarization often follows abnormal pathways in a diseased myocardium causing T-wave inversion.

THE ELECTROCARDIOGRAM

The process of depolarization and repolarization of the heart are reflected in changes of electrical potential at the body surface. These potentials may be amplified and recorded on moving paper or displayed on a cathode-ray tube. Such a record is called an electrocardiogram (ECG).

It must be stressed that, although the electrocardiogram may provide valuable information about the electrical activity of the heart, it gives virtually no information about its pumping ability. It is possible to have a normal ECG when cardiac output is, for practical purposes, zero. Such uncoupling between electrical and mechanical events is said to occur, for example, as a result of overdose with local anaesthetic agents.

Generation of ECG potentials

When the ventricular muscle is electrically inactive, the exterior of its cells is all at the same potential. This happens twice in each cardiac cycle: during diastole the cell membrane is polarized with a transmembrane potential of approximately

70 mV; during the plateau of the action potential the membrane is completely depolarized, and the transmembrane potential is approximately zero (*see* page 33). Between these two states the ventricular muscle is partly polarized and partly depolarized; that is the exterior of the cells in one region is positive with respect to that of the cells in another region. To be more specific, when the depolarization process has spread throughout the interventricular septum and wall of the right ventricle, but has not yet spread throughout the left ventricle, the exterior of the cells in the septal region is negative with respect to that of the apical cells. (This is, of course, the same as saying that the exterior of the apical cells is positive with respect to that of the septal cells. It is potential difference which is important, not absolute potential.)

At certain phases of the cardiac cycle, therefore, part of the myocardium is positive with respect to the remainder. This separation of positive and negative charges forms a source of electromotive force within the chest, and causes current to flow through the extracellular fluids. These are electrolyte solutions and form what is known as a volume conductor, that is, a conductor in which electric current can flow in any direction (compared with, for example, a linear conductor like a wire). This flow of current results in electrical potential differences between different regions of the body surface; and the variation of these potentials with time forms the electrocardiogram.

Potential differences at body surface

Looked at diagrammatically (*Figure 2.6*), the polarized and depolarized regions of the myocardium may be represented as discrete electrical charges separated by a certain distance. These charges form a *dipole*, and current flows through the body fluids from the positive to the negative pole as shown. (Electric current is composed of electrons flowing from a negative to a positive pole. It is common practice, however, to speak in terms of a conventional current which, by

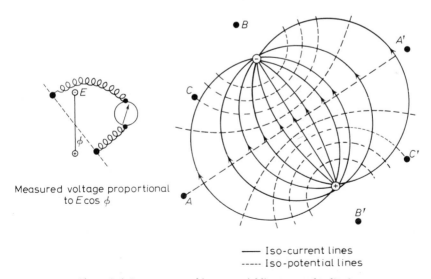

Measured voltage proportional to $E \cos \phi$

——— Iso-current lines
----- Iso-potential lines

Figure 2.6. Iso-current and iso-potential lines around a dipole

definition, flows from the positive to the negative pole.) These lines of current flow are crossed at right angles by equipotential lines, linking all points with the same electrical potential.

As can be seen in *Figure 2.6,* the potential difference between any two pairs of electrodes around the dipole depends on their spacial relationship to it. The potential difference between B and B' is maximal, between A and A' it is minimal, and between C and C' it is of an intermediate value. This is of course the reason for the different size of the ECG deflections as measured by the various leads: the QRS complex in the limb leads is typically maximal in lead II or aV_F, and minimal in lead I or aV_L.

The configuration of the recorded ECG deflection depends on the strength and direction of the cardiac dipole (which of course varies from moment to moment) and on the relative orientation of the recording electrodes to the dipole.

The ECG is usually recorded via an amplifier with a balanced input (*Figure 2.7*), in which case the measured surface potentials must be symmetrical about zero. This is achieved by connecting the right leg of the patient to earth.

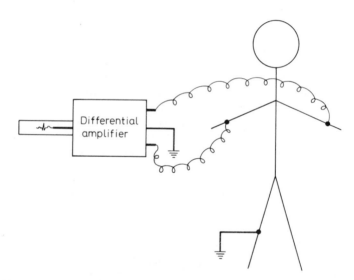

Figure 2.7. Measurement of electrocardiogram (lead I) with a differential amplifier

This type of amplifier considerably reduces the effect of electrical interference from external sources because the balanced input responds only to a *difference* of electrical potential applied to its two inputs, and not at all (or, in practice only to a minor extent) to the same potential applied to each lead. Interfering signals from outside the body are injected into each lead equally; they are therefore considerably attenuated in comparison with ECG signals which, by virtue of the right leg earth connection, are balanced about zero.

The ECG is normally recorded so that 1 mV gives a deflection of 1 cm; and the standard paper speed is 1 cm s^{-1}.

The six limb leads

The six limb leads used in clinical electrocardiography respond maximally to dipoles orientated in the directions shown in *Figure 2.8a*.

Lead I is taken between the right arm and the left arm in such a way that the deflection is upwards when the left arm is positive with respect to the right. Lead II is between the right arm and the left leg; the deflection is upwards when the left leg is positive. Lead III is taken between the left arm and the left leg with an upward deflection when the left leg is positive. The remaining leads are taken between an indifferent electrode (*see* below) and either the left arm (lead aV_L), the right arm (aV_R), or the left leg (aV_F).

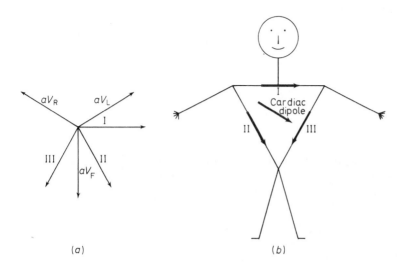

(a) (b)

Figure 2.8. (a) Direction of maximal response of the six ECG limb leads. (b) Simplified derivation of the directions of maximum response of limb leads I, II and III (for explanation see text). The left arm, right arm, and left leg are assumed to lie at the points of an equilateral triangle

In the case of the bipolar limb leads, the dipolar direction to which they respond maximally may be deduced if the simplifying assumption is made that the two arms and left leg are attached to the body at the points of an equilateral triangle in the centre of which lies the cardiac dipole (*Figure 2.8b*). (This is not, in fact, too severe a departure from reality since potentials recorded from the wrists and ankles do not differ greatly from those taken where the limbs join the trunk. The limbs behave as linear conductors which attenuate the potentials slightly, but do not alter them otherwise. It may easily be demonstrated experimentally that the form of the ECG is not altered by changes in the relationship of the limbs to the trunk.)

The maximal response of the unipolar limb leads may be deduced similarly. The indifferent electrode is formed by connecting together the three active limbs—left arm, left leg and right arm. Therefore lead aV_L records, in effect, the potential difference between the left arm and the mean potential of the left leg and right arm. It responds maximally to a dipole pointing to the left, 30° above the horizontal. Similarly, lead aV_F responds maximally to a vertical dipole, and lead aV_R to a dipole pointing to the right and 30° above the horizontal.

The chest leads

The standard clinical ECG comprises also six unipolar chest leads arranged around the left side of the chest from just to the right of the sternum to the posterior axillary line. Although these leads also reflect the spacial relationship of the recording system to the direction of the instantaneous cardiac dipole (*see* above) it is not possible to express this relationship in simple terms, as it is with the limb leads.

A typical recording of the six chest leads from a normal subject is shown in *Figure 2.9.*

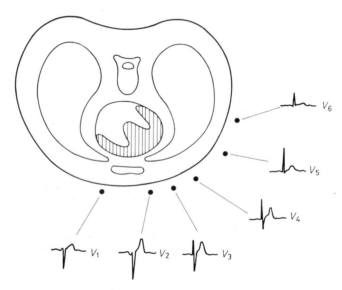

Figure 2.9. The six-lead chest electrocardiogram

The ECG deflections

By combining the above (somewhat simplified) account with a knowledge of the pathway taken by the wave of electrical depolarization through the myocardium (*see* page 32), it is possible to deduce the physiological basis of the ECG deflections in the different leads.

The P wave

Activity starts in the S-A node and spreads via the atrial muscle to the A-V node, thus producing the P wave. The pathway taken by atrial depolarization is such that this wave is positive in all leads except aV_R. The average P wave duration is 90 ms; its amplitude is less than 0.25 mV.

The PR interval

During the PR interval the atrial cells are completely depolarized, while the atrio-ventricular conducting tissue is just becoming depolarized. The potentials generated by this latter process are, however, small and not recordable at the body surface. The ECG therefore remains isoelectric between the end of the P wave and the start of ventricular depolarization.

The QRS complex

Depolarization of the ventricle is a continuous process; the dipole representing the instantaneous state of ventricular depolarization varies continuously in both magnitude and direction. For descriptive purposes, however, it is possible to consider depolarization as occurring in three relatively distinct phases, which respectively give rise to the Q, R and S waves of the ECG.

The first phase involves depolarization of the interventricular septum. This results in a dipole directed from left to right and slightly anteriorly, causing a downward deflection (Q wave) in most leads. Depolarization of the right ventricular wall at a time when the apex is not yet depolarized causes a dipole pointing from the base of the heart towards the apex. This dipole causes a large positive deflection (R wave) in most limb leads, although the deflection may be inverted in aV_R and aV_L. The final phase of ventricular depolarization occurs when the entire myocardium is depolarized except for the base of the septum and the posterior part of the left ventricular wall. The resultant dipole is directed from left to right, slightly upwards and posteriorly and is responsible for the S wave of the electrocardiogram.

It should be understood that there is nothing fundamental about the sequence of deflections Q, R and S seen in the 'normal' electrocardiogram. The polarity of a deflection depends purely on the orientation of the resultant cardiac dipole in relation to the recording electrodes. A positive deflection in one lead may become a negative deflection in another; an R wave in lead II may be an S wave in lead aV_R. The appearance of the normal electrocardiogram in the six limb leads is shown in *Figure 2.10*. Since lead aV_R is almost $180°$ out of phase with lead II its deflections are approximately the mirror-image of those in the latter lead; the main deflection in lead aV_R is negative, accompanied by small positive deflections on either side (RSR$'$ complex).

The normal duration of the QRS complex is 0.12 s. In conditions such as bundle-branch block, where conduction through a major branch of the A-V bundle is impaired, the complex may be considerably prolonged because electrical depolarization may have to reach part of the myocardium via normal myocardial cells, which have a relatively low conduction velocity (0.3 m s^{-1}).

The T wave

Ventricular repolarization is represented by the T wave. The normal interval between the start of the QRS complex and the end of the T wave is approximately 0.4 s, but it varies considerably with heart rate. As mentioned on page 32, the T wave normally has the same polarity as the main deflection of the QRS complex. Atrial depolarization normally coincides with the start of ventricular depolarization; it is therefore buried in the QRS complex.

The ST segment

The QRS complex is followed by an isoelectric period during which the ventricular muscle is completely depolarized. This is, of course, the segment of the electrocardiogram which shows ST segment elevation after a myocardial infarction. Since the myocardium is completely depolarized at this time the ST segment cannot truly be elevated; it is actually the remainder of the waveform which is depressed due to a current of injury flowing between the normally polarized resting muscle and the depolarized dead muscle of the infarct.

Electrical axis of the heart

From a study of the relative sizes of the QRS complex in the various limb leads it is possible to calculate the electrical axis of the heart. This is given approximately by the direction of the limb lead with the largest R wave. It may be determined more accurately by calculation (*see* Recommended Further Reading). In *Figure 2.10* the largest R wave occurs in lead II, indicating that the electrical axis points, in this case, approximately 60° below the horizontal, downwards and to the left.

If the heart becomes rotated clockwise or anticlockwise its electrical axis changes. A horizontal heart shows left axis-deviation and produces a large R

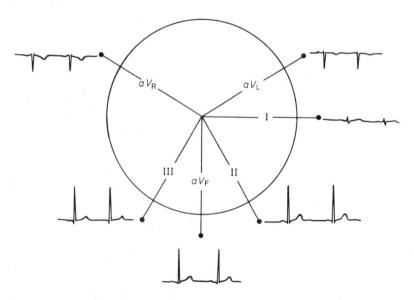

Figure 2.10. Normal six-limb lead electrocardiogram

wave in lead I or aV_L and a large negative deflection in lead III. Conversely, a vertical heart shows right axis-deviation; the maximum positive deflection then occurs in lead III, with negative deflections in leads I and aV_L.

Vectorcardiography

By the use of special lead systems it is possible to calculate the magnitude and direction of the instantaneous cardiac dipole. This is the technique of vectorcardiography (Lamb, 1965). Very approximately, information about the vector's horizontal component is given by limb lead I, about its vertical component by lead aV_F, and about its anterior component in lead V_1 or V_2.

MECHANISM OF CARDIAC CONTRACTION

It is the function of the heart to convert chemical energy contained in complex organic substances into mechanical energy as represented by the potential and kinetic energy of the blood in the large arteries. The majority of myocardial energy production is expended in pumping blood round the body, that is, in overcoming intravascular friction. If the heart is stopped suddenly its oxygen consumption falls to between 20 and 35 per cent of its previous value (Beuren, Sparkes and Bing, 1958).

The efficiency of the heart is low. Only a small proportion (about 15 per cent) of its total energy expenditure is productively utilized; this proportion may, however, be increased during exercise. If the energy which is used just to keep the heart alive without doing physical work is subtracted from the total energy production, the calculated efficiency rises to approximately 18 per cent. This is considerably below the efficiency of many man-made energy converters,

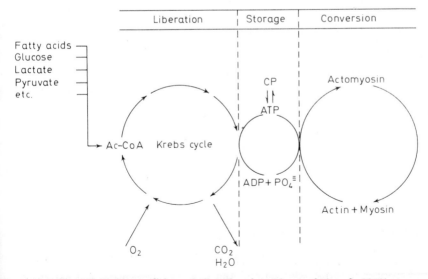

Figure 2.11. Myocardial metabolism (based on Olson and Piatnek, 1959)

although, of course, the reliability of the heart far exceeds that of any artificial device.

The metabolism of cardiac muscle may be considered to occur in three stages: energy liberation, energy storage, and energy conversion (Olson, 1964). Chemical energy is liberated by the breakdown of complex organic molecules, stored as high-energy phosphate bonds in adenosine triphosphate (ATP) and creatine phosphate (CP), and then converted into mechanical energy by the contractile proteins (*Figure 2.11*).

Energy production

The myocardium is fairly omnivorous and can metabolize fatty acids, glucose, lactate, pyruvate and ketone bodies (Opie, 1965). In general, the rate at which any particular substance is metabolized is roughly proportional to its concentration in the arterial blood, although it is affected to some extent by the availability of alternative substrates. At normal blood concentrations, glucose and lactate are utilized about equally.

During hypoxia the heart is unable to utilize lactate, whereas the rate of glucose consumption is increased. Under hypoxic conditions, therefore, coronary venous blood contains an increased concentration of lactate (*see* page 220).

In the post-absorptive state some 60 per cent of myocardial energy production is provided by the metabolism of esterified and unesterified fatty acids. In diabetic ketosis the proportion of total energy supplied by the breakdown of such ketone bodies is increased.

Whatever the substrate being used it ultimately enters the Krebs tricarboxylic acid cycle and is there oxidized to carbon dixoide and water, with the production of ATP from adenosine diphosphate and inorganic phosphate. The enzymes involved in this process are located in the mitochondria.

The precise role of ATP in cardiac contraction is not known. It is known, however, that the addition of ATP to actomyosin from human cardiac muscle causes it to contract; myosin has adenosine triphosphatase activity. Calcium ions also are involved in the generation of the cardiac contraction. It appears that the chief role of ATP is as a source of energy, whereas calcium ions are concerned mainly with the control of the contraction process.

Excitation-contraction coupling

Although most of the experimental work which has been done on muscular contraction has been on skeletal muscle, there is no evidence to suggest any fundamental difference between the mechanism of contraction of skeletal and of cardiac muscle.

Role of Calcium

It has been known for more than 50 years that calcium is necessary for satisfactory myocardial contraction. And it is well recognized that externally-applied calcium ions increase myocardial oxygen consumption and have a positive inotropic* (stimulatory) action on the heart. Conversely, if myocardial cells are placed in a calcium-free solution, depolarization of the cell membrane fails to initiate mechanical contraction (Niedergerke, 1956).

Most experimental evidence suggests that depolarization of the cell membrane is accompanied by an influx of calcium ions into the cell. These ions are thought to 'turn on' the contractile process—to cause interaction between the proteins actin and myosin, thus inducing myocardial contraction. Muscular relaxation seems to be due to a (hypothetical) 'relaxing substance' which combines with free intracellular calcium ions, thus rendering them unavailable, and therefore 'turning off' the contractile process.

The entry of calcium into the cell is aided by the ramifications of the sarcoplasmic reticulum (*see* page 25). This increases the effective area of the cell membrane, and allows calcium ions to enter the cell in the immediate vicinity of the contractile proteins.

MYOCARDIAL CONTRACTILITY

The pumping ability of the heart depends fundamentally on the ability of its myocardial cells to shorten. This ability is influenced both by intrinsic factors such as the Frank-Starling mechanism (*see* page 49), and by the biochemical environment of the heart. Myocardial contractile force is, for example, increased by an increased cardiac filling pressure, by a raised extracellular calcium concentration, and by sympathomimetic amines; it is depressed by an increased extracellular potassium concentration.

The heart's efficiency as a pump depends on how well it can impart energy to the contained blood; and this ability is affected by two separate and distinct mechanisms: the Frank-Sterling mechanism and the myocardium's ability to develop tension from a given end-diastolic fibre-length. The latter is usually called the *myocardial contractility*.

The force-velocity curve

The concept of a force-velocity curve was originally developed by A. V. Hill for skeletal muscle and several workers (for example, Abbott and Mommaerts, 1959; Sonnenblick, 1962) have applied this concept to cardiac muscle.

The conceptual model which Hill developed to explain the known facts about muscular contraction (*Figure 2.12*) consists of a contractile element *A* connected in series with a stiff spring *B*, and in parallel with a second, much weaker spring *C*. The resting tone of the muscle is due to extension of the parallel spring *C*. When the muscle contracts, however, this spring is relaxed and the active tension is provided by the much stiffer spring *B*.

*It is customary to describe the action of various factors on the heart as either affecting the force of myocardial contraction (inotropic influences) or affecting the heart rate (chronotropic influences). Inotropic and chronotropic influences may be either positive or negative. Here the use of the term 'inotropic' without qualification means 'positive inotropic'.

The anatomical basis of the elements described in the previous paragraph is uncertain. Although, in the model, they are considered to be discrete, the elastic components may, in fact, be different properties of the same cellular element. It is permissible for many purposes to ignore the parallel element; this practice is followed in the present, simplified account of the model.

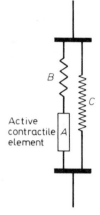

Figure 2.12. Diagrammatic representation of a contractile unit in cardiac or skeletal muscle (see text)

Active contractile element

When the muscle contracts, its contractile element shortens. Activation of the muscle is therefore accompanied either by stretching of its series elastic element, or by external shortening, or by both. When the series elastic element is stretched, the muscle develops external tension, the magnitude of which depends on the elastic modulus of the series elastic element and on the extent to which it is stretched.

At the start of contraction the muscle is generally under some degree of tension, the preload. In the case of cardiac muscle, this is provided by the distending force of the ventricular end-diastolic pressure. The greater the preload, the greater is the external length of the muscle fibres, and because of the Frank-Starling relationship (*see* page 49), the greater is the force of subsequent contraction.

When the muscle is activated, the contractile element shortens until the tension generated by the series elastic element is equal to the external tension applied to the muscle, the *afterload*. Up to this point the contraction is isometric, thereafter the muscle begins to shorten externally. Once the internal tension is equal to the afterload, further shortening of the contractile element is accompanied by external shortening; the tension which is developed then remains constant, that is, the contraction is isotonic.

Experimentally, it is found that if the afterload is progressively increased, the time interval before the muscle begins to shorten increases, whereas the initial rate of shortening decreases (*Figure 2.13a*). The relationship between the initial velocity of shortening and afterload is hyperbolic (*Figure 2.13b*). This curve is the *force-velocity relationship*.

It is generally agreed that the heart's contractile ability is best described by the shape and position of the myocardial force-velocity curve. And simplifying matters very considerably, it seems that an increase of preload increases the maximum isometric tension which the muscle can develop, but has little effect on its maximal velocity of shortening (*Figure 2.14a*). (A good analogy here is

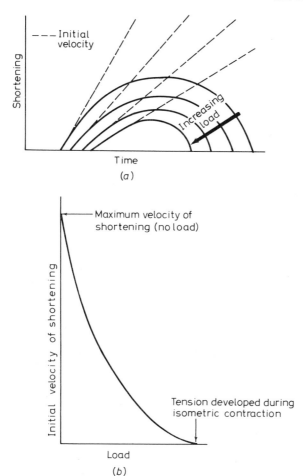

Figure 2.13. The force-velocity curve of cardiac muscle. (a) As the load (afterload) increases the initial velocity of shortening falls, resulting in (b) a hyperbolic relationship between initial velocity of shortening and afterload

that of two horses tethered to a stake: their pull is double that of a single horse, but their speed of movement is the same.) An increase of myocardial contractility, on the other hand, increases both the muscle's maximum isometric pull *and* its maximal velocity of shortening (*Figure 2.14b*). (In the horse analogy stimulating a single horse by whipping him increases both his pull and his speed of movement.)

It may be shown theoretically (Sonnenblick et al., 1970) that changes in the speed of contraction of the contractile element in the Hill model—that is *changes in myocardial contractility*—are reflected in the parameter $(dP/dt_{max})/P$, where dP/dt_{max} is the maximum rate of rise of intraventricular pressure during the isometric phase of ventricular contraction, and P is the instantaneous intraventricular pressure at that time. This was the parameter adopted by Prys-Roberts and Gersh (*see* below) in their studies on myocardial contractility during various forms of anaesthesia.

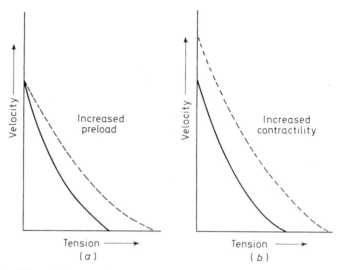

Figure 2.14. Effect of changes of preload and of myocardial contractility on myocardial force-velocity curve

Intercepts of the force-velocity curve

It is not, in fact, necessary to determine the whole force-velocity curve; information about myocardial contractility may be obtained by measuring the intercepts which it makes on the x and y axes respectively. When the afterload is zero the initial rate of contraction is maximal; when the external load is increased until the muscle is unable to shorten the contraction becomes isometric. Measurement of the tension developed by cardiac muscle during an isometric contraction therefore gives an indication of the intercept of the force-velocity curve with the abscissa; measurement of the rate of myocardial shortening at the start of systole (when the afterload is virtually zero) gives an indication of the curve's y intercept.

The x intercept—the tension of isometric contraction. The tension developed by cardiac muscle during an isometric contraction may conveniently be measured by a Walton-Brodie strain-gauge arch (Boniface, Brodie and Walton, 1953). This is shown diagrammatically in *Figure 2.15*. It consists of a semi-rigid arch which is sutured to the ventricular muscle; the bridge of the arch is connected to a strain-gauge which measures the deforming force applied by myocardial contraction. The arch is sufficiently rigid for the contraction to be effectively isometric.

Most of the commonly-used general anaesthetic agents decrease the isometric tension generated by a segment of myocardium (*see* Chapter 7). Sympathetic stimulation or exposure to an increased concentration of sympathomimetic amines increases the isometric tension. There may also be an increase of tension during tachycardia (an example of so-called homeometric autoregulation—*see* page 51). The Walton-Brodie strain-gauge is now less used than formerly because,

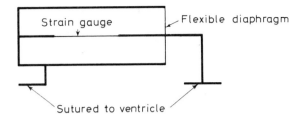

Strain gauge

Flexible diaphragm

Sutured to ventricle

Figure 2.15. Walton-Brodie strain-gauge arch (diagrammatic)

as indicated above, it is sensitive to changes of preload as well as to changes in myocardial contractility.

The y intercept—the initial rate of shortening and dP/dt_{max} It is difficult to measure directly the initial rate of myocardial shortening; an indication of the value of this parameter may, however, be obtained by determining the rate of rise of intraventricular pressure at the start of systole, before the semilunar valves open. The quantity so measured is known as dP/dt_{max}. It may be shown that positive inotropic influences increase dP/dt_{max}, while factors which cause myocardial depression decrease this parameter (Furnival, Linden and Snow, 1967).

The usefulness of dP/dt_{max} as a quantitative index of myocardial contractility is, however, diminished by the fact that this parameter appears to depend on the loading conditions of the ventricular muscle—on the preload and the afterload (Mason, 1969).

Gersh and Prys-Roberts (Prys-Roberts et al., 1972) investigated the value of various indices of myocardial contractility for quantification of the effects of anaesthetic agents on the cardiovascular system; they suggested that the most valuable index was the maximum rate of rise of intraventricular pressure divided by the instantaneous intraventricular pressure at that point in time, i.e. by $(dP/dt_{max})/IP$. This index was first suggested by Veragut and Krayenbühl (1965); and as mentioned above it has a certain theoretical justification (*see also* Appendix III).

Gersh (1970) found that $(dP/dt_{max})/IP$ varied minimally with quite a large change of left ventricular end-diastolic pressure, whereas under the same conditions (dP/dt_{max}) changed by as much as 28 per cent. The index was similarly unresponsive to changes in heart rate induced by atrial pacing; but it changed markedly in response to inotropic influences on the myocardium such as sympathetic stimulation or infusions of isoprenaline or calcium gluconate.

The disadvantage with $(dP/dt_{max})/IP$ and with similar indices is, of course, that they require catherization of the left ventricle and are therefore of little value in intact man. For this reason various workers have sought a non-invasive index of myocardial contractility: one of the most promising of these is the pre-ejection period (PEP), an index which was first proposed by Weissler, Peeler and Roehill (1961). Gersh et al. (1972) however found that PEP was affected by ventricular end-diastolic volume, and by other factors.

PEP is calculated by subtracting the left ventricular ejection time from the total duration of electromechanical systole (the time interval between the ECG Q wave and the start of the first heart-sound measured phonocardiographically (*Figure 2.16*)). Ventricular ejection time is measured by a suitable transducer placed over the carotid artery: it is the time interval between the first upstroke of the carotid pulse and the trough of the dicrotic notch. Always bearing in mind the above *caveat*, the shorter the PEP the greater is the myocardial contractility.

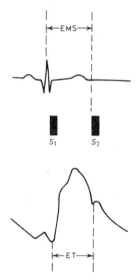

Figure 2.16. Diagram of pre-injection period (PEP). PEP equals duration of electro-mechanical systole (EMS) minus left-ventricular ejection time (ET)

PEP has been used by Forrest, Laurson and Otton (1974) to investigate the effect of epidural block on cardiac function; and a related parameter (PEP^{-2}) has been used by Blackburn et al. (1972) to investigate the cardiovascular effect of changes of Pa_{CO_2}.

Pressure-flow-volume diagram of Fry

It is possible to relate the various techniques for assessing ventricular function during anaesthesia by means of the pressure-flow-volume diagram of Fry (1962) (*Figure 2.17*). Unfortunately, the concepts involved are difficult to grasp and, since the place of this diagram in cardiovascular physiology is not yet well established it is mentioned here but briefly. With this diagram the state of myocardial contractility at any given moment is represented by a surface, plotted in a co-ordinate system consisting of three mutually-perpendicular axes. These represent respectively (*a*) intraventricular pressure—horizontally to the right; (*b*) ventricular volume—horizontally downwards and to the left; and (*c*) velocity of myocardial contraction—vertically. A change of myocardial contractility is represented by a change of the orientation of the surface with respect to one or more of the three axes (for further details *see* Berne and Levy, 1967).

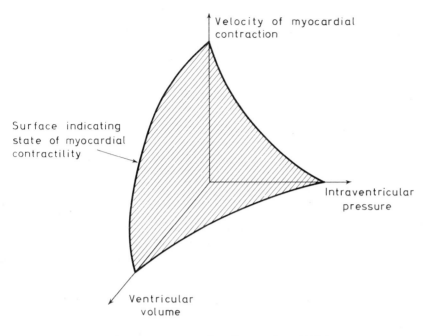

Figure 2.17. Pressure-flow diagram of Fry (1962)

FACTORS AFFECTING STRENGTH OF CARDIAC CONTRACTION

The factors which affect the strength of cardiac contraction are intrinsic and extrinsic.

Intrinsic factors

The Frank-Starling mechanism and Starling's law

The most important intrinsic factor affecting the strength of cardiac contraction is the Frank-Starling mechanism, as a result of which the force of cardiac contraction depends on the length of the muscle fibres at the start of systole. This relationship was described by Starling (1918) in his Linacre lecture of 1915 in the following terms: 'The law of the heart is thus the same as the law of muscular tissue generally that the energy of contraction, however measured, is a function of the length of the muscle fibre'. The relationship was first demonstrated on frog myocardium by Frank in 1895, and on mammalian heart by Patterson, Piper and Starling in 1914. It has more recently been shown to be applicable to man (Braunwald and Ross, 1964).

The relationship between length and passive tension in a segment of relaxed myocardium shows the typical non-linear relationship between stress and strain found with most biological materials (*Figure 2.18a*, lower curve). The upper curve in this figure is the relationship between the pre-contraction length of the

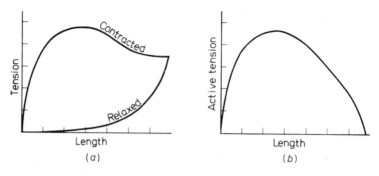

Figure 2.18. Length-tension curves of cardiac muscle

muscle and the tension it generates when contracted. The active tension developed is represented by the vertical distance between the two curves; it is plotted against the length of the relaxed muscle in *Figure 2.18b*. Active tension increases with increasing resting fibre length up to a maximum, and then declines as the muscle becomes overstretched.

Biophysical basis of the Frank-Starling mechanism.   Recent work on the ultrastructure of muscle has suggested a possible biophysical basis for the Frank-Starling mechanism (*Figure 2.19*). Experimentally, a muscle develops its maximum tension when the resting sarcomere length is approximately 2.2 μm. This optimal distance is the same for both skeletal and cardiac muscle, and appears to be the inter-Z distance at which the actin and myosin filaments are able to develop tension most efficiently.

The thick myosin filaments are 1.5 μm in length: the thin actin filaments project 1.0 μm on either side of a Z-line. Since, therefore, the central 0.2 μm of the myosin appears to be devoid of reactive sites, functional overlap between the filaments is maximal when the sarcomere length is 2.2 μm. If the muscle is stretched to increase the sarcomere length beyond this value, overlap is reduced and there are fewer functional bridges between the contractile proteins.

When the inter-Z distance is reduced below 2 μm, the actin filaments overlap in the centre of the sarcomere. The precise way in which this impairs muscular contraction is uncertain; two explanations are commonly suggested. Some workers believe that overlap of the actin filaments reduces the total number of sites available for interaction between the contractile proteins; alternatively, the

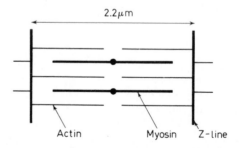

Figure 2.19. Diagram of sarcomere. At an inter-Z distance of 2.2 μm, functional overlap between the myosin and actin filaments is optimal

increase of fibre diameter which occurs when the muscle shortens may separate adjacent contractile elements, thus reducing the mutual longitudinal force they can exert.

Extrinsic factors

Myocardial contractility is influenced by changes of sympathetic stimulation to the heart, and by changes in the composition of the blood. Experimentally, it is increased by stellate ganglion stimulation, and decreased by sympathectomy. In the intact animal it is increased when cardiovascular sympathetic tone is enhanced during shock and exercise, and decreased in response to baroreceptor stimulation (*see* page 97). Ventricular muscle appears to receive no direct nerve supply from the vagus (*see* page 115), therefore changes of parasympathetic tone have no direct effect on myocardial contractility, although they may have a secondary effect mediated via changes of heart rate (*see* below).

Myocardial contractility is depressed by most (probably all) of the commonly-used general anaesthetic agents (*see* Chapter 7), although with some there may be a compensatory increase of sympatho-adrenal activity which compensates for the primary myocardial depression. Carbon dioxide has a similar effect; hypercapnia decreases the contractility of the isolated heart, but, in the intact animal, it is accompanied by increased sympatho-adrenal activity, which counteracts its primary effect on the heart. Myocardial contractility is also depressed by hypoxia.

An increase of myocardial contractility also occurs in response to an increased load on the heart, and sometimes to an increase of heart rate. These responses occur without any increase of myocardial diastolic fibre length; they are therefore termed 'homeometric autoregulation' (Sarnoff and Mitchell, 1962), in contrast to the Frank-Starling mechanism which depends on change of fibre length ('heterometric autoregulation').

Experimentally, in the intact animal, an increase of arterial blood pressure may be accompanied by an increase of ventricular performance. This occurs even in the absence of an increase of coronary perfusion, and without any increase of ventricular end-diastolic pressure. The response therefore differs fundamentally from the increase of ventricular performance which occurs when arterial resistance is increased in the isolated heart-lung preparation. In the latter case the increased arterial pressure causes a transient inability of the ventricle to expel all the blood it receives from the veins; the resulting ventricular distension causes an increase of myocardial contractile force by the Frank-Starling mechanism.

MECHANICAL EVENTS OF THE CARDIAC CYCLE

Atrial systole

Atrial systole follows immediately after the onset of the P wave of the electrocardiogram. Contraction of the two atria is normally slightly asynchronous; right atrial systole normally precedes contraction of the left atrium by approximately 0.02 s. Atrial systole is accompanied by a small rise of intra-atrial pressure (5–6 mm Hg on the right, 7–8 mm Hg on the left) which forces a small, additional quantity of blood into the ventricle, and causes a small increase of ventricular end-diastolic pressure.

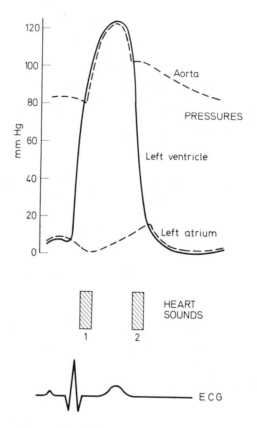

Figure 2.20. Mechanical events in cardiac cycle (traditional)

The atrium is sometimes regarded as analogous to a supercharger* on a petrol engine although, in fact, atrial contraction does not appear to be of great importance except during exercise, when ventricular filling time is seriously curtailed. It is said that, during heavy exercise, as much as 40 per cent of ventricular filling may depend on atrial contraction. Atrial fibrillation has little effect on normal life, but does limit exercise tolerance.

Ventricular systole

Ventricular systole occurs 0.12–0.20 s after contraction of the atria, immediately after the start of the QRS complex of the electrocardiogram. Systole is initially isometric because the A-V valves are closed, and the intraventricular

*A supercharger on a petrol engine forces the petrol-air mixture into the cylinders, thus increasing the quantity of mixture entering the engine over that possible if induction depended on atmospheric pressure alone.

pressure has not risen sufficiently to overcome the end-diastolic pressure in the pulmonary artery or aorta (about 7 and 80 mm Hg respectively).

Although ventricular volume is constant during this phase of contraction, small changes of ventricular shape may still occur; these may be detected by certain recording techniques and incorrectly interpreted as changes of ventricular volume. It is, therefore, probably more correct to describe this phase of ventricular contraction as isovolumetric rather than isometric.

When ventricular pressure exceeds the diastolic pressure in the aorta or pulmonary artery, the semilunar valves open and ventricular ejection starts. This period of the cardiac cycle is divided (rather arbitrarily) into two phases—an initial rapid and a later reduced phase. The end of the maximum ejection phase coincides with the start of the T wave of the electrocardiogram.

Ventricular ejection

It was formerly thought that the maximum rate of systolic ejection coincides with the peak of ventricular pressure. Electromagnetic flowmeter studies by Spencer and Greiss (1962) have shown, however, that peak blood flow velocity occurs about 0.1 s after the start of ventricular systole, while the pressure peak does not occur until about 0.08 s later (*Figure 2.21*). By the time ventricular pressure has reached its maximum, aortic flow velocity has declined to perhaps half its peak value.

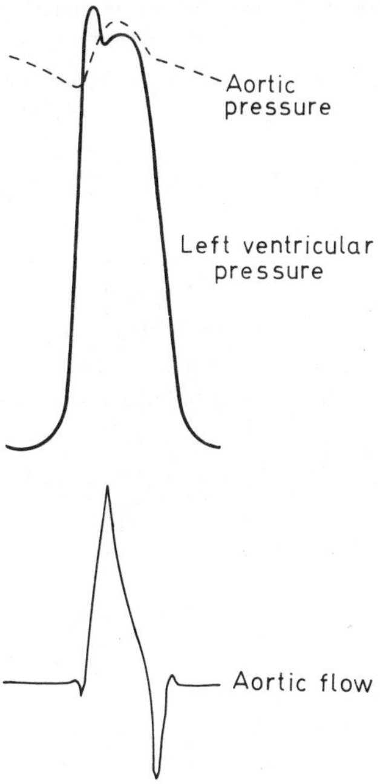

Figure 2.21. Aortic and left-ventricular pressures and aortic blood flow (semi-diagrammatic, based on Spencer and Greiss, 1962)

The period during which aortic flow velocity is increasing is very short (*see Figure 2.21*). During this time intraventricular pressure must exceed the pressure in the aortic root. When flow velocity begins to decrease, however, the pressure gradient must be in the opposite direction, that is, in a direction to oppose blood flow out of the ventricle. Contrary to what might be expected, therefore, aortic pressure during this phase of the cardiac cycle actually exceeds intraventricular pressure, although the difference is only a few mm Hg. Ventricular pressure is greater than aortic pressure for only about 50 per cent of the ejection phase of the cardiac cycle.

This apparent contradiction to the rule that flow is proportional to the pressure gradient (*see* page 5) is explained by the fact that this relationship applies only to steady flow—when pressure energy is dissipated by viscous resistance, but is not converted into kinetic energy. Under unsteady (pulsatile) conditions blood is accelerated first in one direction then in another, that is, pressure energy is converted into kinetic energy and *vice versa*. Under these conditions the relationship $\Delta P = \dot{Q}R$ must be replaced by an equation which contains an inertial component:

$$\Delta P = \dot{Q}R + \rho l/A \, d\dot{Q}/dt$$

where $\dot{Q}$ is the blood flow,
  R is the resistance to flow,
  ρ is the density of blood,
  l is the length of the blood vessel,
  A is its cross-sectional area, and
  $d\dot{Q}/dt$ is the rate of change of blood flow.

Under most conditions it may be shown that pressure differences due to the second term are unlikely to exceed 1 mm Hg.

The phase of rapid systolic ejection merges imperceptibly into the phase of reduced ejection. This transition coincides in time with ventricular repolarization, that is, with the T wave of the electrocardiogram. The reason for this reduction of systolic ejection is a decrease of generated tension as the myocardial fibres shorten; this occurs because part of the force of myocardial contraction is expended in overcoming myocardial viscosity, an effect which is partially offset by an increase of mechanical efficiency at low ventricular volumes (the Laplace relationship, *see* page 12).

At the end of systole the ventricles relax. The intraventricular pressure falls below arterial pressure and the aortic and pulmonary valves close. The subsequent period of isometric ventricular relaxation is terminated by opening of the A-V valves, allowing blood, stored in the atria during ventricular systole, to enter the relaxed ventricles.

Ventricular filling

Early ventricular filling is extremely rapid, particularly during heavy exercise. It is therefore necessary to enquire into the nature of the force which drives blood into the ventricles so rapidly. Linden (1965) calculates that, during exercise at a heart rate of 180 beats min^{-1} (diastole 0.13 s, systole 0.20 s) and with a cardiac output of 25 l min^{-1}, ventricular filling must occur at the rate of 65 l min^{-1}, which is considerably greater than the rate of ventricular ejection (42 l min^{-1}).

Ventricular suction

It has been suggested that, during early diastole, the ventricles 'suck' blood from the atria, that is, the ventricular pressure during this phase of the cardiac cycle falls below the intrathoracic pressure. The evidence for such ventricular suction has been reviewed by Brecher (1958). Bloom (1955) showed that an excised rat heart in a beaker of saline moved about as fluid was expelled from the ventricles during each contraction. He argued that, as the heart was continually expelling fluid, it must be taking in fluid at the same rate, and that this could only be due to ventricular suction. More direct evidence is given by the experimental fact that intraventricular pressures of 10 cm H_2O below the surrounding intrathoracic pressure have been measured in the closed left ventricle of dogs (Brecher, 1956).

Ventricular suction appears to be greatest when the heart is small, or when it is stimulated by sympathetic activity or sympathomimetic amines. Rushmer (1961) suggests that the recoil arises because ventricular contraction stretches the connective tissues between various bands of cardiac muscle, with the result that this stored energy is released during early diastole. If this is so, diastolic ventricular recoil is analogous to the expansion of the chest which occurs when it is released from a position below functional residual capacity. The ventricular volume corresponding to minimal tension in the intermuscular connective tissue has not, however, been established.

Jugular venous pulse

The hydrostatic pressure in the jugular venous system (JVP) provides a valuable index of pressure in the right atrium because there is normally little obstruction to blood flow between the superior vena cava and the heart. JVP is measured clinically either by a manometer connected to a central venous catheter introduced percutaneously through an arm vein—central venous pressure (CVP—*see* page 278) or is assessed by measuring the height of the internal jugular column of blood above the sternal angle.

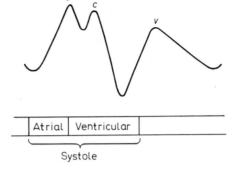

Figure 2.22. The venous pressure pulse (semi-diagrammatic)

Quite apart from providing an index of CVP, clinical assessment of the way in which jugular pressure varies with respiration may give valuable information about cardiac function. JVP normally falls with inspiration as the increasingly sub-atmospheric intrathoracic pressure is transmitted to the extrathoracic veins.

In constrictive pericarditis or cardiac tamponade, however, inspiration may impede cardiac filling, therefore there is a paradoxical increase of venous pressure on inspiration. The interpretation of CVP in relation to cardiac output is considered in Chapter 4.

The normal jugular venous pulse-wave has three positive peaks—*a, c* and *v*—and two intervening troughs (*Figure 2.22*). The *a* wave is due to atrial contraction; it is increased when outflow from the right heart is impeded as in pulmonary stenosis or pulmonary hypertension. The *c* wave is probably due to pulsation transmitted from the ventricles. The *v* wave is due to atrial filling at a time when the tricuspid valve is closed during ventricular systole.

Intracardial pressures

Average values for the pressures in the various chambers of the heart are given in *Table 2.2*.

Table 2.2 NORMAL INTRACARDIAC PRESSURES IN MAN (ADAPTED FROM BRAUNWALD AND CHAPMAN, (1963)

Site	Mean	Range
RA (mean)	3 mm Hg	1–5 mm Hg
RV (peak-systolic)	26 mm Hg	19–31 mm Hg
(end-diastolic)	4 mm Hg	2–6 mm Hg
PA (mean)	14 mm Hg	10–18 mm Hg
(peak systolic)	23 mm Hg	16–29 mm Hg
(end-diastolic)	9 mm Hg	5–13 mm Hg
LA (mean)	8 mm Hg	2–12 mm Hg
('wedge')	8 mm Hg	5–13 mm Hg
LV (end-diastolic)	9 mm Hg	5–12 mm Hg

THE HEART VALVES

The valves which guard the entrances and exits of the two ventricles enable the rhythmic contraction and relaxation of the myocardium to produce a one-way flow of blood through the heart. The demands made on these valves are severe; artificial prostheses compare very unfavourably with the natural product. Not only must the valves open widely to present a small forward resistance, but they must also close promptly and efficiently to prevent regurgitation. They do this some 100 000 times a day for up to 100 years, usually without the development of any serious wear and tear.

The heart valves are of two types, atrio-ventricular (A-V) and semilunar.

Atrio-ventricular valves

The mitral valve has two large cusps of unequal size—an anteromedial and a smaller posterolateral. The tricuspid valve has two large cusps and an additional smaller cusp situated medially.

The area of the cusps is considerably greater than that of the A-V valve ring, therefore they overlap considerably during ventricular systole. Eversion is prevented by the *chordae tendinae* and the papillary muscles which contract at the start of systole, before intraventricular pressure has risen appreciably. The upper parts of the cusps are joined at the commissures so that the area of the orifice is reduced to little larger than that of the aortic valve (Brock, 1952).

The mechanism of closure of the (A-V) valves is worthy of comment. It is often taught that atrial systole is essential if regurgitation is not to occur. Although recent work by cineradiography has cast doubt on the absolute validity of this statement, it is probably substantially correct. Atrial systole causes a surge of blood into the ventricle at the end of diastole. When the atrium relaxes, inertia causes this blood to continue flowing into the ventricle, producing a region of reduced pressure between the valve cusps which are therefore pulled into apposition. Valvular closure is also facilitated by eddy currents behind the cusps and by the fact that a single papillary muscle sends chordae to more than one cusp, thus tending to close the valve when the heart contracts. If ventricular systole is delayed, the cusps tend to float apart again and there may be some regurgitation at the start of systole. Inefficient closure of the valves may therefore occur in atrial fibrillation, when there is no effective atrial contraction, or when A-V conduction is impaired.

Semilunar valves

The competence of the aortic and pulmonary valves depends on the mechanical construction of their cusps rather than on a system of guy-ropes as is the case with the A-V valves. The semilunar valves consist of three symmetrical cusps attached to the fibrous skeleton of the heart at the origins of the aorta and pulmonary artery. This tricuspid arrangement permits the valves both to open and close completely; the condition of bicuspid aortic valve may produce symptoms of aortic stenosis because, as a result of its bicuspid construction, it may not be able to open completely.

The openings of the coronary arteries are protected by the sinuses of Valsalva. Eddy currents in these dilatations prevent the valve cusps occluding the coronary ostia during systolic ejection; they may also be concerned with valvular closure. It has been shown in model systems that considerable regurgitation may occur in early diastole if the sinuses of Valsalva are obliterated (Bellhouse and Talbot, 1969).

Timing of valve opening and closure

The timing of opening and closure of the heart valves (based on Braunwald, Fishman and Cournand, 1956) is shown in *Figure 2.23*. The two sides of the heart do not contract absolutely synchronously, therefore heart sounds due to valvular closure may be slightly split (*see* page 59).

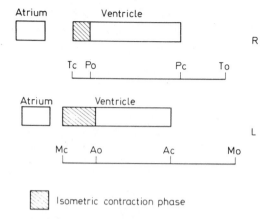

Figure 2.23. *Timing of opening and closure of heart valves (based on Braunwald, Fishman and Cournand, 1956)*

Artificial heart valves

Surgical replacement of an irreparably damaged heart valve was first described by Murray, Roschlan and Lougheed (1956), who replaced a damaged mitral valve with an aortic homograft obtained from a cadaver. Since that time numerous workers have described the use of aortic homografts and heterografts (typically pig valves) to replace damaged mitral and aortic valves. But, although the short-term function of these biological valve replacements is good, they tend to deteriorate with time; and for this reason the modern tendency is to use some form of mechanical valve replacement.

Such prosthetic valves are of five general types (Wright, 1972): the flap valve, e.g. the Abrams; the tricuspid leaflet valve; the ball valve, e.g. the Starr-Edwards; the disc valve; and the pivoting disc valve. Of these the most generally satisfactory at the present time would appear to be the Starr-Edwards ball-in-cage valve, which has of course undergone considerable development since its original description (Starr, 1960).

With all these devices the area available for forward flow is considerably less than with a normal valve; this reduction of cross-sectional area becomes particularly important during exercise. In addition, inertia of the moving part of the valve, for example the ball of a Starr-Edwards prosthesis, causes slight hesitation on closure and some degree of regurgitation. Thrombosis is also an ever-present hazard with all forms of artificial heart valve. The haemodynamic performance of a typical prosthetic valve has been investigated in detail by Rockoff et al. (1966).

HEART SOUNDS AND MURMURS

Some of the mechanical events of the cardiac cycle produce sounds which are transmitted to the body surface where they may be heard either by the unaided ear, or via a stethoscope, or microphone, amplifier and loudspeaker. The output of the amplifier system may also be recorded on moving paper as a phonocardiogram. Phonocardiography has very considerably increased our understanding of the timing of cardiac murmurs, and of abnormal sounds such as the 'opening snap' of mitral stenosis.

At least four heart sounds may be demonstrated by phonocardiography, but only two (or, in younger subjects, three) are normally audible by clinical auscultation.

Heart sounds

First sound

The first heart sound marks the commencement of ventricular systole and coincides with the R wave of the electrocardiogram (*Figure 2.24*). It is due mainly to rapid development of tension in the cusps of the A-V valve, as a result of the rapid rise of intraventricular pressure which occurs at the start of systole. Vibrations from the valve cusps are reinforced by vibrations from the walls of the ventricles, pulmonary artery and aorta, giving rise to the characteristic low-pitched 'lub'. The tricuspid sound is best heard in the fifth intercostal space, just to the left of the sternum; the mitral sound in the fifth space at the cardiac apex.

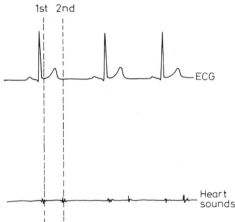

Figure 2.24. Timing of first and second heart sounds in relation to electrocardiogram

Contraction of the two ventricles is normally slightly asynchronous, therefore the first sound may be slightly split, even in normal subjects. Splitting may also occur when the sound has two components corresponding respectively to the isometric and rapid ejection phases of ventricular systole, and, of course, it is widely split in bundle branch block.

The intensity of the first sound depends on the force of myocardial contraction, on the physical characteristics of the valve cusps, and on the degree to which they are apposed at the start of systole. This last factor depends in turn on heart rate and the force of atrial contraction. In mitral stenosis left ventricular filling is impeded; and the first sound is characteristically loud because the valve cusps are still widely separated at the start of ventricular systole. (Closure of the mitral valve is probably initiated by a rapid flow of blood into the ventricle at the end of diastole; *see* page 57).

Changes of the intensity of the first sound have been used as an indication of myocardial function during anaesthesia (Rence, Cullen and Hamilton, 1956). Theoretically, its loudness might just give an indication of the value of dP/dt_{max}, which is an index of myocardial contractility (*see* page 47), although, in view of the many factors which affect the loudness of the first sound, such deductions should be made with care, or possibly not at all.

Second sound

The second heart sound is caused by vibrations set up by aortic and pulmonary valves at the start of ventricular diastole. It normally coincides with the end of the T wave of the electrocardiogram (*Figure 2.24*). The loudness of the second heart sound depends on the arterial pressure distal to the valve. In adult life the aortic component is normally the louder; the reverse is the case during early post-natal life. The loudness of the pulmonary component is increased by pulmonary hypertension; that of the aortic sound is increased by systemic hypertension.

Splitting of the second heart sound.   Normally, the pulmonary and aortic components of the second sound are almost synchronous in expiration. Inspiration, however, increases blood flow through the right side of the heart, thus delaying closure of the pulmonary valve and causing splitting of the second sound. In left bundle branch block, closure of the aortic valve is delayed, therefore splitting occurs during expiration, but not inspiration (paradoxical splitting). In right bundle branch block, and in conditions such as atrial septal defect in which blood flow through the right side of the heart is increased, the second sound is widely split.

Third sound

The rapid flow of blood into the ventricles at the start of diastole may cause vibrations which give rise to a third heart sound that can readily be recognized by phonocardiography, but which is rarely audible except when the circulation is hyperdynamic, for example in severe anaemia or thyrotoxicosis. There is dispute about the cause of this sound: some workers believe it to be due to vibration of the ventricular walls, but Fleming (1969) suggests that it is due to vibration of the mitral valve as this is pulled upon by the *chordae tendinae*. A third heart sound may be considered physiological up to the age of 40.

Fourth (atrial) sound

A fourth sound can be demonstrated phonocardiographically, although it cannot normally be heard by auscultation; it is due to atrial contraction. An audible fourth sound (pre-systolic triple rhythm) is always abnormal and indicates forceful atrial contraction. It is said to be due to rapid blood flow into the ventricle, rather than to actual contraction of the atrial walls.

Murmurs

Cardiac murmurs are, of course, abnormal sounds which may be heard on auscultation. They are generally considered to be due to turbulent blood flow (*see* page 5); but Bruns (1959) suggested that they are more likely to be due to the physical phenomenon of 'vortex shedding' (the phenomenon which is responsible for the sound of an aeolian harp).

Leatham (1958a) describes the three mechanisms which commonly give rise to cardiac murmurs: abnormally high flow through a normal valve, as in anaemia; normal flow through a constricted or irregular valve, as in mitral stenosis, or in subacute bacterial endocarditis; or abnormal flow either through an incompetent valve, e.g. aortic regurgitation, or through an abnormal channel such as a patent ductus arteriosus or septal defect.

Auscultation (Leatham, 1958b)

The first heart sound is low-pitched; most of its vibrational energy lies in the frequency range 30–100 Hz. The second sound is of a higher pitch and consists of frequencies within the range 50–200 Hz. The duration of the first sound is between 50 and 100 ms; that of the second sound between 25 and 50 ms.

Heart sounds heard via a stethoscope are considerably distorted by the non-linear response of the human ear to different frequencies, and by distortion introduced by the stethoscope itself. Distortion due to the latter factor varies considerably with the type of instrument: a bell attenuates the high frequencies, whereas a diaphragm tends to attenuate the high frequencies. There is therefore a considerable difference between the sounds heard with a stethoscope and those heard via a chest microphone and electronic amplifier with a uniform frequency response. (It is, however, possible to modify the response of such an amplifier to make it mimic the transmission characteristics of various types of stethoscope.)

THE CARDIAC PUMP

It is the function of the heart to pump blood round the body at a rate sufficient to maintain the tissues in a healthy state. In other words, the heart must generate a cardiac output sufficient to supply the body's nutritional needs, particularly of oxygen, and also to remove its metabolic waste products from the tissues, where they are produced.

As discussed in Chapter 4, cardiac output is normally determined to a large extent by the state of the peripheral circulation, that is, by the factors which influence the flow of blood back to the heart. Guyton (1968) points out that the heart normally plays a 'permissive role' in the regulation of cardiac output; it permits cardiac output to attain high values when sufficient blood is able to return from the peripheral circulation, although normally output is limited by the rate at which blood can return to the heart from the periphery (the venous return).

The output of the heart is given by the equation:

cardiac output = heart rate x stroke volume.

Stroke volume is equal to the difference between ventricular end-diastolic volume and ventricular end-systolic volume. That is:

cardiac output = heart rate x (v. end-diastolic vol. − v. end-systolic vol.)

It is sometimes convenient to discuss the regulation of cardiac output in terms of the three parameters: heart rate, ventricular end-diastolic volume and ventricular end-systolic volume; but it is often better to use Guyton's holistic approach (*see* Chapter 4).

Heart rate

Heart rate depends on the rate at which the sino-atrial (S-A) node generates its centrifugally-spreading wave of electrical depolarization. This node receives fibres from both the sympathetic and parasympathetic divisions of the autonomic nervous system (*see* next chapter). The sympathetic preganglionic fibres arise in the upper thoracic cord (T1-T5), synapse in the cervical sympathetic ganglia, and then pass to the heart as postganglionic fibres via the cardiac nerves. Although the S-A node receives fibres from both sympathetic chains, its innervation is mainly from the right side. The parasympathetic preganglionic fibres arise in the dorsal motor nucleus of the vagus and synapse in the immediate vicinity of the pacemaker cells.

Effects of cardiac denervation on heart rate

Both divisions of the autonomic nervous system exert a continuous influence on the heart rate. The sympathetic division is stimulatory; the parasympathetic, inhibitory. In experimental animals denervation of the S-A node causes tachycardia, indicating that parasympathetic inhibition is normally more important than sympathetic stimulation.

In humans the heart may be denervated chemically by blocking its parasympathetic supply with atropine and its sympathetic innervation, which is almost entirely β-adrenergic, with propranolol. The intrinsic heart rate is then found to be approximately 110 beats min^{-1} (Sutton et al., 1967), which indicates that, in man as in lower mammals, parasympathetic tone is more important than sympathetic tone in the control of resting heart rate. The changes of heart rate which occur as part of the body's response to physiological stimulation are normally mediated by simultaneous, and opposite, changes of sympathetic and parasympathetic activity. Changes of heart rate caused by mesenteric traction are not completely abolished by the administration of normal doses of atropine.

During exercise, heart rate is increased not only by changes of autonomic activity but also by changes of body temperature and of plasma catecholamine concentration. It is interesting that changes of heart rate still occur in the completely denervated heart (Donald and Shepherd, 1963). Indeed, the exercise tolerance of greyhounds is not greatly diminished by cardiac denervation. Presumably the increase of heart rate which occurs under these conditions is mediated either by increase of blood temperature or by increased secretion of catecholamines from the adrenal medullae.

Relationship between heart rate and cardiac output

An increase of heart rate normally results in an increase of cardiac output. Such an increase is, however, usually accompanied by a decrease of ventricular stroke volume. The relationship between cardiac output and heart rate is, therefore, not linear; the increase tends to fall off at high heart rates. At very high rates diastolic filling is seriously curtailed and cardiac output may actually fall, as happens, for example, during paroxysmal tachycardia.

Changes of heart rate are accompanied by little alteration of systolic duration; they encroach mainly on the period of diastolic filling. At heart rates below 90 beats min^{-1} an increase causes little decrease of stroke volume because the decrease of filling time encroaches mainly on the period of diastasis (*see* page 54); at higher rates, however, the curtailment of diastole encroaches on the period of rapid filling with the result that stroke volume is reduced. Rushmer (1959) stimulated the right atrium of unanaesthetized dogs and showed that increasing the frequency of stimulation caused a progressive decrease of ventricular end-diastolic diameter and of the change of diameter which occurred during systole (*Figure 2.25*). Tye latter parameter is, of course, related to the stroke volume.

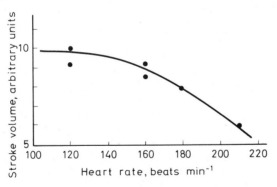

Figure 2.25. Relationship between heart rate and ventricular stroke volume in unanaesthetized, intact dogs (figures from Rushmer, 1959)

In intact man, an increase of heart rate is normally accompanied by an increase of sympathetic tone to the entire cardiovascular system. This increases the force of myocardial contraction (*see* page 51), and raises the mean systemic pressure (*see* page 119); it therefore tends to maintain the stroke volume constant even at high heart rates. During exercise, ventricular filling is aided also by the muscular pump, which tends to force blood back to the heart from the periphery (*see* page 123).

The Bainbridge reflex

It has been shown experimentally that heart rate is influenced by the pressure in the right atrium and great veins. This response was originally described by Bainbridge (1915) who reported that the infusion of saline or blood into the venous side of the circulation caused an increase of heart rate. This response could be abolished by atropine. Some workers have apparently confirmed Bainbridge's findings, others have been unable to do so; and it has been shown by Ahmad and Nicoll (1963) that the magnitude and direction of the response depends on the pre-existing heart rate. At rates below 140 beats min^{-1} venous distension usually causes cardiac acceleration; if the rate is initially high, however, an increase of venous pressure induces bradycardia. The physiological importance of this response in man is unknown.

Ventricular end-diastolic volume

Ventricular end-diastolic volume is determined by the pre-existing ventricular end-systolic volume, the effective ventricular filling pressure, the distensibility of the ventricle and the time available for cardiac filling. The effective ventricular filling pressure is the pressure difference between the interior of the ventricle and its exterior (the intrathoracic pressure).

The intraventricular pressure is normally almost identical to that in the corresponding atrium because the flow resistance provided by the A-V valves is slight. As explained on page 109, the pressure in the right atrium (r.a.p.) is determined by a balance between, on the one hand, the pressures in the peripheral circulation tending to force blood back to the heart and therefore to raise the r.a.p., and, on the other hand, the effectiveness of the cardiac pump which tends to remove blood from the atrium and therefore to reduce r.a.p. Superimposed on the mean pressure are pressure fluctuations due to the intermittent nature of the heart's action.

If the ventricular muscle were completely flaccid during diastole the intraventricular pressure would be identical to the surrounding intrathoracic pressure. This is not, however, the case because as the ventricle fills with blood its wall becomes stretched, and the resulting increase of tension increases the intraventricular pressure above that of its surroundings. The relationship between ventricular volume and transmural pressure is non-linear; the distensibility of the ventricle decreases as it becomes distended. Ventricular filling continues until the back pressure generated by stretch of its walls just balances the distending transmural pressure, at which point ventricular filling ceases.

Very little is known of the factors which affect ventricular distensibility. There is some evidence that sympathomimetic amines may reduce myocardial viscosity, although they probably have little effect on the static compliance of the ventricle. The factors which may influence the diastolic distensibility of the ventricle have recently been reviewed by Levine (1972).

At high distending pressures, ventricular expansion may be limited by the relatively inextensible pericardium. This membrane may, however, become stretched when the heart is dilated, as in chronic heart failure (*see* Chapter 10).

As discussed on page 49, ventricular end-diastolic volume is important in determining the vigour of myocardial contraction. Other things remaining constant, an increase of ventricular end-diastolic volume leads, by the Frank-Starling mechanism, to an increase in the force of cardiac contraction.

Ventricular end-systolic volume

During ventricular systole the heart contracts and expels blood into the arterial system until the pressure generated by the ventricle just equals the pressure in the arterial reservoir, at which point ventricular ejection ceases. (This simple analysis neglects the momentum of the blood as it leaves the heart. As explained on page 53, blood continues to flow out of the ventricle even when the aortic pressure exceeds that in the left ventricle. The reversed pressure gradient due to this cause is, however, small and for most purposes may be ignored.)

The relationship between tension in the ventricular wall and the intraventricular pressure or, strictly, the ventricular transmural pressure, depends on the geometrical arrangement of the myocardial muscle fibres. If the ventricle is considered as a roughly spherical chamber, Laplace's law (*see* page 12) predicts that the intraventricular pressure should be inversely proportional to its radius of curvature. At low ventricular volumes, therefore, ventricular muscle is able to generate a greater pressure for a given wall tension than at larger volumes. Therefore, if the tension generated by ventricular contraction remained constant, intraventricular pressure would rise continually during ventricular ejection. This is not, however, the case, and intraventricular pressure falls during systolic ejection until finally cardiac emptying ceases. The reason appears to be that, as the ventricle contracts, the tension generated by its muscle fibres decreases; therefore the intraventricular pressure is declining at the same time as the arterial pressure is rising, and, bearing in mind the above *caveat* about the momentum of blood leaving the ventricle, ventricular ejection ceases when the two pressures are equal.

This fall of developed tension during myocardial contraction appears to be due mainly to myocardial viscosity which prevents rapid changes of ventricular shape. Part of the energy of cardiac contraction is expended in overcoming internal friction within the myocardium, and is therefore not available for the generation of intraventricular pressure.

Ventricular end-systolic volume, therefore depends on aortic pressure, ventricular end-diastolic volume, and the tension which the myocardium can generate from a given end-diastolic volume. This latter factor depends on the biochemical environment of the myocardial cells and on the amount of autonomic stimulation which they receive (*see* page 49). The force of myocardial contraction is increased by sympathetic stimulation, increased concentrations of sympathomimetic amines, and, in the failing heart, by digitalis. It is decreased by circulating toxins, including most general anaesthetic agents (*see* Chapter 8), acidosis and hypoxia.

RECOMMENDED FURTHER READING

Anon (1970). 'Atrial Function in Man.' *Br. med. J.* **1**, 189
Anon (1976). 'Which Prosthetic Valve?' *Lancet* **i**, 619
Bing, R. J. (1965). 'Cardiac Metabolism.' *Physiol. Rev.* **45**, 171
Blake, T. M. (1972). *'Introduction to Electrocardiography'*, 2nd edn. London; Butterworths

Blinks, J. R. (1967). 'On the Measurement of Myocardial Contractility.' *Anesthesiology* **28**, 800

Braunwald, E., Ross, J. Jr and Sonnenblick, E. H. (1967). 'Mechanisms of Contraction of the Normal and Failing Heart.' *New Engl. J. Med.* **277**, 794, 853, 910, 962, 1012

Gabe, I. T. (1974). 'Starling's Law of the Heart and the Geometry of the Ventricle.' In *The Physiological Basis of Starling's Law of the Heart.* Ciba Foundation Symposium 24, 193

Gibson, D. G. (1975). 'Assessment of Left Ventricular Function in Man by Non-invasive Techniques.' In Oliver, M. F., *Modern Trends in Cardiology,* 3rd edn., ch. 8. London; Butterworths

Hoffman, I. (1973). *ZXY in the ABC of ECG.* Chicago; Year Book Medical Publishers

Hoffman, B. F. and Cranefield, P. F. (1964). 'The Physiological Basis of Cardiac Arrhythmias.' *Am. J. Med.* **37**, 670

Hollins, P. J. (1971). 'The Stethoscope: Some Facts and Fallacies.' *Br. J. Hosp. Med.* **5**, 509

Jewell, B. R. (1974). 'Introduction: The Changing Face of the Length Tension Relation.' In *The Physiological Basis of Starling's Law of the Heart.* Ciba Foundation Symposium 24, 7

Kerkut, G. A. and York, B. (1971). *The Electrogenic Sodium Pump.* Bristol; Scientechnica (Publishers) Ltd

Krikler, D. M. (1974). 'A Fresh Look at Cardiac Arrhythmias.' *Lancet* i, 851, 913, 974, 1034

Leatham, A. (1958). 'Auscultation of the heart.' *Lancet* ii, 703

Linden, R. J. (1968). 'The Heart-ventricular Function.' *Anaesthesia* **23**, 566

Marsden, J. D. (1970). 'Why do cells pump ions?' *New Scientist* **45**, 152

Martinez-Mojares, Gudbjarnason, S. and Bing, R. J. (1969). 'Myocardial Metabolism.' In Morgan Jones, A. *Modern Trends in Cardiology,* 2nd edn. London; Butterworths

Naylor, W. G. (1975). 'The Ionic Basis of Contractility, Relaxation and Cardiac Failure.' In Oliver, M. F., *Modern Trends in Cardiology,* 3rd edn. ch. 6. London; Butterworths

Olson, C. B. and Wand, D. R. (1970). 'On Looking at Electrical Activity of Heart Muscle.' *Anesthesiology* **33**, 520

Reitan, J. A., Smith, N. T., Bonson, V. S. and Kadis, L. B. (1972). 'The Cardiac Pre-ejection Period. A Correlate of Peak Ascending Aortic Blood-flow Acceleration.' *Anesthesiology* **36**, 76

Sonnenblick, E. H., Parmley, W. W., Urschel, C. W. and Brutsaert, D. L. (1970). 'Ventricular Function: Evaluation of Myocardial Contractility in Health and Disease.' *Prog. cardiovasc. Dis.* **12**, 449

Taylor, R. R. (1970). 'Theoretical Analysis of the Isovolumic Phase of Left Ventricular Contraction in Terms of Cardiac Muscle Mechanics.' *Cardiovasc. Res.* **4**, 429

Westbury, D. R. (1971). 'Electrical Activity of the Heart.' *Br. med. J.* **4**, 799

Wright, J. T. M. (1972). 'The Heart, its Valves and their Replacement.' *Bio-med. Eng.* **7**, 26

Chapter 3   The Peripheral Circulation and its Control

The function of the cardiovascular system is to provide blood flow through the capillaries of various tissues at a rate sufficient for their immediate metabolic needs. The metabolic requirements of a given tissue vary considerably from moment to moment; the body must therefore be able to adjust tissue blood flow rapidly in accordance with these changing requirements.

The rate of blood flow through a given tissue equals the quotient of the driving pressure (the difference between arterial and venous blood pressures) divided by the resistance to flow (*see* Chapter 1). Under most circumstances homeostatic mechanisms maintain the arterial and venous pressures relatively constant; therefore blood flow through a given tissue depends mainly on its vascular resistance, that is, on the calibre of its blood vessels, particularly the arterioles and precapillary sphincters. These vessels receive a constant vasoconstrictor tone from the sympathetic division of the autonomic nervous system; and changes of vascular calibre in response to events occurring elsewhere in the body are mediated mainly by changes of this sympathetic tone. With the exception of the external genitalia, the parasympathetic division of the autonomic nervous system is not directly concerned with the regulation of tissue blood flow.

Under conditions of stress, for example during severe exercise or after acute haemorrhage, sympathomimetic catecholamines are secreted by the adrenal medullae. These hormones cause alterations of vascular calibre and redistribute blood flow away from organs such as the skin and gut to more immediately essential organs such as the heart, brain and (during exercise) skeletal muscles (*see* Chapters 7 and 9).

The calibre of the resistance vessels is determined also by the local concentration of various (mainly unspecified) tissue metabolites. If blood flow through a tissue becomes temporarily insufficient for its needs, these substances accumulate, induce vasodilatation and increase blood flow until it is again sufficient for the tissue's requirements. This regulatory mechanism acts at a more local level than the generalized regulation provided by the sympatho-adrenal system, which, because of its anatomical arrangement, tends to have a rather diffuse action.

The phenomena of reactive hyperaemia and autoregulation (*see* page 92) are also thought to be due, partly at any rate, to the action of such vasodilator metabolites.

In some tissues the physiological gases, oxygen and carbon dioxide, have a marked action on the resistance blood vessels. The cerebral vessels, for example, are exquisitely sensitive to changes of arterial $P\text{CO}_2$ (*see* page 139), while increases of $Pa\text{O}_2$ may cause renal vasoconstriction (*see* page 149). Carbon dioxide is generally considered to be one of the hypothetical vasodilators responsible for the phenomena discussed in the previous paragraphs.

If cardiac output remains constant, an increase of blood flow to one tissue must be accompanied by decreased flow to the remaining tissues. An increased blood flow requirement by several tissues simultaneously is, however, normally accompanied by a simultaneous increase of cardiac output; this prevents the remainder of the body being deprived of blood. The control of cardiac output is discussed in Chapter 4.

Decrease of energy round the circulation

Blood leaves the heart at a relatively high energy level. As it flows through the peripheral circulation this energy, both kinetic and potential, is converted into heat; therefore the blood returns to the right atrium with much less energy than when it leaves the left ventricle. Except perhaps during exercise, the kinetic component of the total energy in the large arteries is small in comparison to the pressure energy, and may therefore be ignored for most purposes.

In the great veins the blood pressure is almost zero, although the blood still possesses some kinetic energy. Since the total cross-sectional area of the venae cavae is approximately four times that of the aorta, the flow velocity is only about one-quarter as great, therefore the kinetic energy which is proportional to mass $\times$ velocity^2 is less by a factor of 16. (This simple analysis ignores the fact that blood flow in both the aorta and vena cava is pulsatile. Because of the square law relationship between kinetic energy and flow velocity, the mean kinetic energy under pulsatile conditions is not directly proportional to the square of the mean flow velocity.) The decline of mean pressure down the aorta is very slight, and amounts to only 1–2 mm Hg (McDonald and Taylor, 1959). The pressure drop along the large arteries is similarly only a few mm Hg. The mean pressure at the start of the arterioles is therefore in the region of 80 mm Hg, whereas at their capillary ends it has fallen to approximately 30 mm Hg.

THE AUTONOMIC NERVOUS SYSTEM

To understand the role of the sympathetic and parasympathetic nervous systems in cardiovascular regulation, it is necessary to have at least a basic knowledge of the anatomy of the autonomic system. The present account should be supplemented, if necessary, by a standard textbook.

Anatomically, the autonomic outflow from the central nervous system is classified as either thoraco-lumbar or cranio-sacral. Physiologically, these two divisions correspond respectively to the sympathetic and parasympathetic systems.

The autonomic system differs from the somatic nervous system in that a synapse is interposed between the central nervous system and the innervated effector organ. A description of the nerve supply to a given organ must therefore include: the site of origin of the preganglionic neurones, the pathway taken by these neurones after they leave the central nervous system, the location of the synapses between pre- and postganglionic neurones and the pathway taken by the latter as they pass to the appropriate peripheral effector organ.

Sympathetic system

The sympathetic preganglionic fibres are myelinated (B fibres) and arise from cell bodies in the intermedio-lateral column of grey matter of the thoracic and upper lumbar regions of the spinal cord. They leave the cord by ventral nerve roots and pass via white *rami communicantes* to the sympathetic trunk. This consists of a chain of interconnected ganglia lying on either side of the vertebral column.

In the neck, there are three ganglia on each side—the superior, middle and inferior cervical ganglia. The middle and inferior are often fused together; the inferior may be fused with the first thoracic to form the stellate ganglion. There are usually four lumbar and four sacral ganglia on each side. The sympathetic chain ends in front of the coccyx as the unpaired ganglion *impar*. Most preganglionic fibres synapse in the sympathetic trunk; some, however, pass straight through to synapse in prevertebral ganglia. These latter consist of collections of nervous tissue situated around the origins of the three anterior branches of the abdominal aorta, and are called, respectively, the coeliac, superior mesenteric and inferior mesenteric ganglia.

Some preganglionic fibres synapse immediately after entering the sympathetic chain; others pass up or down for a variable distance before synapsing. A single preganglionic fibre synapses with more than one (as many as 200) postganglionic neurones; a single postganglionic neurone receives many preganglionic fibres. This arrangement accounts, in part, for the diffuse nature of sympathetic activity, which contrasts with the localized action of the parasympathetic system (*see* below).

The postganglionic fibres are non-myelinated (C fibres). They either return to the mixed spinal nerve via a grey *ramus communicans,* or pass directly to large blood vessels in the immediate vicinity of the sympathetic ganglia. They are distributed to all types of blood vessel with the exception of the capillaries, which are not innervated.

The preganglionic neurones to the arm arise in the second to the eighth thoracic segments of the spinal cord. The postganglionic fibres arise in the middle and inferior cervical and first two thoracic ganglia. They are distributed to the limb via the branches of the brachial plexus. The preganglionic supply of the leg arises from the last two thoracic and first two lumbar segments; the postganglionic fibres arise in the lumbar and sacral ganglia and are distributed via the lumbosacral plexus.

The sympathetic supply to the heart arises in the upper four or five thoracic segments; the synapses occur in the superior cervical to the fifth thoracic ganglia of the sympathetic trunk. The postganglionic fibres pass directly to the cardiac plexus which lies between the aortic arch and the bifurcation of the trachea. Branches from this plexus supply the sino-atrial and atrio-ventricular nodes (mainly from the right side), and the conducting tissues and ventricular muscle (mainly from the left side).

PARASYMPATHETIC SYSTEM

The parasympathetic nerve supply to the cardiovascular system is functionally much less important than its sympathetic innervation. Most blood vessels receive no parasympathetic innervation. The only exception to this rule is the blood vessels of the external genitalia, which receive a parasympathetic supply via the *nervi erigentes*. The preganglionic neurones of these nerves arise in the second and third sacral segments of the spinal cord, and synapse in the immediate vicinity of the vascular smooth muscle cells which they supply. These nerves are responsible for vasodilatation of the genital erectile tissue during sexual excitement.

Stimulation of the parasympathetic supply to the salivary glands causes vasodilatation as well as salivary secretion. This vasodilatation is, however, not blocked by atropine and appears to be due to local release of the vasoactive polypeptide, bradykinin, rather than to the activity of parasympathetic vasodilator fibres (Hilton and Lewis, 1955).

The vagus nerve provides a resting inhibitory tone to the sino-atrial and atrio-ventricular nodes of the heart (*see* page 30). The synapses occur in the immediate vicinity of the nodal cells. The ventricular muscle itself, however, appears to be devoid of parasympathetic innervation.

Autonomic reflexes

Although it is customary to exclude afferent nerve fibres from descriptions of the autonomic nervous system, it must be remembered that most autonomic activity is reflex in origin, and that cardiovascular adjustments occur in response to stimulation of both somatic and visceral receptors. In each case, the cell bodies of the afferent neurones lie in the dorsal root ganglia of spinal nerves or their cranial homologues. The modified afferent nerve endings found in the aortic arch and carotid sinus and in the carotid and aortic bodies are discussed on pages 97 and 100, respectively.

CHEMICAL TRANSMISSION

Transmission between pre- and postganglionic neurones, and between post-ganglionic nerve endings and various effector organs is mediated by chemical transmitters. The nature of these substances at different sites in the autonomic nervous system is of considerable physiological and pharmacological importance.

Cholinergic and adrenergic transmission

Transmission between preganglionic and postganglionic neurones in both divisions of the autonomic nervous system is mediated by acetylcholine (cholinergic transmission). This substance is also responsible for the actions of the parasympathetic nervous system on its peripherally-situated effector organs. The more central actions of acetylcholine at the synapses between pre- and postganglionic neurones of both divisions of the autonomic nervous system resemble those of nicotine; its peripheral actions mimic those of muscarine. Only the muscarinic actions are blocked by atropine.

The peripheral transmitter of the sympathetic nervous system is, at most sites, the catecholamine noradrenaline (adrenergic transmission). Some peripheral organs are, however, supplied anatomically by the sympathetic system, although the transmitter is, in fact, acetylcholine; transmission at these sites is blocked by atropine. The blood vessels in skeletal muscle receive both adrenergic and cholinergic sympathetic fibres. The latter are responsible for the vasodilatation which occurs at the start of exercise (*see* page 169) and during a fainting attack. In addition, the coronary arteries may receive sympathetic cholinergic fibres, although this has not been definitely proved.

The transmitters are stored in nerve endings as granules or in small vesicles. From time to time small amounts of transmitter are spontaneously released from the nerve ending, but not at a rate sufficient to cause an overt physiological response. The arrival of a nerve action potential, however, causes the release of a relatively large amount of transmitter which reacts with the postsynaptic receptor sites and causes a physiological response. Acetylcholine appears to be stored as such; noradrenaline is stored in the form of a complex with adenosine triphosphate.

Termination of transmitter activity

It is, of course, necessary for released transmitter to be removed rapidly from the receptor sites, otherwise its action would be prolonged, and fine adjustments of autonomic activity would not be possible. Acetylcholine is rapidly destroyed locally by the enzyme acetylcholinesterase (true cholinesterase); in addition, a small amount diffuses away from the nerve endings to be destroyed in the blood by the enzyme butyrocholinesterase (pseudocholinesterase). Although there are analogous enzymes which destroy noradrenaline—catechol-O—methyltransferase (COMT) and monoamine oxidase (MAO)—the duration of action of released noradrenaline is limited mainly by the rate at which it diffuses away from the receptor sites and by the rate at which it re-enters the nerve terminals. The administration of monoamine oxidase or catechol-O-methyltransferase inhibitors has little effect on the body's response to sympathetic stimulation (Crout, 1961). The re-uptake of noradrenaline is, however, an active process which can be blocked by drugs such as cocaine, and the tricyclic antidepressant agents.

Sympatholytic and parasympatholytic drugs

Ganglion blocking drugs

The actions of the autonomic nervous system may be modified pharmacologically in several ways. Ganglionic blocking drugs, such as hexamethonium, block cholinergic transmission between pre- and postganglionic neurones; they therefore paralyse both the sympathetic and parasympathetic systems. Their use as antihypertensive agents is generally unsatisfactory, because their sympatholytic action is complicated by serious side effects due to concomitant parasympathetic paralysis.

Parasympatholytic drugs

The peripheral actions of the parasympathetic system are blocked by atropine. This drug also abolishes the effects of stimulation of the cholinergic neurones of the sympathetic system, and therefore abolishes sweating. When anticholinergic drugs are used to reverse the action of non-depolarizing muscle relaxants, the body must first be protected against the peripheral autonomic effects of acetylcholine by the administration of atropine.

Sympatholytic drugs

There are many types of peripherally-acting sympatholytic agent (Moran, 1966). Only a brief survey is possible here. Many of these drugs are, or have been, used for the treatment of hypertension. They may be classified into drugs which prevent the release of noradrenaline from sympathetic nerve endings and drugs which block the sympathetic receptor sites.

Reserpine depletes the nerve endings of noradrenaline because it prevents binding of this amine in the cell, thus allowing it to diffuse out to be destroyed by monoamine oxidase. Bretylium prevents the release of noradrenaline without preventing its storage. Guanethidine has a complex action which is mainly due to inhibition of noradrenaline release. α-Methyl dopa is synthesized into α-methyl noradrenaline, as compared with dopa which is converted into noradrenaline as part of the normal synthesis of this agent. α—Methyl noradrenaline is stored in the nerve endings and released by sympathetic stimulation; it is, however, less potent than noradrenaline in stimulating adrenoreceptive sites, therefore it causes little peripheral sympathetic stimulation.* The response of the body to circulating catecholines is not impaired by the administration of any of the above agents.

The peripheral adrenoreceptive sites may be classified as α or β (*see* page 73). Drugs which block the α receptors include various ergot alkaloids, phenoxybenzamine, tolazoline and phentolamine. The most important β blocking agents, at present, are propranolol and practolol. The latter has the advantage that it is relatively cardiospecific (that is, it has little effect on the bronchi); but it is now under a cloud because of undesirable side-effects.

Sympathomimetic amines

The response of the cardiovascular system to stress consists in part of a generalized increase of sympathetic activity to the heart and peripheral circulation, and in part to increased secretion of sympathomimetic amines from the adrenal medullae. The adrenal medullary cells are physiologically analogous to sympathetic postganglionic neurones. In man, however, they secrete two hormones, adrenaline and noradrenaline, whereas the adrenergic neurones of the sympathetic system proper produce only noradrenaline. The ratio of adrenaline to noradrenaline secreted by the human adrenal medulla is roughly 4 : 1.

---

* This is certainly an oversimplification; and it has now been shown that α-methyl dopa has considerable agonist activity. α-Methyl noradrenaline may, however, reduce catecholamine synthesis or inhibit catecholamine release.

α and β receptors

The actions of naturally-occurring sympathomimetic amines and of their synthetic analogues may best be explained in terms of the receptor theory of drug action. Briefly, this theory proposes that the membrane of effector cells contains specialized regions (receptor sites) which react with physiologically or pharmacologically active substances, and that the process of biochemical combination between drug or hormone and receptor is responsible for the observed change of physiological activity in the effector organ. This concept is now well established, although it should be stressed that the physico-chemical identity of the hypothetical receptors has not yet been demonstrated.

There appear to be at least two distinct types of adrenoceptive site. This is suggested by the fact that the potency ratio of two drugs is not identical throughout the body, as it would be if there were only one type of receptor. Experimentally, it is found that the relative potency of a series of sympathomimetic amines in the body varies from region to region. If the three agents, noradrenaline, adrenaline and isoprenaline, are compared as regards their ability to cause contraction of vascular smooth muscle, the order is noradrenaline, adrenaline, isoprenaline; if these same drugs are compared with regard to cardiac stimulation the order is isoprenaline, adrenaline, noradrenaline.

Ahlquist (1948) proposed that the adrenoceptive sites be classified as α and β. Stimulation of α receptors causes contraction of vascular smooth muscle and consequent vasoconstriction; stimulation of β receptors causes smooth muscle relaxation and vascular dilatation. The receptors of the heart are predominantly β in type.

The type of receptor present in any individual organ may be identified by observation of the effects of specific sympathomimetic amines, the action of which is predominantly on one or other type of receptor. Isoprenaline acts almost entirely on the β receptors; drugs such as phenylephrine stimulate mainly the α receptors. Information may also be obtained by observation of the effects of specific blocking agents such as phenoxybenzamine (α) or propranolol (β). (The latter agent has, however, additional local anaesthetic activity which accounts in part for its anti-dysrhythmic activity on the heart.)

The action of the normal sympathetic transmitter, noradrenaline, is predominantly on α sites. It does, however, have some β activity, otherwise sympathetic stimulation would have little effect on the heart.

THE ARTERIES

The main function of the large and medium-sized arteries is to conduct blood from the heart to the capillaries, where exchange of nutrients and waste products can occur between the tissue cells and the blood. The larger arteries also form an elastic reservoir ('Windkessel') which stores part of the energy of cardiac contraction, and so helps to convert intermittent systolic ejection from the heart into a steady flow of blood through the capillaries. The smallest arteries (arterioles) act in conjunction with the precapillary sphincters (*see* page 79) to form a variable resistance which controls the rate of blood flow through the tissues.

Histology

Histologically, the wall of a typical artery consists of three layers, named from within out the *tunica intima,* the *tunica media,* and *tunica adventitia* (*Figure 3.1*).

The intima is lined by a layer of endothelial cells which is continuous with both the endocardium and the capillary endothelium. This layer is water-repellent and helps to prevent intravascular thrombosis. The intima is separated from the media by the internal elastic lamina.

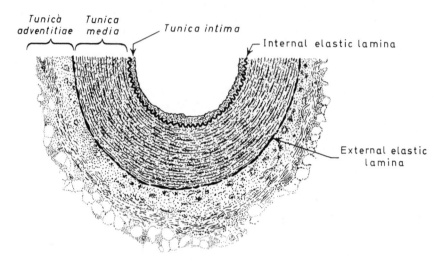

Figure 3.1. TS typical artery (semi-diagrammatic)

The *tunica media* contains both elastic tissue and circularly-arranged smooth muscle fibres. The media of the large (elastic) arteries contains much elastic tissue but relatively little smooth muscle; it is this elastic tissue which enables the artery to store blood during systole, and then to force it at a relatively constant rate through the capillaries during systole. With increasing age the elastic fibres are partially replaced by fibrous tissue, with the result that the arteries become less distensible; systolic pressure therefore rises. The media of the medium-sized (muscular) arteries contains a large amount of circularly-arranged smooth muscle.

The wall of the arterioles consists of little more than a layer of smooth muscle surrounding a tube of vascular endothelium. This muscle receives a copious sympathetic nerve supply and, by its contraction or relaxation, it is responsible for the fine control of tissue blood flow (*see* page 90).

The *tunica adventitia* is composed of intermingled elastic and collagen fibres, which surround the media and merge with the surrounding connective tissues. The innermost layer of adventitia is a layer of elastic material called the external elastic lamina.

Arterial blood pressure

The arterial pressure is generated by the systolic ejection of blood into the arterial tree. If the pressure waveform were symmetrical, its mean would lie

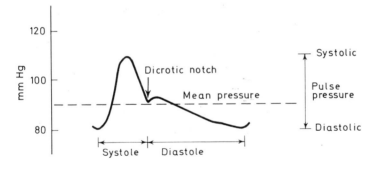

Figure 3.2. Aortic pressure waveform

midway between the systolic and diastolic extremes. This is, however, not the case because the waveform is asymmetrical (*Figure 3.2*), and the mean pressure lies nearer to the diastolic than to the systolic pressure. With a normal pressure waveform, the mean aortic pressure lies approximately one-third of the distance between diastolic and systolic pressures. That is:

$$\text{mean pressure} = \text{diastolic pressure} + \tfrac{1}{3}\ (\text{sys.} - \text{dia.})\ \text{pressure}$$

Ignoring the right atrial pressure, which is only a few mm Hg, aortic blood pressure is related to cardiac output by the formula:

$$\text{mean aortic pressure} = \text{cardiac output} \times \text{total peripheral resistance.}$$

It is easiest to regard this equation as being analogous to Ohm's law:

$$\text{electrical pressure, i.e. volts} = \text{current flow} \times \text{resistance.}$$

Total peripheral resistance (TPR) is the resistance of the entire systemic vascular network lying between the aortic root and the right atrium. It is less than the resistance provided by any single vascular bed because the various organs of the body are all connected in parallel between the arterial and venous sides of the circulation (*Figure 1.11*, page 19). The value of TPR is approximately 20 mm Hg min l^{-1} or 1.2 PRU or 160 000 N s m^{-2} (*see* page 18).

Under normal conditions blood pressure is pulsatile as far as the capillary ends of the arterioles. Flow through the capillaries is, however, almost constant.

The pulse pressure

Pulse pressure is the difference between the systolic and diastolic blood pressures. Although there is obviously a correlation between the aortic pulse pressure and the left ventricular stroke volume, estimation of stroke volume from aortic pressure measurement is fraught with difficulty (*see* page 267). Notwithstanding the lack of a strict quantitative relationship, however, pulse pressure may, at times, give valuable information about cardiac function; and the clinician should have some knowledge of the factors which affect it.

To a first approximation the rate at which blood leaves the arterial reservoir through the peripheral circulation is proportional to the pressure inside the reservoir. During the upstroke of the arterial pressure waveform, left ventricular ejection occurs faster than blood can leave the reservoir; arterial pressure

—

therefore rises. Towards the end of systole the rate of pressure rise declines, and ultimately pressure begins to fall. This occurs partly because of decreased systolic ejection during the latter half of systole (*see* page 53), and partly because of increased peripheral run-off when arterial pressure is high.

The end of systole, which may be defined as the time of aortic valve closure, is indicated by the dicrotic notch on the aortic pressure tracing (*Figure 3.2*). After this time the arterial reservoir is a chamber with only one exit—the peripheral circulation—and the rate of fall of arterial pressure is roughly proportional to the instantaneous pressure, from which it follows that during this part of the cardiac cycle, pressure falls in an approximately exponential manner, with a time constant which is inversely related to the peripheral resistance.

Aortic pulse pressure therefore depends on two factors: left ventricular stroke volume and the distensibility (compliance) of the arterial reservoir. Other things being equal, an increase of stroke volume or a decrease of arterial distensibility causes an increase of pulse pressure. Analysis of the situation is, however, confused by the fact that arterial distensibility depends not only on the physical properties of the arterial wall but also on the height of the mean arterial pressure (*see* page 14).

Left ventricular stroke volume   The factors which affect ventricular stroke volume were discussed in Chapter 2 (*see* page 64). At constant heart rate an increase of cardiac output is accompanied by an increased stroke volume; an increase of heart rate when cardiac output remains constant is, however, accompanied by a decrease of ventricular stroke volume.

Arterial distensibility   In common with many other living tissues, the arterial wall becomes less distensible when stretched. For a given stroke volume, therefore, the pulse pressure is greater when the mean arterial pressure is high. This dependence of pulse pressure on mean pressure is clearly of great clinical importance, yet it is a fact which is often poorly appreciated. The low volume 'thready' pulse of shock is due partly to a decrease of left ventricular stroke volume and partly to a low mean arterial pressure.

In old age, the arterial walls lose their elasticity, becoming less distensible, therefore a given stroke volume causes a larger pulse pressure than it would in a younger person.

The arterial pulse wave

During systole, blood is ejected from the left ventricle into the aorta; and because of the inertia (resistance to acceleration) of the blood already there, much of this newly-ejected blood has to be temporarily accommodated in the proximal end of the arterial reservoir, where it causes localized distension and a consequent localized increase of pressure. This region of increased pressure then travels down the aorta and its branches as a centrifugally-spreading wave, which successively distends the more peripheral parts of the arterial tree. Its passage gives rise to the peripheral pressure pulse which is felt clinically.

Pulse wave velocity

The velocity of the pulse wave in large arteries is approximately 5 m s^{-1} although it varies somewhat with the physical properties of the arterial wall, and with the arterial pressure. The less distensible the arterial wall the greater is the pulse wave velocity; and the velocity is greater in the smaller arteries because they are less distensible than the aorta. (In a completely rigid tube the pulse wave velocity would equal the speed of sound in blood—approximately 1500 m s^{-1}.)

The pressure pulse takes approximately 0.03 s to travel from the aortic root to the carotid artery, and 0.1 s from the carotid to the radial arteries.

(Discussion about pulse wave velocity is complicated by the fact that the different frequency components (*see* page 274) of the aortic pressure wave travel at different velocities, therefore the concept of a single pulse wave velocity is to some extent an approximation, albeit for many purposes a useful one.)

Pulse wave velocity versus blood flow velocity

It is important not to confuse pulse wave velocity with actual blood flow velocity; the latter is much less than the former. In the aorta the mean velocity of blood flow is approximately 1 m s^{-1}, but, as a result of the marked increase of cross-sectional area due to peripheral branching, the velocity declines rapidly down the arterial tree. Flow velocity in the capillaries is only about 0.005 m s^{-1}.

Change of shape of arterial pressure waveform as it passes peripherally

There is a marked change in the shape of the arterial pulse wave as it passes peripherally (*Figure 3.3*). This change consists of an increase of pulse pressure (systolic minus diastolic pressure) due mainly to an increase of systolic pressure. Despite this increase of systolic pressure, however, the area under the curve and, therefore, the *mean* arterial pressure, remains almost constant. Systolic pressure in the femoral artery is 15–25 mm Hg above that in the aorta, but the mean pressures are almost identical.

The cause of this alteration of waveform as the pressure pulse passes peripherally is not known with certainty. One explanation is that the pulse wave is reflected at the periphery—particularly from the origins of the precapillary resistance vessels (*see* below)—and that the incident and reflected waves then interact to cause pressure variations (standing waves) throughout the arterial system. In some regions (antinodes) the two waves summate to cause large pressure fluctuations; elsewhere (nodes) the waves cancel and the fluctuations are minimal.

It has been shown in mathematical models of the arterial system that reflections may occur wherever the diameter or the distensibility of the arterial tree changes. The most important site where such reflections may occur is probably the origin of the arterioles. McDonald (1960) suggests that the coefficient of reflection (ratio of the respective magnitudes of reflected and incident waves) lies between 0.3 and 0.5 in most parts of the systemic circulation.

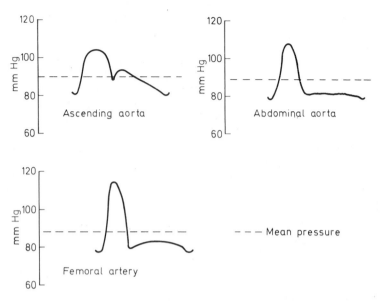

Figure 3.3. Pressure waveforms in ascending aorta, abdominal aorta, and femoral artery (based on McDonald, 1960)

Another explanation for the peripheral change of shape of the arterial pressure wave is that the arterial wall attenuates some frequency components of the pressure pulse preferentially. As a result, the relative proportions of different components of the pressure waveform vary throughout the arterial tree, and the shape of the overall pressure waveform varies also.

The practical consequences of the change of systolic pressure which occurs down the arterial system are obvious: the significance of a given pressure must be considered in relation to its site of measurement. Systolic pressure is higher in the peripheral arteries than in the aorta; the mean pressures are, however, almost identical.

THE CAPILLARIES AND THE MICROCIRCULATION

Capillary blood is separated from the interstitial fluid, the *milieu intérior* of Claude Bernard, by only a single layer of endothelial cells. This is permeable to small molecules such as oxygen, carbon dioxide and glucose, and thus permits the ready exchange of nutrients and metabolites between the blood plasma and the tissue fluid. Neglecting small concentration differences due to the Donnan effect (*see* page 86), the concentration of such substances is almost identical on the two sides of the capillary membrane.

The capillaries, together with the smallest arterioles and venules, constitute the microcirculation, a region of the circulation which is becoming of increasing clinical importance as our understanding of the pathogenesis of such conditions as irreversible shock increases (*see* Chapter 9; also Recommended Further Reading). The anatomical arrangement of the microcirculation has been extensively investigated by Zweifach (1959; 1974). (It must be stressed that Zweifach did not, and obviously could not, investigate all tissues in detail; his findings, therefore, may not necessarily apply to all organs.)

Histology

According to Zweifach the true capillaries arise, not directly from the arterioles, but from channels which are intermediate in structure between an arteriole and a post-capillary venule. These channels are called 'metarterioles', and differ from true arterioles in having only a partial coating of smooth muscle. The true capillaries arise at right angles from the metarterioles, their point of origin being guarded by a ring of smooth muscle called a precapillary sphincter (*Figure 3.4a*).

In certain tissues, there are arterio-venous anastomoses which link the small arteries and veins, thus allowing blood to pass directly through the tissue, without entering the capillaries. In the skin these vessels form a low-resistance pathway, through which a large flow of blood can pass when the body needs to dissipate heat rapidly (*see* page 151). The presence of such anastomoses makes

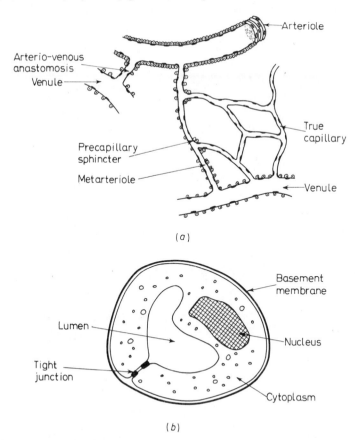

Figure 3.4. (a) The microcirculation (semi-diagrammatic, based on Zweifach, 1959). (b) TS typical capillary (semi-diagrammatic)

the interpretation of tissue blood flow measurements difficult; most techniques measure total blood flow rather than capillary flow, whereas it is the latter which is usually of most physiological importance.

In tissues which do not possess actual arterio-venous anastomoses, there may be *thoroughfare channels*. These form links between the small arteries and veins, and are rather larger than metarterioles, but not as large as the true arterio-venous anastomoses.

It is obviously difficult to calculate accurately the amount of blood contained in the capillaries. The figure usually quoted is approximately 5 per cent of the total blood volume, although Wiedeman (1963) suggests that the amount may be less, and that most of the blood in the microcirculation is held in the post-capillary venules (*Figure 3.5*).

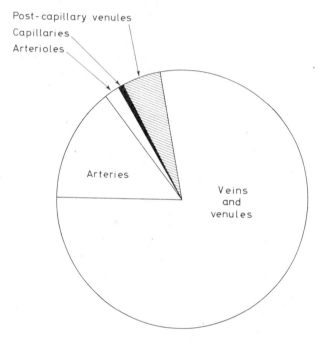

Figure 3.5. Distribution of total blood volume throughout the circulation (from Wiedeman, 1963)

The cross-sectional area of the vascular bed increases considerably as the circulation branches; and the blood flow velocity is correspondingly reduced. Rough calculations suggest that the total surface area of capillary endothelium is approximately 60 square metres in the systemic capillary bed and 40 square metres in the pulmonary circulation (*see* also *Figure 3.6*).

Dimensions

The length of an average capillary is between 0.4 and 0.7 mm, although the path taken by an individual erythrocyte between an arteriole and the

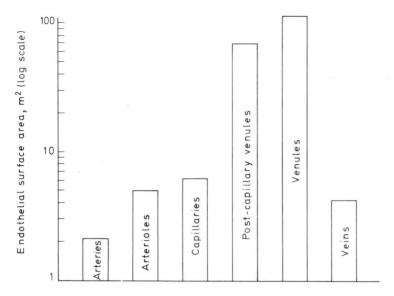

Figure 3.6. Endothelial surface area in various regions of the systemic circulation (figures from Wiedeman, 1967)

corresponding venule may be longer if the cell follows a tortuous path. The normal capillary transit time at rest is approximately 0.7 s. The capillaries vary in diameter from 20 μm down to 5 μm or less. The smallest capillaries are, therefore, smaller than the erythrocytes; these cells are, however, not rigid but can undergo deformation to enable them to pass easily through the narrowest capillaries.

Control of capillary flow

The capillaries themselves appear to have no power of independent contraction. Their endothelial cells are passive, and blood flow is regulated by contraction or relaxation of the metarterioles and precapillary sphincters. At any one time only part of the total number of capillaries in a given tissue is patent; this is the phenomenon of vasomotion.

Examination of living tissue under the microscope reveals that, as some capillaries open, others close. This rhythmic response is called 'vasomotion' and is due to periodic contraction and relaxation of the precapillary sphincters, presumably in response to local changes in the concentration of vasodilator metabolites (*see* page 91). There is a gradient of such vasomotor activity throughout the microcirculation, it being greatest in the smallest vessels; and this quantitative difference of smooth muscle activity is reflected in differences in the cells' electrical activity (Akers and Lee, 1953).

In tissues such as the skeletal muscles where the oxygen demand is very variable, the majority of capillaries are shut during periods of inactivity; and there is a great increase in the number of open capillaries when metabolic activity increases. This expansion of the capillary bed greatly reduces the distance over which oxygen must diffuse between the erythrocytes and the cellular mitochondria. In skeletal muscle Krogh (1919) calculated that there were 100 times more capillaries open during exercise than during rest; and although subsequent studies have suggested that he probably overestimated the difference, there is no doubt that the ratio is considerable.

Methods of studying the microcirculation

It is possible to get a rough, although at times rather inaccurate, picture of the state of the microcirculation of an organ by measuring its overall perfusion in relation to the perfusion pressure. It is also possible to measure the optical density of a superficial tissue and to infer changes in the microcirculation from changes of light transmission. The optical density of the ear pinna, for example, is reduced during induction of anaesthesia with both cyclopropane and ether (Neff, Stiles and Michelson, 1938), suggesting that these agents cause microcirculatory vasoconstriction.

The difficulty with this type of technique is that it estimates overall tissue perfusion, and therefore does not necessarily give a valid indication of blood flow through the capillaries. An increase of tissue flow may by-pass the exchange vessels via thoroughfare channels or arterio-venous anastomoses (*see* page 79).

Direct observation techniques

More significant information may be obtained by direct microscopic observation of small blood vessels, and of the way in which they respond to various physiological stimuli. These techniques are, unfortunately, not applicable to man. It is possible, for example, to study newly-formed vessels in a rabbit's ear with a Clark chamber or, by using Sandison's modification of the original technique, to observe naturally-innervated vessels in the same situation (van den Brenk, Cass and Chambers, 1956). More recently, observations have been made of the microcirculation in dog omentum or rat mesoappendix.

Except for possible species differences these preparations give valid information about the response of the small vessels to changes of their physiological environment, including the effects of general anaesthesia (*see* page 198).

Capillary permeability

The structure and permeability of the capillary wall varies from tissue to tissue. The capillaries of the renal glomeruli are relatively permeable and permit the passage of fairly large molecules; the epithelium of the cerebral capillaries is relatively impermeable, and constitutes the so-called 'blood-brain barrier'.

It is thought that lipid-soluble substances such as the respiratory gases and general anaesthetics can diffuse through the bodies of the capillary endothelial cells; water-soluble molecules, e.g. glucose are, however, thought to diffuse through 'pores' in the intercellular cement substance.

The structure of a typical capillary as it appears in cross-section under the electron microscope is shown semi-diagrammatically in *Figure 3.4b*. Its wall is composed of thin endothelial cells with nuclei which bulge into the capillary lumen. The junction between adjacent cells is a tortuous channel, 90–150 Å in width, bridged by dark areas known as tight junctions. These are thought to be regions where the membranes of adjacent cells are fused; they therefore help to hold the tissue together but, at the same time, limit the area available for diffusion.

The inner surface of the capillary endothelium is coated by a layer of proteinaceous material which helps to prevent intravascular thrombosis. The outer surface is surrounded by an electron-dense basement membrane approximately 300 Å thick, which is itself surrounded by connective tissue composed of collagen, reticular and elastic fibres embedded in an homogenous ground substance.

In tissues such as the endocrine organs and gastro-intestinal mucosa, the thickness of the endothelial cells is in places reduced, producing localized areas called 'fenestrations' which are closed by only a thin cytoplasmic membrane. This type of endothelium is relatively permeable to water-soluble molecules, even of quite large size. The capillaries of the renal glomeruli have similar fenestrations, but the openings are completely devoid of endothelial tissue, being closed only by the basement membrane. In the central nervous system the capillaries are invested by glial cells, this increases their effective thickness and considerably reduces their permeability, so constituting a 'blood-brain barrier'. In the liver, spleen, bone marrow and lymph glands there are no true capillaries; the arterioles and venules here are linked by tortuous channels up to 40 μm in diameter called sinusoids which are lined by phagocytic reticulo-endothelial cells. The walls of such sinusoids contain gaps of up to 5 μm between adjacent cells and there is no basement membrane.

These differences of capillary permeability are reflected in differences in the protein content of lymph from various organs (*Table 3.1*).

Table 3.1   PROTEIN CONCENTRATION IN LYMPH FROM VARIOUS ORGANS (FIGURES FROM RUSHMER, 1961)

Organ	*Lymphatic protein concentration (per cent)*
Lungs	3.2
Heart	3.4
Liver	6.0
Kidney	3.5
Gut	3.5
Skeletal muscles	0.8
Skin	0.7

Pappenheimer (1953) investigated the permeability of capillary membranes to substances of varying molecular weight. He concluded that the observed permeability of an average capillary could be explained on the assumption that its wall contained pores 35–40 Å in diameter. Electron microscopy has, however, as yet failed to confirm the existence of such pores.

Capillary exchange

The exchange of substances between plasma and interstitial fluid occurs mainly by diffusion. For a given membrane area and permeability the rate of diffusion is proportional to the concentration gradient, or, in the case of a charged particle, to the electrochemical potential gradient of the substance under consideration.

An uncharged molecule moves down a concentration gradient from a region of high concentration to one of low concentration. If the substance under consideration is charged—is an ion—the driving force is the *algebraic* sum of the concentration gradient and the electrical potential gradient, rather than the concentration gradient alone. Charged particles may, therefore, move down a gradient of electrical potential against a concentration gradient.

The precise pathway taken by different substances through the capillary membrane is uncertain. At the molecular level the membrane appears to consist of three layers—a middle, lipid layer surrounded by inner and outer layers composed of protein or mucopolysaccharide (Robertson, 1960). Lipid-soluble substances, such as respiratory gases or anaesthetic agents are able to pass freely through the membrane, but the lipid barrier impedes the passage of water-soluble substances such as glucose. Such molecules probably traverse the membrane via the intercellular junctions which, of course, form but a small percentage of the total membrane area.

The passage of substances through capillary membranes is aided also by the constant exchange of water and solutes which occurs between the plasma and interstitial fluid (*see* below). Fluid leaves the capillary at its arterial end and returns at the venous end, thus considerably enhancing the exchange of substances between the cells and the blood.

The Starling hypothesis

In 1896 Starling proposed his explanation for the exchange of fluid between plasma and interstitial fluid. He suggested that this was determined by, on the one hand, the difference of hydrostatic pressure between the capillary lumen and the interstitial fluid and, on the other hand, by the difference of colloid osmotic pressure (oncotic pressure) between these compartments. Since the capillary membrane is, to a greater or lesser extent, permeable to small molecules, the crystalloid osmotic pressure is the same on both sides of the capillary membrane, and differences of crystalloid osmotic pressure therefore play no part in determining fluid exchange across the capillary wall.

At the arterial end of the capillary, the hydrostatic pressure inside the vessels is considerably greater than that in the interstitial space. Fluids and electrolytes therefore move into the extravascular compartment, despite the tendency of the plasma oncotic pressure to hold fluid intravascularly. At the venous end, however, intravascular pressure is reduced by the fall of pressure which occurs along the length of the capillary, while, at the same time, the intravascular protein concentration is increased by fluid loss at its arterial end; as a result fluid and electrolytes re-enter this part of the capillary. Any fluid not returned in this way is removed via the lymphatics, and ultimately re-enters the intravascular compartment via the thoracic duct and right lymphatic duct.

The values of intra- and extra-capillary hydrostatic pressures, and colloid osmotic pressures usually quoted in support of Starling's hypothesis are given in *Table 3.2.* Although subsequent work has amply confirmed the general validity of Starling's hypothesis, some of the figures in this table now appear to be rather inaccurate.

Table 3.2   TYPICAL FIGURES USED IN SUPPORT OF THE STARLING HYPOTHESIS

Hydrostatic pressure, capillary (arterial end)	32 mm Hg
capillary (venous end)	15 mm Hg
tissue	0–10 mm Hg
Colloid osmotic pressure, plasma	25 mm Hg
tissue	? 5 mm Hg

Hydrostatic pressure   Most of the decline of hydrostatic pressure round the systemic circulation occurs in the arterioles (*see* page 74); there is also a decrease of approximately 20 mm Hg between the arterial and venous ends of the capillaries (*Figure 1.10,* page 17). Capillary pressures have been measured directly in various vascular beds, including the skin capillaries of man. The pressure at the arterial end is usually in the region of 30 mm Hg and at the venous end approximately 15 mm Hg. It must be remembered, however, that these are average figures, and considerable variation may occur from tissue to tissue. In the renal glomeruli, for example, the capillary pressures are considerably higher, thus enhancing the formation of glomerular filtrate. When there is wide dilatation of the precapillary resistance vessels, as in a metabolically active tissue, the pressure drops across the capillaries and the arterioles may be more nearly equal.

In the pulmonary circulation, which is a low-pressure system (*see* Chapter 6), the hydrostatic pressures are much less than those in the systemic circulation, thus favouring re-absorption of fluid from the alveoli, and helping to prevent the formation of pulmonary oedema.

Accurate estimation of hydrostatic pressure in the interstitial fluid compartment is more difficult. Most workers who have attempted to make this measurement have inserted a small hypodermic needle percutaneously, and have then measured the pressure required just to force fluid into the tissue. Pressures determined in this way are about 5 mm Hg above atmospheric. However, as Guyton (1963) points out, this technique is unphysiological in the extreme because the diameter of the needle is several hundred times larger than the tissue space into which it is inserted. Moreover, the system fails to respond to changes of interstitial pressure, and the injection of fluid into the tissue has very little effect on its apparent hydrostatic pressure.

Guyton therefore devised a more physiological technique. He implanted a perforated hollow sphere under the skin (*Figure 3.7*) and then, when the wound had healed, measured the pressure inside the sphere. He argued that this was the same as the interstitial fluid pressure because the interior of the sphere was in direct contact with the tissue spaces. Pressures measured in this way are sub-atmospheric by approximately 5 mm Hg.

Surprising though this result seems at first sight, Guyton's argument is cogent, and his experimental technique has the advantage that the apparent tissue pressure is readily altered by minor degrees of venous occlusion, which is certainly not the case with the standard technique.

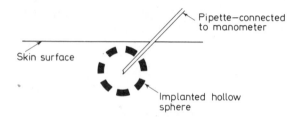

Figure 3.7. Guyton's technique for measuring interstitial fluid pressure

Osmotic pressures   The osmotic pressure of the plasma proteins is approximately 25 mm Hg. Osmotic pressure depends on the number of particles present in a given volume of solution, rather than on the actual mass of solute present. The molecular weight of albumin (70 000) is approximately half that of globulin (150 000), therefore a given concentration of albumin generates twice the osmotic pressure as does the same concentration of globulin. In addition, there is normally twice as much albumin as globulin in the plasma, therefore the majority of the plasma colloid osmotic pressure is due to albumin.

The presence of protein molecules on one side of a semipermeable membrane causes a small difference of crystalloid concentration across the membrane due to the Donnan effect, and thus enhances the osmotic effect of the protein. Negatively-charged protein anions attract positively-charged cations to maintain electrical neutrality, thus increasing the total osmolarity of the protein-containing fluid. This effect becomes increasingly important at high protein concentrations (von Ott, 1956), therefore the relationship between colloid osmotic pressure and protein concentration is curvilinear (*Figure 3.8*).

This increase is of physiological importance. Plasma protein concentration increases as fluid leaves the arterial end of the capillary; the resulting increase of oncotic pressure helps to draw interstitial fluid back into the vascular compartment at its venous end. Similarly, in the kidney, the colloid osmotic

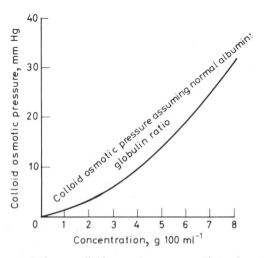

Figure 3.8. Increase of plasma colloid osmotic pressure with total protein concentration (based on von Ott, 1956)

pressure of blood leaving the glomeruli is increased because approximately 20 per cent of its plasma has been filtered into Bowman's capsule. The resulting increase of peritubular colloid osmotic pressure aids re-absorption of fluid from the convoluted tubules.

It is difficult to assess quantitatively the interstitial fluid oncotic pressure. It is not possible to obtain uncontaminated samples of interstitial fluid, so that its composition is not known precisely, and its chemical structure is so complex that calculations of its osmotic pressure must be very imprecise. In addition, the protein concentration varies from tissue to tissue (*see* page 85). The value which is usually assumed is 5 mm Hg.

The other assumptions on which the Starling model is based are that the permeability of the capillary membrane is uniform throughout its entire length, and that the area available for fluid exchange is similar at the arterial and venous ends of the capillary. Both of these assumptions have been challenged.

Wiederhielm (1967) has shown that the permeability of the endothelium is approximately 60 per cent less at the arterial than at the venous end of the capillaries, and also that the venules, as well as the capillaries, may be involved in fluid exchange. The tendency for water and electrolytes to return to the intravascular compartment is therefore probably greater than has usually been assumed in the past. Against this, however, must be set the increased hydrostatic pressure gradient suggested by Guyton's work, which tends to increase filtration out of the capillary, and thus to compensate for the increased re-absorption postulated by Wiederhielm.

THE VEINS

It is important to appreciate that the veins have two physiological roles. They are not merely passive conduits which conduct blood back to the heart from the tissues, and provide a convenient source of blood for the haematologist and chemical pathologist; they act also as a low-pressure reservoir of blood which can be called upon during physiological emergencies, such as acute haemorrhage. The venoconstriction which occurs under these conditions increases the mean systemic pressure (*see* page 119), and thus tends to restore output to normal (*see* Chapter 9).

Histology

The histological structure of the veins is similar to that of the arteries, except that the former have thinner walls and a muscular coat which is virtually devoid of elastic tissue. They are considerably more distensible than the corresponding arteries, and can therefore hold a larger volume of blood at a given intravascular (or, strictly, transmural) pressure. The veins are thus well adapted to act as a low-pressure reservoir of blood (*see* previous paragraph).

Like the arteries, the veins receive a copious nerve supply from the sympathetic, but not from the parasympathetic, division of the autonomic nervous system. When these nerves are stimulated the veins constrict, causing a rise of venous pressure and a consequent translocation of blood from the veins to the systemic arteries and vessels of the pulmonary circulation. The veins constrict also in response to circulating sympathomimetic amines, such as adrenaline and noradrenaline. The venous sympathetic receptors are probably mainly α in type (Wood, 1968), although there is dispute on this point (probably due to species differences); *see also* White and Udwadia (1975)

RESISTANCE VERSUS CAPACITANCE VESSELS

Folkow (1960a) points out that the systemic circulation consists of a number of 'parallel-coupled' vascular beds connected in parallel between the arterial and venous sides of the circulation, and that each of these parallel-coupled beds comprises a number of different types of blood vessel interconnected in series ('series-coupled'). Folkow divided the vessels of any given bed into five categories. These correspond roughly with obvious anatomical subdivisions, although the classification is essentially physiological rather than anatomical:

1. vessels which form the arterial reservoir (the 'Windkessel', *see* page 73)—the large elastic arteries:
2. vessels which provide the majority of resistance to blood flow through the tissues—the arterioles and precapillary sphincters;
3. exchange vessels—the capillaries, and perhaps the post-capillary venules;
4. vessels, the main function of which is to store blood—the veins;
5. shunt vessels which exist in some tissues and permit blood to flow from the arterial to the venous sides of the circulation, by-passing the exchange vessels—the arterio-venous anastomoses.

Folkow also classified the vessels into *resistance* vessels and *capacitance* vessels. The function of the former is to control blood flow through individual capillary beds or, acting in concord throughout the body, to control total peripheral resistance and arterial blood pressure. The function of the capacitance vessels is to act as a store of blood which can be called upon in an emergency, for example, to minimize the effects of acute hypovolaemia.

To a large extent, the resistance vessels comprise the arterioles and precapillary sphincters, while the capacitance vessels are formed mainly by the veins. However, some resistance to flow is provided by the post-capillary venules, which thus have some resistance function; while the arteries act, to some extent, as a blood reservoir, although one which is much smaller than the venous reservoir (*Figure 3.5*, page 80). (Because the walls of the arterial reservoir are relatively inextensible the loss of a small amount of blood from this site causes a pronounced fall of arterial pressure. In haemorrhage therefore, the majority of the lost blood comes from the venous, not the arterial, reservoir.)

In the present context this division into resistance and capacitance vessels is important because their control is not identical. Constriction of the capacitance vessels tends to occur uniformly throughout the body, whereas constriction of the resistance vessels tends to occur more locally, in response to local changes in metabolic demand. Venous constriction induced by nervous or hormonal stimulation tends to be generalized throughout the body. The response of the resistance vessels, however, varies from tissue to tissue; it may be constriction in some tissues and dilatation in others. Venous sympathetic receptors appear to be (mainly) α in type; the receptors of the resistance vessel are both α and β (*see* page 73).

CONTROL OF THE SYSTEMIC CIRCULATION

Control of blood vessel calibre depends on both neural and hormonal mechanisms. During local variations of tissue activity, local changes of resistance vessel calibre occur, mediated to a large extent by chemical factors such as changes in the local concentration of tissue metabolites (*see* page 91); but there is in addition usually a neurally-mediated change in resistance vessel calibre in other regions of the body (*see* page 95). In haemorrhage, increased sympathetic activity causes constriction of both resistance and capacitance vessels, and so helps to maintain the cardiac output and arterial blood pressure (*see* Chapter 9).

The capillaries appear to have no power of independent contraction; and blood flow through the capillary bed is controlled by the smooth muscle tone of the arterioles, precapillary sphincters and post-capillary venules.

Control of arteriolar resistance

The degree of smooth muscle tone in the arteriolar walls depends on:

1. its inherent tone;
2. autonomic nervous stimulation;
3. the concentration of circulating sympathomimetic amines and other hormones; and
4. the local concentration of various vasodilator metabolites.

Inherent tone

In many tissues the arteriolar smooth muscle has an inherent tone, even in the absence of external nervous or chemical stimulation. This inherent tone varies markedly from tissue to tissue; in general, it is greatest where the vessels receive a poor sympathetic innervation. In skeletal muscle, the myocardium and brain, the tone is relatively great; whereas it is almost non-existent in the cutaneous arterio-venous anastomoses. Resting blood flow to skeletal muscle is 3–5 ml $100 \text{ g}^{-1} \text{ min}^{-1}$; this figure is merely doubled by sympathetic blockade, whereas complete smooth muscle paralysis by accumulation of vasodilator metabolites (*see* page 155) increases it to as much as 50 ml $100 \text{ g}^{-1} \text{ min}^{-1}$.

The cause of this inherent tone is uncertain. It has been suggested that it is due to blood-borne vasoconstrictor substances. However, if this were the case, the vessels with the greatest tone would be the ones most sensitive to such agents, whereas, in fact, the reverse appears to be the case. It is known that, even in the absence of external stimuli, smooth muscle cells contract spontaneously and Folkow (1960b) suggests that the observed tone may be due to the uncoordinated contraction of these cells; at any given moment some cells contract while others relax, thus causing partial contraction of the muscle as a whole. Bayliss (1902) suggested that mechanical stretching of the vessel wall by internal pressure was sufficient to cause it to contract; and modern views of smooth muscle physiology are to some extent in agreement with this hypothesis (Folkow and Neil, 1971).

Nervous stimulation

Three nervous mechanisms need to be considered:

1. sympathetic adrenergic vasoconstrictor nerves;
2. sympathetic *cholinergic* vasodilator nerves; and
3. parasympathetic cholinergic vasodilator nerves.

The last two are concerned chiefly with local control of blood flow. The general control of the circulation is mediated mainly by changes of sympathetic vasoconstrictor tone. Most cardiovascular reflexes, with the exception of the so-called defence reactions, also act via changes of this vasoconstrictor tone. (Some workers, for example, Beck and Brody (1961), have postulated the existence of sympathetic adrenergic vasodilator nerves. The evidence for these is, however, tenuous, and they will not be considered here.)

Sympathetic vasoconstrictor fibres   These are considered on page 95 in relation to the integration of cardiovascular responses to various stimuli.

Sympathetic vasodilator fibres   The function of the sympathetic cholinergic vasodilator fibres is reviewed by Uvnäs (1960). Their distribution is limited to the arterioles of the skeletal muscles, and possibly of the myocardium. They are concerned chiefly with the body's cardiovascular responses to emotion, and with preparation of the body for 'fight or flight'. The muscular vasodilatation which occurs at the start of, or even before, exercise is mediated via these cholinergic fibres (*see* page 169). In addition, they appear to be responsible for the muscular vasodilatation which occurs during a fainting (vaso-vagal) attack. Contrary to what is the case with the sympathetic vasoconstrictor fibres, the blood vessels appear to receive no resting vasodilator tone.

   These sympathetic cholinergic fibres are represented centrally in the cerebral cortex, with relay stations in the anterior hypothalamus and mesencephalon; the descending neurones by-pass the medullary vasomotor centres on their way to the spinal cord. Stimulation of the appropriate region of the hypothalamus causes an alerting reaction with muscular vasodilatation accompanied by arteriolar constriction in the skin, gastro-intestinal tract and spleen, and by cardiac acceleration and increased secretion of catecholamines from the adrenal medullae. Such stimulation causes a marked redistribution of cardiac output with but little change of arterial blood pressure, and prepares the body for physical activity—for fight or flight.

Parasympathetic vasodilator fibres   The parasympathetic system plays a minor role in the control of the peripheral circulation. There appear to be true parasympathetic vasodilator fibres only to the pial vessels, and to the vessels of the external genitalia. It was at one time thought that the vasodilatation which occurs in the salivary glands in response to parasympathetic stimulation is due to parasympathetic vascular innervation; it now appears, however, that this response is due to local liberation of the vasodilator polypeptide, bradykinin (Hilton and Lewis, 1955). This response is not blocked by atropine. Bradykinin release also appears to be responsible for cutaneous vasodilatation during sweating (Fox and Hilton, 1958); *see also* page 153.

Chemical control

Blood vessel calibre is regulated also by the concentration of various chemicals in the immediate vicinity of the vascular smooth muscle cells. These substances may either be produced locally, or in distant organs and then transported to the target tissue by the blood. Of the latter type, adrenaline and noradrenaline are the most physiologically important, but vascular resistance in certain tissues is influenced also by changes of oxygen or carbon dioxide tension. The respiratory gases are, in this case, acting as hormones. It has been suggested that, during intense generalized sympathetic activity, noradrenaline may enter the circulation from the sympathetic nerve endings to cause alterations of vascular smooth muscle tone in distant organs. It should be appreciated that the physiological response to vasodilator chemicals injected into the blood stream is not necessarily the same as when these substances are produced locally; injected substances affect vascular smooth muscle tone only after they have diffused out of the capillaries into the tissue spaces.

The relative importance of nervous and chemical factors in the control of vascular calibre varies considerably from tissue to tissue. In tissues such as the skin, the vessels are primarily under the control of the sympathetic nervous system; in other tissues they are more influenced by changes of chemical environment. The cerebral vessels are unresponsive to sympathetic stimulation but are extremely sensitive to changes of Pa_{CO_2} (*see* page 139).

Changes of Pa_{O_2} and Pa_{CO_2}   In most tissues an increase of Pa_{CO_2} or a decrease of Pa_{O_2} causes a decrease of vascular resistance; opposite changes induce vasoconstriction. In the pulmonary circulation, however, hypoxia causes vasoconstriction (*see* Chapter 6). This response is important in the pathogenesis of pulmonary hypertension and *cor pulmonale*. Teleologically, the reason for this paradoxical response appears to be that, in the systemic circulation, hypoxia causes increased blood flow which tends to restore tissue oxygenation, whereas in the lungs, hypoxically-induced vasoconstriction tends to maintain the ventilation/perfusion ratio of a given region within normal limits (*see* page 161).

Autoregulation   The dependence of tissue blood flow on the local concentration of various metabolites is probably largely responsible for the phenomena of autoregulation and reactive hyperaemia.

Experimentally, blood flow through certain organs is found to remain almost constant despite wide variations of arterial blood pressure (*Figure 3.9*); this is 'autoregulation'. Selkhurt (1946), for example, found that renal blood flow was virtually independent of arterial pressure, provided this was above a critical level of about 80 mm Hg, although, below this level, flow declined precipitously. Autoregulation is known to occur in experimental animals in the kidney, skeletal muscles, brain, myocardium and intestine; it has also been demonstrated in the renal and cerebral circulations of man. (Although the relative independence of blood flow on arterial pressure is readily demonstrable in the healthy circulation, it is possible that diseased vessels may lose their capacity to dilate beyond a certain size. Autoregulation in such circumstances may be inefficient, and a decrease of arterial pressure for any reason may be accompanied by an unexpectedly large fall of blood flow.)

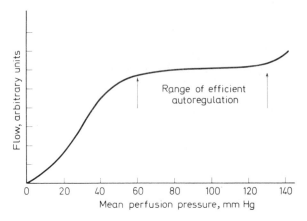

Figure 3.9. The phenomenon of autoregulation (diagrammatic)

Several explanations have been proposed to account for autoregulation (*see*, for example, Johnson 1964). Most workers, however, assume that it is due mainly to local accumulation of vasodilator metabolites. A fall of arterial pressure causes a temporary decrease of tissue blood flow; this permits vasodilator metabolites to accumulate, so inducing vasodilatation and restoring the blood flow to normal.

The precise nature of the hypothetical metabolite (or metabolites) is unknown. A decrease of Po_2, an increase of Pco_2, or an increase of hydrogen ion concentration all relax vascular smooth muscle, as do lactic acid, adenosine diphosphate, adenosine triphospate and potassium ions. It has also been suggested that acetylcholine and histamine may be involved, similarly bradykinin and other polypeptides are known to be potent vasodilators. There is, of course, no *a priori* reason that the metabolite should not vary from tissue to tissue. The coronary circulation is particularly sensitive to oxygen lack; the cerebral circulation is very sensitive to changes of Pco_2.

Other workers suggest that autoregulation is due primarily to plasma skimming (*see* page 11) and is, therefore, dependent on the inhomogenous nature of blood. Bayliss (1902) suggested that vascular smooth muscle could respond directly to an increase of intravascular pressure with vasoconstriction and an increased resistance to blood flow.

Vasomotion   Vasomotion (*see* page 198) is also assumed to be due to the action of vasomotor metabolites. If the flow through part of the capillary bed is interrupted by smooth muscle contraction of the arterioles, metarterioles or precapillary sphincters, metabolites accumulate until they cause the muscle to relax, thus restoring flow through the ischaemic region of the microcirculation. The increased flow then washes out the accumulated metabolites so that the process is repeated, thus accounting for the rhythmic contraction and relaxation of capillaries which can be observed under the microscope.

Control of the capacitance vessels

Relatively little is known about the factors which control venous calibre. The veins receive a copious innervation from the sympathetic division of the autonomic nervous system, therefore generalized sympathetic activity causes venoconstriction throughout the body, thus raising the mean systemic pressure (*see* page 119). This venoconstriction is enhanced by stimulation of venous sympathetic receptors by circulating catecholamines.

The post-capillary venules are in addition controlled by local chemical factors. Tissue hypoperfusion in shock may cause paralysis of the precapillary resistance vessels as a result of local accumulation of vasodilator metabolites at a time when the post-capillary vessels are still constricted. The capillaries then become overfilled with blood with deleterious consequences to the body as a whole (*see* page 226).

Cardiovascular integration

The final common pathway for the vasoconstrictor sympathetic supply to the blood vessels arises in the medullary vasomotor centres. Descending fibres pass thence to preganglionic cell bodies in the thoraco-lumbar region of the spinal cord. It has recently been shown that, although the spinal neurones are normally under the control of higher centres, they are, in fact, capable of some degree of independent action. Section of the cervical region of the spinal cord causes a profound fall of arterial blood pressure and complete abolition of cardiovascular changes in response to afferent stimulation. After a time, however, partial recovery from this condition of 'spinal shock' occurs; the blood pressure returns almost to normal and reflex responses to sensory stimulation reappear. Distension of the bladder in spinal man may cause arterial hypertension (Whitteridge, 1960).

The isolated spinal cord also appears able to induce reflex vasoconstriction in response to a reduction of the circulating blood volume. This response may be mediated by local hypoxia of the cord; and experimentally it can be abolished by artificially increasing the arterial blood pressure or by the administration of oxygen. The value of this response as an emergency mechanism is obvious; but the role, if any, which it plays in normal circulatory homeostasis is uncertain.

The medullary centre

The classical concept of a medullary vasomotor centre (*Figure 3.10*) was a discrete collection of neurones which receive afferent impulses from many regions of the body—the baroreceptors, the chemoreceptors, the hypothalamus, the cerebral cortex, the skin, and so on; these impulses are then 'integrated' (algebraically summed), with due regard to whether they are inhibitory or excitatory, to modify efferent autonomic activity in accordance with the needs of the body as a whole.

ACP—4*

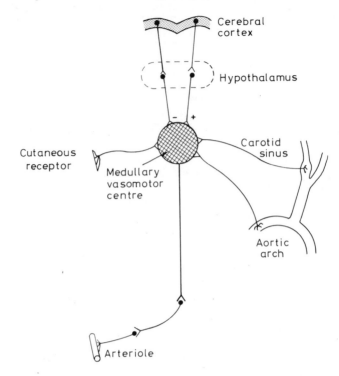

Figure 3.10. Classical concept of medullary vasomotor centre

The evidence on which the existence of medullary centres is based comes from both experimental brain-stem section and the results of electrical stimulation of the medulla. Section of the brain-stem above the level of the upper pons does not affect systemic blood pressure, nor the majority of cardiovascular reflexes (Wang, 1964); section lower down, however, causes hypotension, and some impairment of these reflexes; section at the level of the upper cervical cord causes severe hypotension and the complete abolition of most cardiovascular reflex responses.

While there is little doubt that particular regions of the medulla are of prime importance in the control of the cardiovascular system, it now appears that the medullary cardiovascular centres are less anatomically discrete than was formerly believed; and that the cardiovascular reflexes may relay, not only in the medulla, but also in higher centres such as the mid-brain and hypothalamus. In addition, there is evidence that the higher centres may influence the cardiovascular system via neurones which do *not* act through the medullary centres (Peiss, 1964).

Stimulation experiments reveal that a wide area of the brain-stem is concerned with cardiovascular regulation. This sensitive region extends from the middle of the pons to the level of the obex (at the inferior angle of the fourth ventricle). Stimulation of some regions causes cardiac acceleration and peripheral vasoconstriction (pressor response); stimulation of other regions induces bradycardia and hypotension (depressor response). The anatomical boundaries of the two types of region are, however, somewhat inconstant and there is

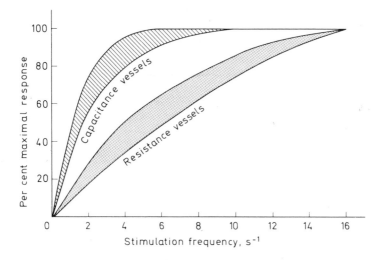

Figure 3.11. Stimulation frequencies required to cause maximal contraction of resistance and capacitance vessels (based on Mellander, 1960)

considerable overlap. The pressor regions tend to lie laterally in the medulla; the depressor areas lie more medially.

Most tissues receive a certain amount of resting sympathetic 'tone', and changes of vascular calibre are brought about by changes in this tone (*Figure 3.11*). However, the importance of sympathetic activity in the control of vascular calibre varies from tissue to tissue (*see* Chapter 5): in general, tissues such as the heart and brain, where the inherent vascular tone is considerable, receive the least sympathetic innervation; conversely, the cutaneous arteriovenous anastomoses which possess little inherent vascular tone are very sensitive to sympathetic stimulation. As a result of this gradation of sympathetic innervation, a generalized increase of sympathetic activity causes a redistribution of cardiac output away from tissues such as the kidney and gut to the brain and heart (*see* page 217).

The higher centres

The classical teaching was that the higher centres—the mid-brain, the hypothalamus, and the cerebral cortex—influence the cardiovascular system purely through the medullary vasomotor centres. It has now been shown experimentally, however, that cardiovascular adjustments can still occur in response to hypothalamic stimulation even after destruction of most of the medulla, including the region which contains the classical vasomotor centres. It appears, therefore, that descending fibres from higher centres may reach the sympathetic preganglionic neurones in the spinal cord, without passing through the medullary vasomotor centres.

Peiss (1964) suggests that there is, in fact, a hierarchy of centres within the central nervous system, all of which are concerned with cardiovascular regulation. These include the classical vasomotor centre(s) in the medulla, plus additional centres in the mid-brain, the diencephalon and the cerebral cortex and limbic system; these centres are all interconnected by neural pathways, both excitatory and inhibitory. Efferent fibres reach the spinal cord by several routes, both direct and via lower centres; and the precise pathway involved in any particular response depends on the area of afferent stimulation. For example, information from the special senses induces changes of blood pressure via centres located in the cerebral cortex, while information from the carotid and aortic baroreceptors causes cardiovascular adjustments mainly via the medullary centres.

Hypothalamus   In lower animals a confusing variety of cardiovascular responses can be elicited by hypothalamic stimulation. Sometimes the response is pressor; sometimes it results in cardiovascular depression. Pitts, Larrabee and Bronk (1941) showed that hypothalamic stimulation caused increased sympathetic tone to the blood vessels, and that this response could be blocked by simultaneous stimulation of medullary depressor areas. Rushmer, Smith and Lasker (1960) showed that stimulation of the hypothalamus of the conscious, unrestrained dog caused cardiovascular responses very similar to those normally seen during exercise.

Cortex   The location of the cortical cardiovascular centres has been investigated by Wall and Davis (1951) who showed that cardiovascular responses could be elicited from three main regions of the primate cerebral cortex: the sensory-motor cortex; the posterior orbital cortex and the insula; and the temporo-cingulate system. The efferent pathways from these regions descend either in the pyramidal tracts, or via relays in the hypothalamus.

Control of arterial blood pressure

In health, reflex mechanisms maintain arterial blood pressure constant within fairly narrow limits, despite changes of body posture and wide variations of vascular resistance in response to changes in the vascular resistance of various organs. This is an example of a homeostatic mechanism or, in engineering terminology, of a negative-feedback control system. The controlled variable is the blood pressure; and the system is arranged so that changes of pressure cause compensatory responses which tend to restore the pressure to its previous level.

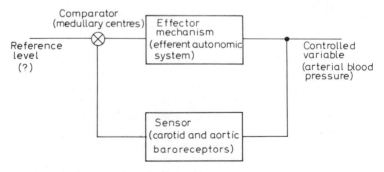

Figure 3.12. Components of a negative-feedback control system

This is negative feedback. (Positive feedback—where the response is in a direction to enhance the initial change—plays little part in the normal control of the cardiovascular system, although it may occur in disease, for example, deteriorating shock—*see* page 222.)

A negative-feedback system requires three elements (*Figure 3.12*): a sensor to measure the level of the controlled variable; a comparator to compare this actual level with the ideal or reference level; and an effector mechanism to adjust the system in such a direction that the error signal (the difference between the reference level and the actual level of the controlled variable) is reduced to a minimum. In the case of the system which controls arterial blood pressure, the sensor comprises the baroreceptors in the walls of the larger arteries; the comparator is a rather ill-defined collection of medullary neurones related to the 'vasomotor centre(s)' (*see* page 94); the effector mechanism is the autonomic nervous supply to the heart, peripheral blood vessels and adrenal medullae.

The baroreceptors

The chief arterial baroreceptors are the carotid sinuses and the pressure receptors which lie in the walls of the aortic arch. In addition, there are probably pressure receptors in the walls of most of the large aortic branches (Heymans and Neil, 1958). It is generally assumed that these baroreceptors all behave similarly, qualitatively at any rate; (*see* however, Kidd and Linden (1975), Recommended Further Reading).

The carotid sinus is formed by a dilatation of the common carotid artery at its bifurcation, and is confined mainly to the origin of the internal carotid artery. In this region the arterial wall is modified so that its muscular media is thinned and partially replaced by elastic tissue. The vessel wall here contains many afferent nerve endings of the glossopharyngeal nerve; and a rise of intra-arterial pressure stretches the relatively thin wall, thus stimulating the afferent endings and causing action potentials to pass to the medulla at an increased rate.

Although the carotid sinus is called a baroreceptor, it is not in fact sensitive to pressure *per se,* only to deformation of the arterial wall. The usual cause of such deformation is, of course, a change of arterial pressure; but the nerve endings may also be stimulated by, for example, external pressure. If the sinus is encased in a rigid plastic collar no cardiovascular adjustment occurs in response to a local change of arterial pressure (Hauss, Kreuziger and Asteroth, 1949).

Relationship between carotid sinus pressure and afferent nervous activity   Experimentally, it is possible to measure the rate at which action potentials pass up the glossopharyngeal nerve, and to investigate how this rate varies with changes of carotid sinus pressure. With steady pressures, the action potential frequency in a single fibre is zero if the carotid pressure lies below a certain threshold value, which varies somewhat from fibre to fibre; but above threshold the action potential frequency increases with increasing pressure until a maximum is reached, above which no further increase occurs. The relationship between pressure and firing rate is, therefore, an S-shaped curve. The increased afferent activity to the medulla as arterial pressure is increased is due partly to an increase of action potential frequency in fibres which were already above

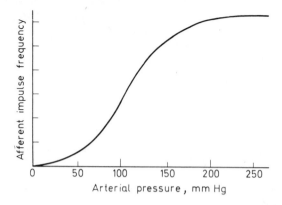

Figure 3.13. Relationship between action potential frequency in glossopharyngeal nerve and blood pressure in carotid sinus (diagrammatic)

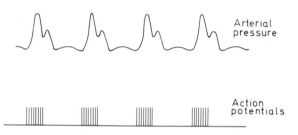

Figure 3.14. Action potentials in glossopharyngeal nerve in relation to arterial pressure waveform (diagrammatic)

threshold, and partly to recruitment of new fibres which were previously below threshold (*Figure 3.13*).

The response of the baroreceptors to pulsatile pressures is more complex. Landgren (1952) found that, at a given pressure the firing-rate was greater when the pressure was rising than when it was falling (*see Figure 3.14*). Mathematically, therefore, the response of the baroreceptors varies, not only with pressure (P), but also with rate of change of pressure (dP/dt). (Such a response is common with many biological receptors. Man-made control systems also are often designed to respond, not only to their actual input, but also to its time rate of change; this enables the system to respond more rapidly to a changing input, because its response is already partially geared to the input's probable future value.)

Central 'integrating' mechanisms

An increase of arterial pressure at the baroreceptors causes action potentials to pass at an increased rate to the cardiovascular centres in the medulla and, possibly, also in higher centres such as the hypothalamus (*see* page 96). These centres 'integrate' information from the baroreceptors with afferent information from other regions of the body, and adjust efferent autonomic activity appropriately. Provided there is no physiological contra-indication, an increase of action potential frequency from the baroreceptors causes cardiovascular changes in a direction which lowers the arterial pressure.

Effector mechanisms

The cardiovascular response to a fall of arterial pressure therefore consists of: constriction of resistance vessels in most tissues (not, however, in the brain or heart, where sympathetic innervation is functionally almost non-existent, *see* page 139); increase of the rate and force of cardiac contraction; and constriction of the capacitance vessels. The last two factors cause an increase of cardiac output* (*see* Chapter 4); and as a result the blood pressure, which approximately equals the product of cardiac output and total peripheral resistance (*see* page 75), is restored towards normal. It appears in general that the resistance vessels in the skin and kidneys play but a minor role in the body's minute-to-minute baroreceptor responses. This is doubtless because these tissues have important functions to perform; and it would be undesirable for these to be continually interrupted in response to barostatic demands. Nevertheless both renal and cutaneous blood flow are severely reduced when there is a marked fall in arterial pressure, as in shock (*see* page 221).

It should be noted that blood pressure can never be restored completely to normal by the baroreceptor reflex; if it were, the compensatory mechanisms on which its restoration depends would, of course, no longer be active. The extent to which a change of blood pressure is attenuated by baroreceptor activity is a measure of the efficiency of the body's cardiovascular homeostatic mechanisms. It may be shown mathematically that the attenuation depends on the 'gain' of the system, that is, on factors such as the sensitivity of the baroreceptors and the sensitivity of the blood vessels to changes of sympathetic tone (*see also* below).

Of course, in some circumstances the maintenance of a constant blood pressure may not be an appropriate physiological response. The baroreceptor reflex is then over-ruled by other cardiovascular reflexes. In the presence of severe hypoxia or cerebral ischaemia, for example, an increase of arterial blood pressure may be essential for survival; under these circumstances maintenance of a normal blood pressure would be totally inappropriate. Similarly, the blood pressure is raised in severe exercise; the carotid and aortic homeostatic mechanisms are then over-ruled, thus preventing the limitation of muscle blood flow which would otherwise occur.

Baroreceptor responses in man

Rather surprisingly, there is a considerable amount of information about the activity of the carotid baroreceptors in man. A decrease of pressure within the carotid sinus, caused by proximal compression of the carotid artery, causes tachycardia and an increase of arterial pressure. Direct stimulation of the sinus

---

*This is not, of course, to say that cardiac output is necessarily increased above normal. This is obviously not the case in hypovolaemic shock, where the cardiac output remains low, but not as low as it would be in the absence of these compensatory responses.

nerve at operation causes bradycardia and hypotension, with a maximal response at a stimulation frequency of about 60 Hz (Carlsten et al., 1958). It is possible also to stimulate the carotid sinus in intact man by application of a sub-atmospheric ('negative') pressure to the appropriate region of the neck (Ernsting and Parry, 1957). The sinus responds, of course, to transmural pressure rather than to the absolute value of arterial pressure. Such stimulation causes bradycardia and hypotension, the heart rate and mean arterial pressure decreasing almost linearly with the degree of applied negative pressure (Bevegård and Shepherd, 1966). After the administration of atropine, the change of heart rate is abolished, but the blood pressure response is unaffected.

A recently-introduced technique for the evaluation of baroreceptor sensitivity in intact man is measurement of the change of heart rate which is caused by intravenous injection of phenylephrine (Smyth, Sleight and Pickering, 1969). Phenylephrine acts almost entirely on the α sympathetic receptors (*see* page 73), whereas the myocardial receptors are almost entirely β. Any change of heart rate induced by phenylephrine must, therefore, be secondary to an increase of arterial blood pressure caused by peripheral vasoconstriction. The sensitivity of the baroreceptor reflex may then be expressed as the slope of the relationship between change of arterial blood pressure and the resulting change of heart rate. This slope is significantly reduced by general anaesthesia with nitrous oxide and/or halothane (Bristow, Prys-Roberts and Fisher, 1969).

OTHER CARDIOVASCULAR REFLEXES

The chemoreceptors

The aortic and carotid chemoreceptors are concerned mainly with the control of respiration. They are therefore considered in detail in the companion volume on respiration by Nunn (1969). Since, however, they are also concerned with adjustments of the cardiovascular system in response to changes of Pa_{O_2}, Pa_{CO_2}, and pH, they are also considered here briefly.

The carotid body lies at the carotid bifurcation, just in front of the carotid sinus. It is copiously supplied with arterial blood from the occipital and ascending-pharyngeal arteries. Afferent nerve fibres run from it to the medulla via the glossopharyngeal nerve. The aortic bodies lie in the vicinity of the aortic arch around the origins of the subclavian arteries. Their afferent nerve fibres pass to the medulla via the vagus.

The chemoreceptors are all histologically similar and consist of epitheloid cells surrounded by a network of sinusoidal blood vessels. Although the chemoreceptor bodies are very small, their blood flow per unit weight is extremely large. It has been estimated that the carotid body, which weighs about 2 mg, has a blood flow of $2 \, l \, min^{-1} \, 100 \, g^{-1}$ of tissue (as compared with renal blood flow which is $400 \, ml \, min^{-1} \, 100 \, g^{-1}$).

Cardiovascular response to changes of blood gas tensions

In experimental animals it is possible to perfuse isolated chemoreceptors with blood of known composition, and to record action potentials in their afferent nerves. Such experiments suggest that the chemoreceptors are stimulated by a fall of Po_2 or by a rise of Pco_2. The work of von Euler, Liljestrand and Zotterman (1939), however, suggests that they have little tonic activity at normal blood gas tensions.

Chemoreceptor stimulation is usually considered to cause a generalized increase of cardiovascular sympathetic activity, and a decrease of cardiac parasympathetic tone. Some workers, however, suggest that the responses which accompany changes of Pao_2 or $Paco_2$ are mediated directly via medullary chemoreceptors, rather than via the carotid and aortic bodies. Peripheral hypoxia or hypercapnia in the absence of such medullary stimulation may cause bradycardia rather than tachycardia. Daly and Scott (1962), for example, found that hypoxic stimulation of peripheral chemoreceptors, at constant Pco_2 , caused bradycardia accompanied by a rise of systemic vascular resistance.

The carotid body appears to be sensitive also to changes of blood flow. Landgren and Niel (1951), for example, found that haemorrhage caused an increase of afferent nervous activity from the chemoreceptors, despite constant levels of Pao_2 and $Paco_2$. This increased activity was reversed by restoration of the blood volume to normal. Such chemoreceptor stimulation is presumably due to stagnant hypoxia although, in view of the enormous blood flow in relation to oxygen consumption of the carotid and aortic bodies, the occurrence of such hypoxia is surprising.

The role of the chemoreceptors in producing the cardiovascular changes which accompany alteration of $Paco_2$ (*see* Chapter 7) is uncertain. There is virtually no information about the relative roles played by central and peripheral mechanisms in the causation of this response.

Other reflexes

In addition to the reflexes already discussed, many others have been demonstrated in experimental animals. But although these reflexes have been extensively studied in cats and dogs, their elucidation in man is far less complete, and the part (if any) which they play in normal cardiovascular homeostasis is unknown. They will be mentioned here but briefly.

Cardiac reflexes

Many mechano-receptors have been described in relation to the heart—at the junction of the venae cavae with the right atrium, at the orifice of the tricuspid valve, in the pulmonary veins and left atrium, in the ventricular walls, and in the walls of the coronary arteries. These receptors are particularly profuse around the atrial openings of the systemic and pulmonary veins (Coleridge, Coleridge and Kidd, 1964). They send afferent impulses to the medulla via the vagus.

The effects of stimulation of these cardiac receptors are complex. Some workers maintain that there are two types of atrial receptor, one discharging at an increased rate during atrial systole, the other during the atrial distension which accompanies ventricular systole; others dispute these findings and maintain that there is only one type of receptor. Distension of the region between the pulmonary veins and left atrium causes tachycardia and, usually, an increase of arterial blood pressure (Ledsome and Linden, 1964). This effect is mediated by an increase of sympathetic tone to the heart. By increasing the efficiency of the cardiac pump it aids the Frank-Starling mechanism to increase left ventricular output when atrial pressure is raised (*see* page 49).

Bainbridge reflex

Atrial receptors may also be concerned in the Bainbridge reflex (*see* page 64). It is known, for example, that intravenous infusions may cause tachycardia in experimental animals, both anaesthetized and conscious, but attempts to relate this response to an increase of atrial pressure have led to conflicting results (*see*, for example, Ledsome and Linden, 1964).

Role of atrial receptors in regulation of blood volume

In addition, it appears that left atrial receptors may be concerned with the regulation of blood volume. An increase of left atrial pressure may suppress ADH (anti-diuretic hormone) release from the posterior pituitary, thereby causing a water diuresis and a consequent reduction of total blood volume (*see* page 128).

Pulmonary receptors

Baroreceptors have also been demonstrated in the pulmonary arteries (Coleridge and Kidd, 1963). Stimulation of these receptors in experimental animals by pulmonary inflation causes a reflex increase of heart rate. In man, however, stimulation of afferent vagal fibres from the lungs appears to have little effect on arterial blood pressure (Guz et al., 1964).

In addition, there may be pulmonary chemoreceptors which are stimulated by a variety of drugs, such as veratridine and mepyramine. The physiological significance of such receptors is, however, completely unknown.

CARDIOVASCULAR EFFECTS OF SPINAL AND EPIDURAL ANAESTHESIA

The role of the autonomic nervous system in the control of the heart and circulation is well illustrated by the cardiovascular changes which accompany spinal and epidural anaesthesia.

The peripheral effects of spinal anaesthesia appear to be due solely to block of preganglionic sympathetic fibres as they leave the thoracic and lumbar regions of the spinal cord. There is no evidence of brain-stem depression due to spread of the local anaesthetic agent through the subarachnoid space to the medulla (Greene, 1958). In the case of epidural anaesthesia, however, sufficient local anaesthetic may be absorbed from the highly-vascular epidural space to cause systemic cardiovascular effects (Bonica, Berges and Morikawa. 1970); these may be confused with direct effects from sympathetic blockade. The anatomical level of sympathetic block under spinal and epidural anaesthesia rarely coincides with the level of sensory loss (Greene, 1962).

Spinal anaesthesia causes dilatation of both capacitance and resistance vessels. There is also relaxation of the vascular smooth muscle of metarterioles and precapillary sphincters, and a decrease of vasomotion. This relaxation is not, however, complete; the vessels retain some degree of inherent tone. Further dilatation can still occur in response to chemical stimulation by hypoxia, acidosis or vasodilator metabolites.

Effect on capacitance vessels

Dilatation of the capacitance vessels reduces mean systemic pressure (*see* page 119) and therefore decreases cardiac output. In high spinal anaesthesia this decrease of cardiac output is accentuated by reduction of sympathetic tone to the heart, with a consequent reduction of myocardial contractile force. Pugh and Wyndham (1950) found, in subjects with sensory block between T3 and T6, that cardiac output was decreased by 21 per cent in the horizontal position and by up to 36 per cent in the head-up position (30–40°). This further decrease of cardiac output on tilting was accompanied by arterial hypotension, and was presumably due to reduction of venous tone, allowing pooling of blood in dependent regions to cause a reduction of mean systemic pressure.

In pregnant women this decrease of venous tone may accentuate the pooling of blood in the lower extremities which occurs when the weight of the gravid uterus rests on the inferior vena cava. This phenomenon may be prevented by suitably positioning the patient.

Effect on resistance vessels

Dilatation of resistance vessels causes a fall of total peripheral resistance (TPR) despite compensatory vasoconstriction in the non-anaesthetized, normally-innervated regions of the body. Sancetta et al. (1952) found that spinal anaesthesia caused TPR to decrease by almost 20 per cent. This decrease, coupled with a fall of cardiac output, causes a fairly severe reduction of arterial blood pressure. The maximum decrease of peripheral resistance during spinal anaesthesia is said to be approximately 20 per cent, therefore a reduction of arterial pressure in excess of this amount must be due to a simultaneous reduction of cardiac output.

A fall of TPR is not, however, a constant finding. Shimosato and Etsten (1969) investigated the effects of spinal and epidural anaesthesia in unpremedicated normal subjects, and found no significant changes of cardiac output, nor of TPR, although there was a considerable redistribution of tissue blood flow. Bonica, Berges and Morikawa (1970), similarly found no change of cardiac output or TPR with epidural anaesthesia up to T4; although with higher levels there was some fall of vascular resistance with arterial hypotension.

The arteriolar dilatation which occurs during spinal anaesthesia reduces the pressure difference between the arterial reservoir and the capillaries, thus allowing capillary pressure to remain relatively constant despite a marked

reduction of arterial pressure. This minimizes shifts of fluid between the intra-
and extravascular compartments.

Effect on tissue blood flow

The effects on spinal anaesthesia on tissue blood flow are complex. Sympathetic
denervation causes vasodilatation in the denervated tissues, accompanied by
compensatory vasoconstriction in the normally-innervated tissues. This vasodilatation tends to increase blood flow through the denervated tissues, but the
extent of this increase is limited by the simultaneous decrease of arterial blood
pressure. In addition, in many tissues there is considerable autoregulation (*see*
page 92), therefore tissue blood flow tends to remain constant despite marked
changes of arterial pressure.

If the percentage decrease of blood pressure is less than the degree of local
vasodilatation, there is an increase of blood flow to the denervated tissues; if the
effects of vasodilatation are quantitatively less than the effects of arterial
hypotension, tissue blood flow is reduced. The relative importance of autoregulation and vasodilatation due to sympathetic denervation varies considerably
from tissue to tissue (*see* Chapter 5).

Brain

The cerebral vessels are under sympathetic control only to a minor extent.
They are, however, capable of a considerable degree of autoregulation, therefore
arterial hypotension during spinal anaesthesia causes only a slight reduction of
cerebral perfusion (Kleinerman, Sancetta and Hackel, 1958). At very low arterial
pressures, however, there may be some decrease of blood flow because
autoregulation is never perfect; this is especially so in previously hypertensive
patients, in whom there may be a severe reduction of cerebral perfusion when
arterial pressure is reduced, even to normal levels.

Heart

Similarly, the coronary vessels are but slightly (or not at all) under the
control of the sympathetic nervous system. The situation differs, however, from
that of the cerebral circulation in that a reduction of arterial blood pressure
reduces the work of the heart, therefore myocardial oxygen consumption falls
proportionately. Coronary vascular resistance tends to remain constant despite a
fall of arterial pressure.

Hackel, Sancetta and Kleinerman (1956) found that myocardial blood flow
and oxygen consumption were both reduced by almost 50 per cent during high
spinal anaesthesia, although coronary vascular resistance was normal. Despite the
marked reduction of coronary perfusion, however, they found no abnormality
of myocardial uptake of glucose, lactate or pyruvate. The situation therefore
differed considerably from that found in shock, when myocardial extraction of
pyruvate was found to be reduced almost to zero. During spinal anaesthesia,

therefore, myocardial perfusion seems to be adequate despite the fact that it may be reduced to almost half its usual value.

Kidney

The renal blood vessels are controlled by both nervous and local factors. The kidney shows a considerable degree of autoregulation, and its blood flow is, therefore, relatively independent of arterial pressure, provided this is above about 80 mm Hg. When arterial pressure falls to very low levels, however, there is a sharp rise of renal vascular resistance, accompanied by a precipitous fall of blood flow. The cause of this phenomenon is uncertain; it may involve the renin-angiotensin mechanism (*see* page 129) or, alternatively, some form of critical vascular closure (*see* page 15).

Splanchnic region

The resistance of the splanchnic vascular bed remains fairly constant during spinal anaesthesia; blood flow is therefore approximately proportional to the mean arterial pressure (Mueller, Lynn and Sancetta, 1952). These workers found that the reduction of splanchnic flow was roughly proportional to the anatomical level of anaesthesia—the mean flow was 590 ml min^{-1} m^{-2} body surface during high (above T4) spinal anaesthesia and 742 ml min^{-1} m^{-2} during low spinal anaesthesia. Despite this decrease of blood flow, splanchnic oxygen consumption remained almost constant, therefore hepatic venous oxygen content is likely to be considerably reduced during spinal anaesthesia.

Skin and Skeletal Muscles

During spinal anaesthesia there is normally an increase of blood flow to the skin and skeletal muscles in the denervated regions, accompanied by compensatory vasoconstriction and decreased flow to the normally-innervated regions. This vasoconstriction helps to maintain arterial blood pressure at fairly normal levels. Provided the mean arterial pressure does not fall below about 40 mm Hg, blood flow to the skin and skeletal muscles of the denervated regions is, therefore, increased.

RECOMMENDED FURTHER READING

Altura, B. M. (1971). 'Chemical and Humoral Regulation of Blood Flow through the Precapillary Sphincter.' *Microvasc. Res.* **3**, 361

Amundsen, E. (1969). 'Plasma Kinins.' *Scand. J. clin. Lab. Invest.* **24**, 301

Bard, P. (1960). 'Anatomical Organization of the Central Nervous System in Relation to Control of the Heart and Blood Vessels.' *Physiol. Rev.* **40** (Suppl. 4), 3

Bülbring, E. (1964). *Pharmacology of Smooth Muscle.* Czechoslovak Medical Press, Prague; Pergamon

Burki, N. and Guz, A. (1970). 'The Distensibility Characteristics of the Capacitance Vessels of the Forearm in Normal Subjects.' *Cardiovasc. Res.* **4**, 93

Eisele, J. H. (1972). 'The Use of Nerve Blocks for Studying Cardiopulmonary Physiology in Man.' *Br. J. Anaesth.* **44**, 606

Folkow, B. and Neil, E. (1971) *Circulation,* chps 15, 16, 17, 18 and 19. Oxford University Press

Gebber, G. L. (1970). 'The Central Organization of the Baroreceptor Reflexes. *Anesthesiology* **32**, 193

Gray, I. R. (1972). 'Control of Blood Pressure.' *Br. med. J.* **2**, 31

Haddy, F. J., Overbeck, H. W. and Daugherty, R. M. Jr. (1968). 'Peripheral Vascular Resistance.' *Ann. Rev. Med.* **19**, 167

Herskey, S. G. (1974). 'General Principles and Determinants of Circulatory Transport.' *Anesthesiology* **41**, 116

Johnson, P. C. (1964). 'Review of the Previous Studies and Current Theories of Autoregulation.' *Circulation Res.* **14** (Suppl. 1), 2

Karnovsky, M. J. (1967). 'The Ultrastructural Basis of Capillary Permeability studied with Peroxidase as a Tracer.' *J. cell. Biol.* **35**, 213

Kidd, C. and Linden, R. J. (1975). 'Recent Advances in the Physiology of Cardiovascular Reflexes, with Special Reference to Hypotension.' *Br. J. Anaesth.* **47**, 767

Lunzer, M. R., Manghani, K. K., Newman, S. P., Sherlock, S. P. V., Bernard, A. G. and Ginsberg, G. (1975). 'Impaired Cardiovascular Responsiveness in Liver Disease.' *Lancet* ii, 382

McDonald, D. A. (1974). *Blood Flow in Arteries,* 2nd edn. London; Edward Arnold

McDowall, D. G. (1969). 'Regional Blood Flow Measurement in Clinical Practice.' *Br. J. Anaesth.* **41**, 761

Mason, D. T. (1968). 'The Autonomic Nervous System and Regulation of Cardiovascular Performance.' *Anesthesiology* **29**, 670

Mellander, S. and Johansson, B. (1968). 'Control of Resistance, Exchange, and Capacitance Functions in the Peripheral Circulation.' *Pharmacol. Rev.* **20**, 117

Michel, C. C. (1972). 'Flows across Capillary Walls.' In Bergel, D. H., *Cardiovascular Fluid Dynamics,* p. 242. London; Academic Press

Needham, T. N. (1972). 'The Measurement of Blood Flow: Strain Gauge Plethysmography.' *Biomed. Eng.* **7**, 266

Peiss, C. N. (1965). 'Concepts of Cardiovascular Regulation; Past, Present and Future.' In *Nervous Control of the Heart.* Baltimore; Williams and Watkins

Rodbard, S. (1971). 'The Burden of the Resistance Vessels.' In *American Heart Association Monograph,* **33**, 2

Sewell, I. A. (1974). 'Circulation in the Tissues (the Microcirculation).' In Scurr, C. and Feldman, S., *Scientific Foundations of Anaesthesia.* London; Heinemann

Shepherd, J. T. and Vanhoutte, P. M. (1975). *'Veins and their Control.'* London; W. B. Saunders

Sleight, P. (1975). 'Neural Control of the Cardiovascular System.' In Oliver, M. F., *Modern Trends in Cardiology,* 3rd edn, ch. 1. London; Butterworths

Stainsby, W. N. (1973). 'Local Control of Regional Blood Flow.' *Ann. Rev. Physiol.* **35**, 151

Torrance, R. W. (1968). *Arterial Chemoreceptors.* Oxford; Blackwell

Webb-Peploe, M. M. and Shepherd, J. T. (1968). 'Veins and their Control.' *New Eng. J. Med.* **278**, 317

Wells, R. (1973). *The Microcirculation in Clinical Medicine.* London; Academic Press

Willenkin, R. L. and Greene, N. M. (1964). 'Circulatory Effects of Spinal and Epidural Anesthesia.' In Fabian, L. W., *Anesthesia and the Circulation,* p. 109. Philadelphia; F. A. Davis

Zanchetti, A. (1975). 'The Nervous Control of Circulation.' In *Physiological Basis of Anaesthesiology.* Padua; Piccin Medical Books

Zweifach, B. W. (1974). 'Mechanisms of Blood Flow and Fluid Exchange in Microvessels: Hemorrhagic Hypotension Model.' *Anesthesiology* **41**, 157

Chapter 4 Regulation of Cardiac Output

Blood flow through the body's peripheral tissues depends to a large extent on the metabolic requirements of those tissues (*see* Chapter 5). It is axiomatic that, if blood flow through a given tissue changes, then this change must be accompanied either by a reciprocal change of flow to other tissues, or by a change of cardiac output. Although redistribution of cardiac output plays some part in the body's response to physiological stress, as in exercise (*see* page 167), and still more in its response to pathological stress such as acute blood loss, most changes of man's internal or external environment are accompanied also by changes of his total cardiac output.

The cardiac output of a normal man at rest is approximately $5 \, \text{l} \, \text{min}^{-1}$; considerable departures, however, may occur from this figure under different physiological circumstances: during certain forms of anaesthesia cardiac output may fall to as low as $2.5 \, \text{l} \, \text{min}^{-1}$ (Prys-Roberts et al., 1968), whereas during severe exercise it may increase to as high as 25 or even $30 \, \text{l} \, \text{min}^{-1}$ (*see* page 170).

A knowledge of the factors which regulate cardiac output is important, both because it illustrates the essential unity of the cardiovascular system, and because it is often necessary clinically to have some idea of a patient's likely cardiac output. Measurement of cardiac output in humans is difficult and time-consuming and is therefore seldom used in the routine treatment of seriously ill patients, even though information about this parameter might improve their clinical management. Fortunately, it is often possible to use a knowledge of the factors which regulate cardiac output to make an informed guess about its probable value under any given set of circumstances, from simple measurements such as central venous and arterial blood pressure. The patient's response to treatment may be assessed similarly.

CARDIAC OUTPUT VERSUS VENOUS RETURN

Attempts to understand the interaction of the various factors which regulate cardiac output are often frustrated by the confusion which exists about the role played by, on the one hand, the factors which affect cardiac output, and, on the other hand, the factors which affect venous return. Cardiac output is the amount of blood pumped out of the left ventricle each minute; it is the flow of blood through the aortic valve. Venous return is the amount of blood which flows back to the heart each minute from the veins; it is the blood flow into the right atrium.

Over any appreciable period of time, cardiac output must equal venous return, since the right and left sides of the circulation are connected in series. The statement that, under certain circumstances, 'cardiac output is reduced because venous return is reduced', is thus tautological. What it means is that cardiac output is reduced because *the condition of the peripheral circulation is such that the forces which return blood to the right side of the heart are reduced and, as a result, cardiac output is reduced.*

EFFICIENCY OF CARDIAC PUMP VERSUS FACTORS AFFECTING VENOUS RETURN

There is confusion also about whether the cardiac output depends primarily on the ability of the heart to act as a pump or on the ease with which blood can flow back to the heart from the periphery, that is, on the state of the peripheral circulation. These two opposing concepts are represented diagrammatically in *Figures 4.1a* and *4.1b.*

In *Figure 4.1a* the heart is considered as a pump connected to a large venous reservoir with no intervening resistance. Under these circumstances cardiac output depends solely on the efficiency of the cardiac pump, and not at all on factors external to the heart. The other situation is represented by *Figure 4.1b* which shows the heart as a pump, the output of which is limited by the rate at which blood can return from the peripheral circulation. This venous return depends on the hydrostatic pressure difference between the venous reservoir and the right atrium, and on the resistance to flow between these points.

In practice, neither of these simplifications explains the experimental facts satisfactorily, and in fact, cardiac output depends on the pumping ability of the heart and on the state of the peripheral circulation. Under most circumstances, however, it is limited more by peripheral than by central factors; a threefold increase of cardiac output may occur as a result of changes in the peripheral circulation without any change in the efficiency of the cardiac pump (Guyton, 1968).

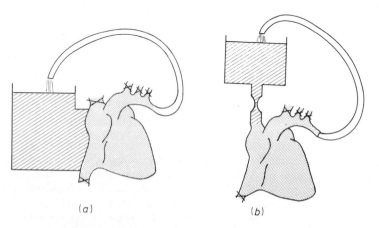

(a)   (b)

Figure 4.1. Regulation of cardiac output (based on Guyton). (a) Concept that output depends solely on pumping ability of heart. (b) Concept that output depends solely on condition of peripheral circulation

It is clear that cardiac output does not depend solely on the pumping efficiency of the heart because it is well recognized clinically that factors quite independent of the heart—such as an increase of blood volume—may cause an increase of cardiac output. Haemorrhage has the opposite effect even when myocardial nutrition is unimpaired. Also, opening an arteriovenous fistula causes an immediate increase of cardiac output, even when the pumping ability of the heart remains constant (Guyton and Sagawa, 1961). On the other hand, there is equally no doubt that a reduction of cardiac efficiency may cause a decrease of cardiac output, for example in valvular heart disease, myocardial infarction and myocarditis.

Cardiac output, therefore, depends on both central and peripheral factors, and an understanding of its regulation must be based on knowledge of both these factors and of the ways in which they interact.

Right atrial pressure

In any discussion about the regulation of cardiac output the right atrial pressure (r.a.p.) plays a central role, because it is involved in the determination of both cardiac output and venous return. On the one hand, an increase of r.a.p. increases diastolic filling of the heart, and therefore causes (by the Frank-Starling mechanism, *see* page 49) a greater force of myocardial contraction and a greater cardiac output; on the other hand, an increase of r.a.p. tends to prevent the return of blood from the periphery, and therefore reduces venous return.

There is thus a paradox, because an increase of r.a.p. tends simultaneously to cause both an increase of cardiac output and a decrease of venous return, but, as explained on page 111, cardiac output and venous return are normally equal. The solution to this paradox lies in the fact that, in any one subject at any one time, there can be but a *single* rate of blood flow through the heart. The system therefore comes to an equilibrium with the r.a.p. at such a level that forward flow of blood out of the heart (cardiac output) is just equalled by the flow of blood back from the veins (venous return).

Changes of either cardiac efficiency or of the peripheral circulation result, in general, in changes of both cardiac output and right atrial pressure. If the efficiency of the heart increases, it can pump more blood at a given r.a.p. However, if the heart pumps more blood, the venous return must also be increased (*see* earlier); and, if the rest of the circulation remains unchanged, this can occur only if r.a.p. falls. An increase of cardiac efficiency is therefore accompanied by a fall of r.a.p. until the increased venous return which this permits is just balanced by the increased cardiac output (which now, of course, occurs at a lower r.a.p.).

In a similar way, an increase of pressure in the peripheral circulation due, for example, to over-transfusion, increases the flow of blood into the heart — the venous return. However, if the efficiency of the cardiac pump remains constant, the heart can expel more blood only if r.a.p. increases. The system, therefore, comes to a new equilibrium with a raised r.a.p. and an increased cardiac output and venous return. Acute hypovolaemia produces the reverse situation; the system comes to equilibrium with a low r.a.p. and a decreased cardiac output and venous return.

The way in which central and peripheral factors interact in the regulation of cardiac output is shown diagrammatically in *Figure 4.2.* With a given cardiac efficiency, the amount of blood pumped by the heart each minute is determined by the pressure in the right atrial reservoir; this in turn depends on the pressure difference between the peripheral circulation and the right atrium, on the resistance to blood flow back into the heart, and on the actual flow through the system.

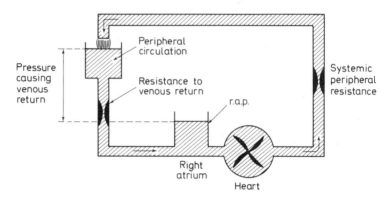

Figure 4.2. Diagrammatic representation of circulation, showing central importance of right atrial pressure (r.a.p.) in determination of both cardiac output and venous return (see text)

Although venous return depends on the pressures in the peripheral circulation, it is not possible to point to the pressure in any single vessel and to say that it is *this* pressure alone which determines the flow of blood back to the heart. The pressure gradients throughout the system are such that they tend to force blood round the circulation towards the right atrium: the arterial pressure forces blood to the capillaries, the capillary pressure forces blood to the veins, and so on. As will be seen later (page 119) the pressure in the venous side of the circulation is of more importance than arterial pressure in determining venous return; therefore the peripheral circulation is represented in *Figure 4.2* by a single reservoir coupled to the right atrium via a single resistance.

In the diagram the heart is represented as a single pump, the output of which is determined entirely by the right atrial pressure. The actual heart, of course, comprises two pumps in series interconnected by the pulmonary circulation. Although a full analysis of the regulation of cardiac output would have to take account of the separate control of the outputs of the two ventricles, the simplified analysis presented here is satisfactory for almost all purposes. The full, more detailed analysis, is considered by Guyton (*see* Recommended Further Reading; also page 125).

Compensatory mechanisms

In the previous paragraphs the interaction of central and peripheral factors in the control of cardiac output was considered on the assumption that these were independent. Changes of cardiac pumping efficiency were considered on the assumption that the peripheral circulation was not affected by changes of cardiac output. This is clearly unjustified: a decrease of cardiac output consequent to a reduction of cardiac efficiency is accompanied by changes in the peripheral circulation which tend to restore cardiac output to normal. These compensatory responses are considered in greater detail on page 125; it is sufficient to consider here one such mechanism.

A decrease of cardiac efficiency causes a decreased cardiac output and increased right atrial pressure. The decreased output causes arterial hypotension, which is detected by the aortic and carotid baroreceptors (*see* page 97) and, as a result, there is a reflex increase of sympathetic tone to the heart, to the peripheral resistance vessels, and to the veins. This increased sympathetic tone improves myocardial efficiency to an extent which depends on the cause of the cardiac depression; the arteriolar constriction increases the total peripheral resistance and so tends to raise arterial blood pressure; the increased sympathetic tone to the veins decreases the capacity of the circulatory system and so increases the pressure available to drive blood back to the heart (*see* page 120). As a result of these compensatory responses, the diminished cardiac output is partially restored to normal, and the system comes to a new equilibrium with a reduced cardiac output which is not, however, as low as it would have been in the absence of compensatory mechanisms.

Guyton's graphical analysis

Guyton (*see* Recommended Further Reading) illustrates graphically the interaction of central and peripheral factors in the regulation of cardiac output by two curves, which represent respectively, the relationships between cardiac output and r.a.p. (*Figure 4.3a*) and between venous return and r.a.p. (*Figure 4.3b*). The former shows cardiac output increasing with increasing r.a.p.; the latter shows venous return decreasing with increasing r.a.p. These two curves, therefore, illustrate the paradox of page 109; an increase of r.a.p. is accompanied simultaneously by an increase of cardiac output and by a decrease of venous return. The solution lies in the fact that the axes in the two figures are identical — over any appreciable period of time venous return is equal to cardiac output — therefore it is possible to superimpose the curves on a single diagram; and when this is done (*Figure 4.3c*), the point where the curves cross (*A*) represents the instantaneous values of cardiac output and r.a.p. It gives the only pair of values of cardiac output and r.a.p. which simultaneously satisfy the equations represented by the two curves shown in the upper figures.

When the physiological state of the body changes, the point of intersection also changes: the system comes to a new equilibrium with a different cardiac output and r.a.p. In *Figure 4.4* the dotted curve represents the relationship between cardiac output and r.a.p. with a hypereffective heart such as might occur as a result of an infusion of isoprenaline. The equilibrium point is now at *A'*: there is a greater cardiac output and a lower r.a.p. than was the case with the normal heart (point *A*).

It is possible with this type of graphical analysis to represent quantitatively the effect of most of the factors which influence cardiac output, and to illustrate the compensatory mechanisms by which the body attempts to restore cardiac output to normal when it has been reduced by pathological processes. This type

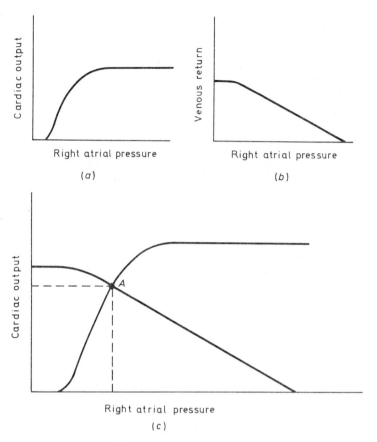

Figure 4.3. Regulation of cardiac output. (a) Relationship between r.a.p. and cardiac output. (b) Relationship between r.a.p. and venous return. (c) Actual values of cardiac output and r.a.p. determined by point A at which cardiac output and venous return curves cross (see text)

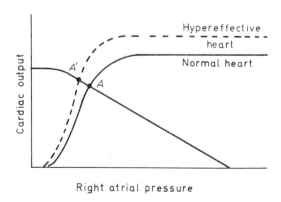

Figure 4.4. Cardiac output with a hypereffective heart and a normal peripheral circulation (point A'). Cardiac output is high, r.a.p. is low

of elegant graphical analysis is described in detail by Guyton, Jones and Coleman (1973).

Unfortunately, however, most doctors find it difficult to think in terms of graphs, therefore the present approach is largely descriptive. Reference will, however, be made from time to time to the rather more elegant graphical approach.

THE CARDIAC PUMP

It is possible to analyse the effect of physiological changes of environment on the efficiency of the cardiac pump in terms of their effect on heart rate, ventricular end-diastolic volume and ventricular end-systolic volume. This approached was outlined in Chapter 2. For the present purpose, however, it is more convenient to consider the overall nature of the relationship between cardiac output and r.a.p., and the factors which affect this relationship. An increase of cardiac output at a constant r.a.p. indicates that the heart has become a more effective pump; conversely, if the heart requires a higher r.a.p. to expel the same amount of blood, this is evidence of decreased cardiac efficiency.

Relationship between cardiac output and right atrial pressure

One of the most important determinants of the amount of blood pumped by the heart each minute is the end-diastolic length of the myocardial fibres (*see* page 64). This parameter is normally closely related to the mean value of the r.a.p. Provided the muscle fibres are not over-stretched, the greater their end-diastolic length the greater is the force of subsequent myocardial contraction and, other things being equal, the greater is the cardiac output. This is the Frank-Starling relationship (*see* page 49).

The relationship between right atrial pressure and cardiac output may conveniently be investigated by the Starling heart-lung preparation. This has the advantage that it represents a carefully-controlled situation, because the heart is completely denervated and free from the action of circulating hormones, and the arterial blood pressure is kept constant by a 'Starling resistance'. (This consists of a flaccid tube surrounded by a pressure reservoir in such a way that the blood pressure proximal to the resistance is kept constant and equal to that in the surrounding reservoir.)

The disadvantage of the heart-lung preparation is, of course, that it is unphysiological. It would, for example, be more realistic to allow the heart to pump against either a constant peripheral resistance or one which varied in response to physiological stimuli. This is what happens in the intact animal, where an increase of cardiac output, due, for example, to an increase of r.a.p., is usually accompanied by an increase of arterial pressure which imposes an increased load on the heart, and thus limits the increase of cardiac output which occurs at high atrial pressures (*see also* page 190). (The tendency for arterial blood pressure to rise in response to an increase of cardiac output is, of course, partially off-set by reduction of peripheral resistance from passive vascular dilatation with the increased intravascular pressure, and from the operation of baroreceptor reflexes — *see* page 96).

The relationship between cardiac output and r.a.p. for a heart of average efficiency, pumping blood against an average peripheral resistance is shown in *Figure 4.5.* It is based on the experimental findings of Fermoso, Richardson and Guyton (1964), but the scale has been adjusted to extrapolate their results, which were in dogs, to man. These workers measured the changes of cardiac output which occurred when r.a.p. was acutely raised or lowered by rapid transfusion or removal of blood from the circulation. Although such comprehensive studies have not been made, and probably cannot be made, in intact man, there is much evidence to suggest that the relationship between human cardiac output and r.a.p. is similar to that shown in *Figure 4.5* (*see* Braunwald and Ross, 1963).

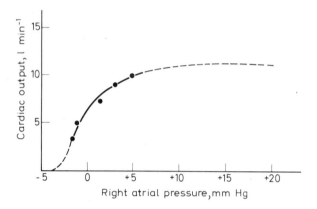

Figure 4.5. Experimental relationship between cardiac output and r.a.p. (redrawn, scaled to apply to man, from Fermoso, Richardson and Guyton, 1964)

The normal cardiac output of 5 l min^{-1} occurs at an r.a.p. of a few mm Hg, cardiac filling, of course, being aided by the sub-atmospheric intrathoracic pressure. At sub-atmospheric atrial pressures cardiac filling is prevented because there is then insufficient pressure difference between the interior and exterior of the heart to cause ventricular distension, and cardiac output therefore falls to zero at an r.a.p. of −2 or −3 mm Hg.

With increasing r.a.p. cardiac output rises because increased ventricular distension increases the force of myocardial contraction by the Frank-Starling mechanism. An increase of r.a.p. can increase cardiac output to between 2 and 3 times its normal value in the absence of external inotropic* influences. At high atrial pressures cardiac output ceases to increase; this plateau is probably due partly to arterial hypertension which causes an increased load on the heart and thus impedes ventricular emptying, and partly to pericardial inextensibility which limits ventricular end-diastolic volume, and therefore ventricular stroke volume.

Starling found that, when r.a.p. was increased above a certain level, cardiac output fell. Crowell and Guyton (1962), however, found no evidence of this fall; and it may be that the decline of cardiac output found by Starling at high filling pressures was an artefact due to non-specific factors causing a time-dependent decrease of myocardial efficiency.

* *See* footnote on p. 43.

Factors affecting the relationship between cardiac output and right atrial pressure

The relationship between cardiac output and r.a.p. is influenced by changes of cardiac pumping efficiency and by changes of intrathoracic pressure (*Figure 4.6*). Changes of cardiac efficiency alter the scale of the ordinate (y-axis); and changes of intrathoracic pressure shift the cardiac function curve bodily sideways without altering its general shape. Increased cardiac efficiency

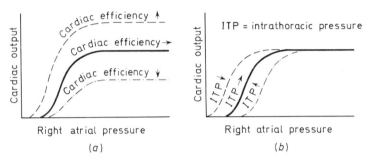

Figure 4.6. (a) Influence of cardiac efficiency on cardiac function curve (diagrammatic). (b) Influence of changes of intrathoracic pressure (ITP) on cardiac function curve (diagrammatic)

means that the heart can expel more blood at a given r.a.p.; decrease of efficiency moves the curves in the opposite direction, downward and to the right (*Figure 4.6a*). A decrease of intrathoracic pressure moves the curve to the left; an increase moves it to the right (*Figure 4.6b*). This shift occurs because the pumping ability of the heart depends, not on the absolute value of r.a.p., but on the effective cardiac filling pressure — the difference between right atrial and intrathoracic pressures.

Cardiac efficiency

The factors which affect the efficiency of the cardiac pump are summarized in *Table 4.1*. Physiologically, the most important factor which increases cardiac efficiency is increased sympathetic stimulation and/or an increased concentration of sympathomimetic amines in the blood going to the heart. Both these factors have a positive inotropic influence on the heart.

Alteration of autonomic tone   When the sympathetic innervation of the heart is maximally stimulated, the maximum output which can be achieved at high atrial pressures is increased by roughly 70 per cent, to approximately 25 l min^{-1}. When sympathetic tone is abolished, cardiac function is depressed, and the maximum cardiac output is decreased by approximately 20 per cent. Changes of parasympathetic tone have the opposite effect, although they are mediated mainly by changes of heart rate and strength of atrial contraction; vagal stimulation is not thought to affect the strength of ventricular contraction directly (Carlsten, Folkow and Hamberger, 1957).

Table 4.1   FACTORS AFFECTING EFFICIENCY OF CARDIAC PUMP

Increased	*Decreased*
Sympathetic stimulation (rate and force of contraction)	Parasympathetic stimulation (probably rate only)
Parasympathetic inhibition	Sympathetic inhibition
Increased concentration of sympathomimetic amines	Ischaemia and myocardial infarction
	Myocarditis
Decrease of arterial blood pressure − afterload	Valvular heart disease
	Increase of arterial blood pressure − afterload
	Hypoxia
	Acidosis

Heart rate   Pure changes of heart rate, without simultaneous changes of myocardial contractility, have a complex effect on the relationship between cardiac output and r.a.p. For any given state of myocardial contractility, there is an optimal heart rate, both above and below which cardiac output may be decreased. Cardiac output is decreased by bradycardia because the extent to which stroke volume can increase to compensate for a decrease of heart rate is limited by pericardial inextensibility (*see* page 64); during tachycardia stroke volume is decreased because insufficient time is available for satisfactory ventricular filling (*see* page 54).

Pathological processes   Myocardial efficiency is reduced by pathological processes, such as myocardial infarction, myocarditis, and valvular abnormalities. Myocardial hypoxia also causes a reduction of cardiac efficiency, irrespective of the cause of the hypoxia.

Afterload   The pumping ability of the heart is altered by changes of afterload (*see* page 44). The less the load presented to the heart the greater is the amount of blood which it can expel at any given r.a.p. and state of myocardial contractility. In the normal heart, however, this effect is minimized by the Frank-Starling mechanism. When the afterload is increased, the heart is momentarily unable to expel its full stroke volume, therefore the ventricular end-diastolic volume is increased, and the resulting increase of myocardial contractile force compensates for the increased load.

Sarnoff (1955) suggested that, at any given r.a.p., cardiac output is inversely related to the systemic total peripheral resistance, and more recently Prys-Roberts has shown the importance of this mechanism in determining cardiac output during halothane anaesthesia. Halothane causes a decrease of myocardial contractility (Prys-Roberts et al., 1972b); but at normal levels of P_{CO_2} it appears to cause little or no peripheral vasodilatation (Gersh et al., 1972), and so no change of systemic vascular resistance. The weakened heart is therefore required to eject blood against a normal peripheral resistance and, as a result, the cardiac output falls. Hypocapnia causes peripheral vasoconstriction, and the greater load which this imposes on the halothane-weakened heart causes a further reduction of cardiac output. Myocardial contractility under these circumstances does not appear to be depressed (Foëx and Prys-Roberts, 1975). Conversely, hypercapnia produces a decrease of peripheral resistance and an increase of cardiac output due mainly to the decreased load presented to the heart by the dilated peripheral circulation.

A similar effect is seen with large doses of morphine. The administration of 2 mg kg^{-1} of morphine, and artificial ventilation with oxygen, results in peripheral vasodilatation and an increase of cardiac output (Wong et al., 1973). But the addition of nitrous oxide causes peripheral vasoconstriction; and this imposes an increased load on the heart, and therefore causes a fall of cardiac output.

Intrathoracic pressure

The factors which affect intrathoracic pressure and shift the cardiac function curve sideways are fairly obvious. The curve is shifted to the right by an increase of intrathoracic pressure due, for example, to pleural effusion, pneumothorax or intermittent positive pressure ventilation, especially with excessive inflation pressures or insufficient expiratory duration (*see* page 193). The curve is displaced in the opposite direction by a decrease of intrathoracic pressure due, for example, to an excessive degree of negative expiratory airway pressure during intermittent positive–negative pressure ventilation.

Cardiac tamponade has a particularly deleterious effect on cardiac output because it increases the pressure in the immediate vicinity of the heart, even though the general intrathoracic pressure may be relatively normal. The effect of tamponade is particularly marked at large cardiac volumes, such as occur at high atrial pressures.

VENOUS RETURN

The factors which affect venous return may be investigated in the experimental animal by replacing the right ventricle with a mechanical pump, which withdraws bloods from the right atrium and re-injects it into the pulmonary artery. The greater the pumping rate the lower is the r.a.p., and the greater is the cardiac output and, therefore, venous return. With this preparation it is easy to measure simultaneously venous return and r.a.p., and hence to plot the experimental relationship between these variables over a wide range of atrial pressures.

Guyton and his co-workers (Fermoso, Richardson and Guyton, 1964), have also investigated the influence of changes of r.a.p. on venous return in relatively intact animals with closed chests. They did this by introducing a balloon into the pulmonary artery in such a way that, by progressively obstructing right ventricular outflow, they were able to reduce venous return, and therefore to investigate the relationship between this variable and r.a.p. There is, in fact, little difference between curves obtained by this technique and by that described in the previous paragraph.

Relationship between venous return and right atrial pressure

The typical experimental relationship between venous return and right atrial pressure is shown in *Figure 4.7*. This is based on results from experimental animals, but the scale is adjusted to make it applicable to man. The curve has two distinct regions, a sloping right-hand segment and a horizontal left-hand segment, linked by a transitional zone around an r.a.p. of zero. The slope of the relationship between venous return and r.a.p. has the units, flow pressure^{-1}; the reciprocal of this slope, therefore, has the units of resistance and is known as the *resistance to venous return* (Guyton, Jones and Coleman, 1973).

On the right-hand segment of the curve, venous return depends on this resistance and on the pressure difference between point *A* and the r.a.p. The pressure represented by point *A* is known as the *mean systemic pressure,* a term to be defined later (*see* next page).

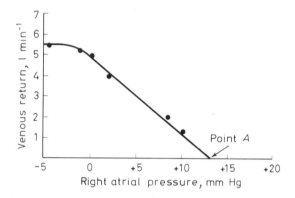

Figure 4.7. Experimental relationship between venous return and r.a.p. (redrawn, scaled to apply to man, from Fermoso, Richardson and Guyton, 1964)

The slope of the venous return curve decreases as r.a.p. approaches zero. At atrial pressures below zero the curve is almost horizontal, and the resistance to venous return is very high. The reason for this increase of resistance is venous collapse when the pressure inside the veins becomes sub-atmospheric; veins have relatively thin walls, and they therefore collapse when the transmural pressure becomes negative. Such collapsed vessels, of course, offer a very high resistance to blood flow.

Pressure gradient causing venous return

The driving force which returns blood to the heart is the pressure difference between the peripheral circulation and the right atrium. It is not, however, possible to indicate the pressure at any single point in the circulation, and to say that it is this pressure alone which is responsible for returning blood to the heart. There is a continuous decline of pressure round the circulation from the aorta to the right atrium; and the pressure gradient is at all points in a direction to force blood round the circulation back to the right heart. (As explained in Chapter 3, blood actually flows, not from a region of high pressure to a region of low pressure, but from a region of high total energy to a region of low total energy. Normally, however, the kinetic component of the total energy is small compared with the hydrostatic pressure component, therefore it is usually permissible to equate pressure energy with total energy, as is done here.)

Mean systemic pressure (Guyton, Jones and Coleman, 1973)

Despite the conceptual difficulty described in the previous paragraph, it is possible to define mathematically a single *virtual* pressure which represents the effective pressure driving blood back towards the heart. This is the mean systemic pressure (m.s.p.) which may be defined as the pressure which would be present throughout the systemic circulation if it were suddenly arrested and blood transferred instantaneously from the arteries to the veins until pressure was uniform throughout the system. (Mean circulatory pressure is the pressure, defined in this way, throughout the entire circulation, pulmonary as well as systemic. Numerically the mean systemic pressure is almost the same as the mean circulatory pressure.)

In experimental animals, m.s.p. may be measured by inducing ventricular fibrillation and transferring blood rapidly from the arterial to the venous side of the circulation until the pressure is uniform. In dogs m.s.p. is approximately 7 mm Hg; for obvious reasons, it has not been determined in man. (The pressure in the human systemic circulation after a cardiac arrest is approximately 20 mm Hg (Sykes, 1967). Under these circumstances, however, reflex changes are likely to have altered the capacity of the system fairly markedly. Guyton, Polizo and Armstrong (1954) showed, in experimental animals, that after arterial and venous pressures had been equalized, there was a period of about 7 seconds during which pressure was constant; after this time m.s.p. began to rise due to sympathetically-induced vasoconstriction.)

The concept of mean systemic pressure is perhaps most easily understood by reversing the argument used to define this quantity. If the heart were at rest, the pressure throughout the cardiovascular system would be uniform, and would depend on the relationship between the volume of blood contained in the system and its capacity. By definition, the pressure would then equal the mean systemic pressure (strictly the mean circulatory pressure which is numerically almost the same). If the heart were then started, blood would be transferred from the venous to the arterial sides of the circulation, with a consequent rise of arterial and fall of venous pressure. Because the compliance of the arterial system is considerably less than that of the venous reservoir, the increase of arterial pressure would be considerably greater than the fall of venous pressure (*see* below). Transfer of blood would continue until the pressure gradients throughout the cardiovascular system were sufficient to permit a flow of blood from the arterial reservoir back to the right atrium, just equal to the rate at which it was simultaneously pumped out of the left ventricle, that is, until venous return equalled cardiac output.

Mathematical derivation of mean systemic pressure It may be shown mathematically that m.s.p. is equal to the sum of the pressures in the various segments of the systemic circulation, each weighted according to the relative capacity of that segment. Consider a very simple model of the circulation consisting solely of an arterial and a venous reservoir interconnected by appropriate vascular resistances (*Figure 4.8*). The volume of blood (V_a) held in the arterial reservoir by virtue of the arterial pressure (P_a) is $P_a C_a$, where C_a is the compliance of the arterial reservoir. Similarly, $V_v = P_v C_v$, where the symbols have the same significance but refer to the venous reservoir. By analogy, the volume of blood (V_s) which would be held in the circulation by virtue of the mean systemic pressure (P_{ms}), if the arterial and venous pressures were equalized, would be $P_{ms} C_s$, where C_s is the compliance of the entire systemic circulation.

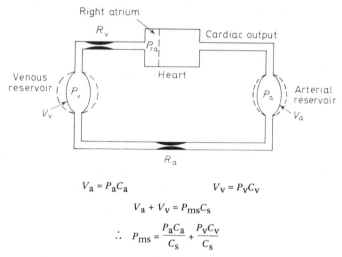

$$V_a = P_a C_a \qquad\qquad V_v = P_v C_v$$

$$V_a + V_v = P_{ms} C_s$$

$$\therefore \; P_{ms} = \frac{P_a C_a}{C_s} + \frac{P_v C_v}{C_s}$$

Figure 4.8. Diagram of circulation used to derive mean systemic pressure (P_{ms}) and resistance to venous return (for explanation see text)

Since, by definition, the volume of blood in the system is identical in the two cases, it is possible to equate V_s to the sum of V_a and V_v. Therefore $P_{ms} C_s = P_a C_a + P_v C_v$. This may be arranged as:

$$P_{ms} = P_a\, C_a/C_s + P_v\, C_v/C_s.$$

(Neglect of the capillaries in this simple analysis is justified because the volume of blood stored in these minute vessels is less than 5 per cent of the total, *see* page 80.)

The venous system is considerably more distensible than the arterial side of the circulation, therefore m.s.p. is much closer to venous than to arterial pressure. Experimentally, the venous reservoir is between 18 and 30 times more distensible than the arterial reservoir (Guyton, Armstrong and Chipley, 1956).

Factors affecting mean systemic pressure   The extent to which the circulatory system is filled with blood determines m.s.p. It therefore depends both on the total amount of blood contained in the system, and on the system's volume. An increase of blood volume increases m.s.p., as does a decrease of circulatory capacity, particularly on the venous side. Richardson, Stallings and Guyton

(1961) showed, in the dog, that there is an almost linear relationship between m.s.p. and blood volume. In the absence of reflex vasoconstriction, a 15 per cent reduction of blood volume reduces m.s.p. almost to zero: an increase of 15 per cent increases it by almost 100 per cent. The regulation of blood volume is considered on page 127.

Since m.s.p. depends not only on actual blood volume, but also on the capacity of the vascular system, it is influenced by changes of vasomotor tone. Total spinal anaesthesia reduces m.s.p.; intense sympathetic stimulation increases it. Quite apart from such active changes of vascular tone, m.s.p. may also be altered passively by changes of extravascular pressure. It is, for example, increased by abdominal compression, positive pressure ventilation and contraction of the skeletal muscles.

Stress relaxation Another factor affecting m.s.p. is the phenomenon of stress relaxation, by which the cardiovascular system adjusts its capacity according to the volume of fluid it is required to contain. The precise physical basis of this phenomenon is uncertain. It has been found experimentally, however, that an increase of intravascular pressure, due, for example, to rapid blood transfusion, is followed by a gradual decline of pressure over the next few minutes. Undoubtedly part of this fall is due to extravasation of fluid into the interstitial spaces, but part appears to be due to progressive relaxation of vascular tone, that is, to the phenomenon of stress relaxation.

Resistance to venous return

Venous return depends on the difference between mean systemic and right atrial pressures and on the resistance to venous return (*see Figure 4.7*). The relationship between venous return and r.a.p. is linear over a wide range of atrial pressures indicating a constant resistance to venous return.

As is the case with m.s.p. the resistance to venous return is not localized to any single point in the circulation, but is distributed (unequally) between the different segments. The simple model of the circulation considered on page 120 (*Figure 4.8*) may also be used to discuss resistance to venous return. If cardiac output is $\dot{Q}$,

$$\dot{Q} = (P_v - P_{ra})/R_v \qquad \text{i.e.} \quad P_v = \dot{Q} R_v + P_{ra},$$
$$\text{and} \quad \dot{Q} = (P_a - P_v)/R_a \qquad \text{i.e.} \quad P_a = \dot{Q} R_a + P_v,$$

where P_v P_{ra}, and P_a are, respectively, the pressures in the venous reservoir, the right atrium and the arterial reservoir, and R_a and R_v are, respectively, the resistance between the arterial and venous reservoirs, and between the venous reservoir and the right atrium. Combining these equations gives $P_a = \dot{Q}(R_a + R_v) + P_{ra}$.

Now $C_s P_{ms} = C_a P_a + C_v P_v$ (*see* page 120), therefore, substituting for P_a and P_v,

$$C_s P_{ms} = C_a\{\dot{Q}(R_a + R_v) + P_{ra}\} + C_v(\dot{Q}R_v + P_{ra}),$$

whence

$$\dot{Q} = \frac{C_s P_{ms} - (C_a + C_v) P_{ra}}{C_a(R_a + R_v) + C_v R_v}$$

$$= \frac{(C_a + C_v)\ (P_{ms} - P_{ra})}{C_a(R_a + R_v) + C_v R_v}$$

Resistance to venous return (pressure difference/flow) is, therefore,

$$\frac{C_a(R_a + R_v) + C_v R_v}{C_a + C_v} = \frac{C_a R_a + (C_a + C_v) R_v}{C_a + C_v}$$

which is the relationship derived by Guyton (1955).

The compliance (C_v) of the venous reservoir is considerably greater than the compliance (C_a) of the arterial reservoir, therefore the above equation may be approximated by the much simpler expression:

$$\text{resistance to venous return} = R_v + R_a C_a / C_v.$$

Resistance to venous return depends therefore, under most conditions, more on R_v (the resistance between the venous reservoir and the right atrium) than on R_a (the resistance between the arterial and venous reservoirs).

This rather difficult mathematical concept is perhaps better derived intuitively. An increase of resistance between the venous reservoir and the right atrium causes blood to be dammed back in the venous reservoir. The compliance of this chamber is, however, sufficiently great for it to be able to accommodate a relatively large amount of blood with but little rise of intravascular pressure. An increase of resistance between the arterial and venous reservoirs, however, causes retention of blood in the relatively uncompliant arterial reservoir; the consequent rise of intravascular pressure then tends to overcome the increased resistance to blood flow between these two chambers.

It should be remembered, however, that arteriolar resistance (R_a) is numerically considerably higher than venous resistance (R_v), therefore it is not possible to dismiss R_a altogether. In fact, under may circumstances, the resistances to venous return provided by the veins and by the arterioles are quantitatively almost the same (Guyton, personal communication). The range of variation of arteriolar resistance is normally much the greater, which increases the physiological importance of this region of the circulation.

Factors affecting resistance to venous return

The factors which affect the resistance to venous return are mainly those which alter the calibre of the vessels lying between the venous reservoir and the right atrium. An increase of sympathetic activity causes venoconstriction, thus increasing the resistance and altering the slope of the venous return curve. (It should be noted, however, that the effect of venoconstriction in increasing m.s.p. is normally much greater than its effect on the resistance to venous return.) Resistance to venous return is increased also by localized constriction of the great veins due, for example, to obstruction by surgical intervention or pressure from a gravid uterus. The venous collapse which occurs when intravascular pressure becomes sub-atmospheric causes a considerable increase of venous resistance and limits venous return at low atrial pressures (*see Figure 4.7*).

The muscular pump

An additional factor which influences venous return is the pumping action of the diaphragm and contraction of the skeletal muscles. The pressure swings which occur between thorax and abdomen during the respiratory cycle aid return of blood towards the heart; rhythmic venous compression by muscular contraction also helps venous return because the veins possess one-way valves, therefore venous compression can force blood onwards towards the right atrium. The effect of these mechanisms is to reduce the resistance to venous return so that the blood flow which occurs with a given mean systemic-to-right atrial pressure difference is increased.

Although the precise quantitative role of the diaphragmatic and muscular pumps is uncertain, there is little doubt that they play an important part in increasing cardiac output during muscular exercise (*see* page 170). During artificial ventilation by intermittent airway pressure, the normal sequence of intrathoracic and abdominal pressure swings is reversed; and this probably accounts for the reduction of cardiac output which occurs, even when mean intrathoracic pressure and Pa_{CO_2} are maintained at the levels found during spontaneous ventilation (Prys-Roberts et al., 1967; *see* page 194).

RECAPITULATION

An understanding of the way in which cardiac output depends both on the state of the peripheral circulation, particularly on the mean systemic pressure, and on the efficiency of the cardiac pump is so important that the basis of the argument will be repeated.

Cardiac output depends on right atrial pressure (r.a.p.). The greater the r.a.p., the greater is the cardiac output. This is the Frank-Starling mechanism. The greater the efficiency of the cardiac pump, the greater is the cardiac output at a given r.a.p. or, alternatively, the lower is the r.a.p. required to expel a given cardiac output. This much is straightforward and easily understood.

The difficulty arises when we come to consider what determines r.a.p., because we immediately encounter the circular argument that, on the one hand, r.a.p. determines cardiac output, but on the other hand, cardiac output determines the difference between mean systemic pressure (m.s.p.) and r.a.p., and therefore the value of r.a.p. itself. Cardiac output depends on r.a.p.: r.a.p. is determined by cardiac output. An increase of r.a.p. causes an increase of cardiac output, but this increase of cardiac output causes an increased difference between m.s.p. and r.a.p. and therefore a fall of r.a.p.; this is a stable situation, and the body comes to an equilibrium with a value of r.a.p. which produces a certain cardiac output and, simultaneously, an identical venous return (flow of blood back to the right side of the heart).

(If the feedback were positive, an increase of cardiac output due to an increase of r.a.p. would be accompanied by a decrease of the difference between m.s.p. and r.a.p., and therefore by a further increase of r.a.p. The system would come to an equilibrium position with a very high cardiac output and, simultaneously, a very high r.a.p. This is a physiologically impossible situation.)

The fact that the pressure difference between m.s.p. and r.a.p. increases with cardiac output is intuitively obvious, although the fact that there is a linear relationship between these variables for positive values of r.a.p. (*see Figure 4.7*) depends on experimental findings, as does the precise shape of the cardiac function curve shown in *Figure 4.5*. The argument in the previous paragraphs does not, however, depend on the precise nature of the relationships between cardiac output and r.a.p., and between venous return and r.a.p., only on the fact that an increase of r.a.p. causes an increase of cardiac output, while an increase of cardiac output widens the difference between m.s.p. and r.a.p., and therefore lowers r.a.p.

SHOCK

Shock is considered in detail in Chapter 9. The essential physiological defect in shock is, however, a reduction of cardiac output, therefore it is appropriate to consider here the mechanisms by which cardiac output is reduced in this condition, and the compensatory mechanisms which minimize the reduction of cardiac output.

Shock may occur either because of an acute reduction of cardiac efficiency — cardiogenic shock — or because the mean systemic pressure is reduced. The latter condition is commonly due to acute hypovolaemia as in haemorrhagic shock, but may occur also in the presence of a normal blood volume, when the capacity of the vascular system is increased, for example, by the action of circulating toxins.

Pure haemorrhagic shock may, after a time, be complicated by a deterioration of cardiac function; there is then an additional element of cardiogenic shock. This leads to further deterioration of the patient's condition; and may prevent recovery when his blood volume is finally restored to normal, that is, may account in part for the condition of 'irreversible' shock (*see* page 223). The cause of this impairment of cardiac efficiency is complex, but there is little doubt that, in addition to the direct effect of ischaemia and hypoxia on cardiac metabolism, acidosis from anaerobic metabolism in remote, underperfused tissues may cause an additional impairment of cardiac function (*see* page 225).

Haemorrhagic shock

In haemorrhagic shock, m.s.p. is reduced thus causing a reduction of cardiac output. The body reacts to this situation with an increase of sympathetic activity which tends to restore m.s.p. and cardiac output to normal. Although these compensatory responses normally occur *pari passu* with the primary reduction of cardiac output, it is convenient to consider the body's response to haemorrhage as if it occurred in two separate stages — an initial fall of cardiac output, followed by various compensatory responses which restore the output towards normal.

The state of the body immediately after an acute haemorrhage is with a low m.s.p., an almost normal resistance to venous return, and normal cardiac efficiency. This situation is represented by point *B* in *Figure 4.9*; the normal state of the circulation is represented by point *A*. There is, therefore, a low cardiac output and a low r.a.p.

The reaction of the body to this situation takes the form of an increase of sympathetic tone to the heart and the remainder of the cardiovascular system. This increased sympathetic activity increases the efficiency of the cardiac pump, moving the cardiac function curve upwards and to the left; it also causes venous constriction, thus raising the m.s.p. and (slightly) the resistance to venous return. The situation after the occurrence of these compensatory responses is represented by point *C* in *Figure 4.9*.

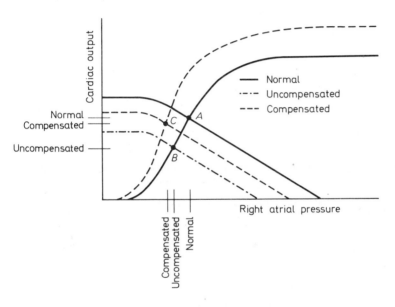

Figure 4.9. Cardiac output and r.a.p. in compensated and uncompensated haemorrhagic shock (for explanation see text)

Provided the initial reduction of m.s.p. is not too great, cardiac output may be restored almost to normal, although the r.a.p. — which is measured clinically as central venous pressure (*see* page 278) — is still below normal as it must be in the presence of a reduced cardiac output and increased cardiac efficiency.

The simultaneous constriction of resistance vessels has virtually no effect on cardiac output; it does, however, increase total peripheral resistance, thus tending to maintain arterial blood pressure. It also tends to divert the reduced cardiac output away from the vasoconstricted tissues to more important regions of the circulation, such as the brain and heart (*see* page 217).

If the efficiency of the cardiac pump is decreased by myocardial hypoxia this produces a combination of haemorrhagic and cardiogenic shock; the cardiac function curve then moves downwards and to the right, causing a severe reduction of cardiac output, accompanied by a rise of r.a.p.

ACP—5*

Cardiogenic shock

The cardiac output and r.a.p. immediately after an acute reduction of cardiac efficiency is shown by point *B* in *Figure 4.10*; cardiac output is reduced, r.a.p. is increased. Point *A* again represents the normal state of the cardiovascular system.

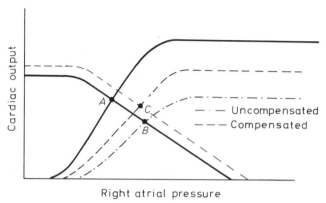

Figure 4.10. Cardiac output and r.a.p. in compensated and uncompensated cardiogenic shock (for explanation see text)

As in the case with haemorrhagic shock, the body responds by an increase of sympathetic tone to the entire cardiovascular system. The increased sympathetic activity to the heart tends to restore the efficiency of the cardiac pump, although the extent to which it can do so obviously depends on the amount of undamaged cardiac muscle present, and on the extent to which the myocardium can respond to positive inotropic influences. If myocardial function is severely depressed by acidosis, the heart's response to increased sympathetic tone may be minimal. Under favourable circumstances, however, increased sympathetic activity moves the cardiac function curve towards normal, upwards and to the left.

The accompanying venoconstriction raises the m.s.p. above normal and causes a small increase of resistance to venous return. This increase of m.s.p. causes a further improvement of cardiac output (point *C*).

The concomitant arteriolar constriction has little effect on cardiac output, but diverts blood from the skin and gut to more immediately essential organs. In fact, there is evidence that an increase of blood pressure may, in the presence of myocardial depression, impose such a load on the damaged heart that it may cause a further reduction of cardiac output (*see* page 116). Treatment of shock with sympathomimetic amines, the action of which is predominantly on the resistance vessels, may so increase the load on a heart damaged by acidosis or hypoxia that their administration may be accompanied by a decrease of cardiac output, and by a paradoxical worsening of the patient's condition, despite the increase of arterial pressure (*see* Chapter 9).

(This analysis applies strictly only to a hypothetical, generalized decrease of myocardial efficiency. In practice, cardiogenic shock is often due to myocardial infarction, when it is the left ventricle which is predominantly affected, initially at any rate. In this case, left ventricular depression causes a decrease of cardiac output, accompanied by an increase of the mean pulmonary pressure, rather than of the mean systemic pressure. Left atrial pressure is then raised, while right atrial pressure may be relatively normal.)

REGULATION OF BLOOD VOLUME

The blood volume of a normal adult is approximately 5–5.5 litres (75 ml kg^{-1}) in the male and 4–4.5 litres (67 ml kg^{-1}) in the female, although the precise value varies somewhat with age and body build. In health, blood volume is maintained within fairly narrow limits, although the site of the receptors which detect departures from normality, and the mechanisms which restore the volume to normal after a change has occurred are disputed.

Short term mechanisms

Short term changes of blood volume can occur as a result of haemorrhage, or of the movement of fluid between the intravascular and interstitial fluid compartments. In certain animals, such as the dog, the spleen may act as a reservoir of red cells which can be moved into the general circulation — with a consequent increase of blood volume — in response to sympathetic overactivity; but this mechanism seems to be of little importance in man.

The interrelationship between, on the one hand, the hydrostatic pressures in the capillaries and interstitial spaces and, on the other hand, the colloid osmotic pressure of the plasma proteins is considered in detail in Chapter 3. A decrease of capillary hydrostatic pressure, due, for example, to constriction of the arterioles or precapillary sphincters, decreases intracapillary pressure and thus allows the osmotic withdrawal of extracellular fluid from the interstitial spaces into the blood. Haemodilution may occur during some forms of hypotensive anaesthesia, even in the absence of excessive fluid administration (Bond, 1969). The haemodilution which occurs soon after acute loss of blood is considered in Chapter 9.

Conversely, during muscular exercise, there is an increase of capillary hydrostatic pressure in the active muscles, with a consequent loss of fluid into the interstitial spaces (*see* Chapter 7). It is said that as much as 15 per cent of the plasma volume can be 'lost' in this way during the first 20 minutes of exercise.

Longer term mechanisms

The longer term mechanisms which control blood volume are less well understood. Blood volume is the sum of the red cell mass (volume) and the plasma volume. The latter is dependent on several factors, of which the most important is the total amount of plasma protein in the body; it is influenced also by the amount of sodium in the body, and by the total body water (*see* below).

Red cell mass (volume)

The precise nature of the system which controls the red cell volume is unknown, but it is known that hypoxia of any sort (hypoxic, anaemic, or stagnant) causes stimulation of the bone marrow, and increased red cell maturation. This appears not to be a direct effect on the narrow but to be mediated via the hormone erythropoeitin which is released from the kidney in response to hypoxia.

Plasma proteins

The plasma volume is dependent principally on the amount of plasma protein present in the body, because the balance between capillary hydrostatic pressure and plasma protein osmotic pressure considered above ensures that the plasma protein concentration is kept fairly constant. The plasma proteins form a 'colloid osmotic skeleton' for the plasma compartment just as sodium chloride forms the 'osmotic skeleton' for the extracellular fluid compartment.

The mechanism(s) which controls the plasma protein volume is unknown; it may be, however, that a fall of plasma protein concentration results in increased protein synthesis in the liver by some sort of mass-action effect. After haemorrhage, the plasma proteins are restored much more rapidly than is the red cell mass.

Water and electrolytes

Blood volume is much less dependent on changes in water and electrolyte balance than on changes in red cell mass or plasma protein concentration. Changes in body water are spread throughout its intracellular and extracellular compartments (total volume about 50 litres), and so have relatively little effect on the intravascular compartment (volume about five litres). Changes in body sodium are accompanied by changes in extracellular fluid volume because the osmolarity of the extracellular fluid is maintained almost constant (*see* below); but the consequent changes of plasma volume are relatively slight because the plasma volume is only about three litres (cf. the total extracellular fluid volume of 15 litres).

Antidiuretic hormone (ADH)

Changes of blood volume which are accompanied by alteration of the plasma crystalloid osmotic pressure as a result of water retention or loss of water unaccompanied by electrolytes, are detected by osmoreceptors in the supra-optic nucleus of the hypothalamus, so causing a change in the rate of secretion of ADH (antidiuretic hormone, vasopressin) from the posterior pituitary. This hormone then adjusts the rate of water re-absorption by the renal tubules so as to restore blood volume to normal.

The precise mode of action of ADH is unknown. One of its chief effects is to increase the water permeability of the distal convoluted tubules and collecting ducts, thus permitting osmotic extraction of water from the tubular lumen into the isotonic renal cortex and hypertonic renal medulla. It has also been suggested that ADH may reduce blood flow through the renal medulla, thus increasing the hypertonicity of this region and causing further urinary concentration.

ADH secretion may also be altered by changes of extracellular fluid volume. This effect is thought to be mediated chiefly via stretch receptors in the walls of the atria and great veins, although changes of arterial baroreceptor activity may also be involved. Henry and Pearce (1956) showed that stretching the canine left atrium caused inhibition of ADH secretion.

Aldosterone

The adrenal cortical hormone, aldosterone is also intimately concerned with the regulation of blood volume. This steroid enhances sodium–potassium exchange in the distal convoluted tubule and therefore induces sodium retention. The resulting plasma hypertonicity stimulates secretion of ADH, thus retaining water and increasing the extracellular fluid volume. There is also some evidence that aldosterone may affect the water permeability of the distal part of the nephron (Giebisch and Lozano, 1959).

Control of secretion   The factors which affect the secretion of aldosterone are only partially understood. ACTH (adreno-corticotrophic hormone) probably influences aldosterone secretion to a minor extent but is far more potent in stimulating the secretion of other adrenal steroids, such as cortisol. Aldosterone release is affected also by changes of plasma electrolyte concentrations, probably by a direct action on the adrenal cortex. Such changes must, however, be fairly large; and they therefore probably play little part in the normal regulation of aldosterone secretion. Plasma potassium concentration must rise by 1 mmol l^{-1}

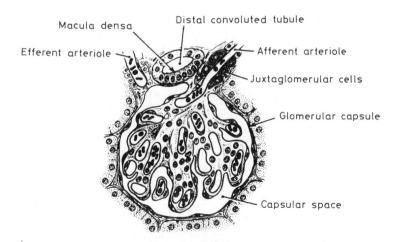

Figure 4.11. The renal juxtaglomerular apparatus (reproduced with permission from Bell, G. H., Davidson, J. N. and Emslie Smith, D., 1972. 'Textbook of Physiology and Biochemistry,' 8th ed.; Churchill Livingstone)

or plasma sodium concentration fall by 20 mmol l^{-1} before stimulation of aldosterone secretion occurs (Ganong, 1973).

Perhaps the most important mechanism controlling aldosterone secretion is the renin–angiotensin system. Renin is produced by the juxtaglomerular apparatus which is composed of granular, modified smooth muscle cells in the media of the afferent glomerular arteriole, *Figure 4.11*; and it is thought that these cells sense the renal arteriolar blood pressure which, of course, tends to vary with renal blood flow, and therefore with total blood volume. A decrease of blood pressure in the afferent glomerular arterioles causes secretion of the enzyme renin into the renal venous blood.

Once released into the blood stream, renin catalyses the breakdown of an α_2-globulin, angiotensinogen, forming the decapeptide angiotensin I. This is then converted into the octapeptide angiotensin II, which causes widespread vasoconstriction and a consequent rise of arterial blood pressure. In addition, angiotensin appears to enhance directly the secretion of aldosterone (Laragh et al., 1960).

There is controversy about the precise nature of the stimulus which causes renin secretion. Many workers consider that renin release occurs in response to changes of blood pressure (either mean or pulse pressure) or of blood flow in the renal artery, and that these haemodynamic alterations are detected by the juxtaglomerular cells which surround the afferent renal arterioles. Alternatively, other workers suggest that renin secretion depends mainly on the composition of the urine in the early distal convoluted tubule which is here closely applied to the juxtaglomerular apparatus of the same nephron in a region called the *macula densa* (*see Figure 4.11*); and it is suggested that this structure may respond to changes of urine osmolarity so as to adjust the secretion of renin by the juxtaglomerular apparatus. Lever (1965) suggests a way in which these two conflicting hypotheses may be reconciled. He proposes that an increase of pressure in the renal medullary capillaries may cause increased ultrafiltration of fluid into the ascending limb of Henle's loop, and that the resulting decrease of osmolarity in the tubular fluid would then be detected by the juxtaglomerular cells. Experimental confirmation of this hypothesis is, however, not yet available.

RECOMMENDED FURTHER READING

Albert, S. N. (1965). 'Blood Volume.' *Anesthesiology* **24**, 231

Gauer, O. H. and Henry, J. P. (1963). 'Circulatory Basis of Fluid Volume Control.' *Physiol. Rev.* **43**, 423

Gauer, O. H., Henry, J. P. and Behn, C. (1970). 'The Regulation of Extracellular Fluid Volume.' *Ann. Rev. Physiol.* **32**, 572

Gregersen, M. I. and Rawson, R. A. (1959). 'Blood Volume.' *Physiol. Rev.* **39**, 307

Guyton, A. C. (1963). 'Venous Return.' In *Handbook of Physiology Circulation*, Vol. II. Washington; American Physiological Society

Guyton, A. C. (1968). 'Regulation of Cardiac Output.' *Anesthesiology* **29**, 314

Guyton, A. C., Jones, C. E. and Coleman, T. G. (1973). *Cardiac Output and its Regulation*, 2nd edn. Philadelphia; W. B. Saunders

Guyton, A. C., Taylor, A. E. and Granger, H. J. (1975). *Circulatory Physiology. II. Dynamics and Control of the Body Fluids*. Philadelphia; W. B. Saunders

Kelman, G. R. (1969). 'Cardiac Output in Shock.' *Int. Anesth. Clin.* **7**, 4

Linden, R. J. (1965). 'The Regulation of the Output of the Mammalian Heart.' *Sci. Basis Med. Ann. Rev.*, p. 164. London; Athlone Press

Mason, D. T. and Bartter, F. C. (1968). 'Autonomic Regulation of Blood Volume.' *Anesthesiology* **29**, 681

Milnor, W. R. (1974). 'Blood Volume.' In Mountcastle, V. B., *Medical Physiology*, 2nd edn, p. 1019. St Louis; C. V. Mosby

Pearce, J. W. (1961). 'A Current Concept of the Regulation of Blood Volume.' *Br. Heart J.* **23**, 66

Rushmer, R. F. (1970). *Cardiovascular Dynamics*, 3rd edn, ch. 3. Philadelphia; W. B. Saunders

Salem, M. R., Yacoub, M. H. and Holaday, D. H. (1968). 'Interpretations of Central Venous Pressure Measurements.' In Jenkins, M. T., *Common and Uncommon Problems in Anesthesiology*, p. 135. Oxford; Blackwell

Samet, P., Fritts, H. W., Fishman, A. P. and Cournand, A. (1957). 'The Blood Volume in Heart Disease.' *Medicine* **36**, 211

Sarnoff, S. J. (1955). 'Myocardial Contractility as Described by Ventricular Function Curves: Observations on Starling's Law of the Heart.' *Physiol. Rev.* **35**, 107

Sarnoff, S. J. and Mitchell, J. H. (1962). 'The Control of the Function of the Heart.' In *Handbook of Physiology, Circulation*, Vol. I, p. 489. Washington; American Physiological Society

Chapter 5   Tissue Blood Flow

The metabolic rate of any given tissue varies widely under different physiological circumstances, and this variability of metabolic requirement is reflected in a similar variability of tissue blood flow. Tissue perfusion must be sufficient both to supply essential nutrients and also to remove metabolic waste products before they can accumulate sufficiently to cause tissue damage. Normally, a tissue's oxygen supply is more vulnerable than its supply of other nutrients, and its blood flow is adjusted in the main to ensure an adequate oxygen supply.

The details of blood flow regulation vary considerably from organ to organ, depending on the precise physiological demands which the body makes on the particular tissue under consideration. Cerebral blood flow, for example, must be maintained relatively constant because the metabolic rate of this organ varies but slightly under widely different physiological conditions; blood flow to the skin or skeletal muscle, however, varies considerably in response to changes of the physiological load imposed on these tissues.

The distribution of total cardiac output between the various body tissues at rest (based on Wade and Bishop, 1962) is shown in *Figure 5.1a*; the relative oxygen consumptions of the different regions are shown in *Figure 5.1b*; and the disparity between the oxygen consumption of a given region and its blood flow — as reflected in variation of the arterio-venous oxygen content difference — is shown in *Figure 5.2*.

The distribution of total cardiac output at rest, compared with its distribution during moderately severe exercise is shown in *Figure 5.3*. The most

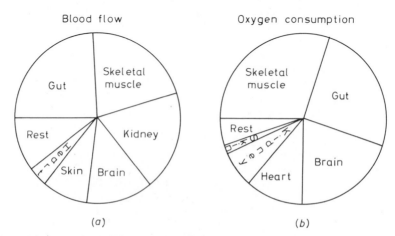

Figure 5.1. *Proportional distribution between body tissues of (a) total cardiac output and (b) total body oxygen consumption (from Wade and Bishop, 1962)*

striking change is the large increase of blood flow to the skeletal muscles, with smaller increases to the skin and myocardium; blood flow to the gut and kidney is decreased; cerebral blood flow is virtually unchanged. Such a redistribution of cardiac output is due to sympathetic over-activity and increased secretion of sympathomimetic amines from the adrenal medullae (*see* Chapter 7). This cardiovascular response to exercise should be compared with the redistribution of blood flow which occurs in, for example, congestive cardiac failure (*see* *Figure 10.1,* page 236).

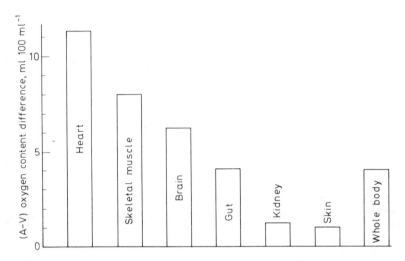

Figure 5.2. *Arterio-venous oxygen content difference in various tissues (figures from Wade and Bishop, 1962)*

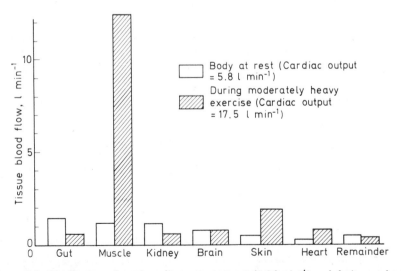

Figure 5.3. *Distribution of total cardiac output at rest (5.8 l min⁻¹) and during moderate exercise (17.5 l min⁻¹) (figures from Wade and Bishop, 1962)*

Mapleson's standard man

Modelling of anaesthetic uptake by computer simulation requires accurate knowledge about the rate of blood flow to the body's various organs and tissues. Mapleson (1973) has performed a valuable service by analysing the data which is available in the literature on this subject. The parameters of his standard man are given in *Table 5.1*.

Table 5.1   MAPLESON'S STANDARD MAN (MAPLESON, 1973)

	Tissue		*Perfusion*		
	Mass (kg)	*Volume* (l)	(ml min^{-1}) 100 g^{-1}	(ml min^{-1})	percent (of cardiac output)
Lung parenchymal tissue	0.50	0.50			
Visceral compartment					
Adrenals	0.02	0.02	508	102	1.6
Thyroid	0.02	0.02	500	100	1.5
Kidneys	0.30	0.28	396	1188	18.3
Heart	0.30	0.28	81	243	3.7
Brain	1.50	1.43	53	795	12.3
Prostate	0.02	0.02	49	10	0.2
Splanchnic tissue	3.92	3.73	39	1529	23.6
Salivary glands, eyes, thymus	0.09	0.09	30	27	0.4
Testes	0.04	0.04	23	9	0.2
Spinal cord	0.03	0.03	16	5	0.1
Lean compartment					
Red marrow	1.40	1.33	10	140	2.2
Skin and non-fat subcutaneous tissue	6.10	5.81	5	305	4.7
Lymphoid tissue, blood vessels, cartilage, nerves	1.09	1.04	5	55	0.8
Non-parenchymal lung tissue	0.50	0.50	5	25	0.4
Muscle and bladder	30.15	28.71	2	603	9.3
Fat compartment					
Fatty marrow	2.20	2.32	2.8	62	1.0
Fat tissue	10.00	10.52	2.4	240	3.7
Bone cortex	6.40	3.42	0	0	0.0
Teeth	0.02	0.01	0	0	0.0
Arterial blood	1.08	1.03	–	–	–
Venous blood	4.32	4.11	–	–	–
Peripheral shunt	–	–	∞	1042	16.0
Total	70.00	65.24		6480	100.0

THE BRAIN

Compared with other tissues, the brain has a high metabolic rate. Despite this fact, however, it has little in the way of stores of either oxygen or of glucose; interruption of cerebral blood flow for more than a few seconds, therefore, results in loss of consciousness. Cerebral oxygen consumption is virtually constant during wide variations of cerebral function, ranging from intense intellectual activity on the one hand to deep sleep on the other. The main physiological requirement is thus for a constant cerebral blood flow, and in keeping with this requirement for a constant blood flow, the cerebral vascular bed exhibits a considerable degree of autoregulation (*see* page 92).

Symptoms of cerebral ischaemia occur when blood flow is reduced to approximately 60 per cent of normal (Finnerty, Witkin and Fazekas, 1954). Cerebral vascular resistance is controlled mainly by the local concentration of vasoactive metabolites, and by the tensions of oxygen and carbon dioxide in the blood, rather than by changes of sympathetic tone.

Anatomy

In man, the blood supply to the brain comes from the internal carotid and vertebral arteries. These interconnect at the base of the brain in the circle of Willis, which distributes its six large branches to the cerebral tissues. The anterior and middle parts of the brain are supplied mainly by the internal carotid arteries, the posterior part mainly by the vertebral arteries. Although the communicating branches which link the two sides of the circle are readily demonstrable anatomically, they do not form a functionally adequate anastomosis; and in elderly patients, particularly, cerebral blood flow may be seriously impaired by unilateral carotid occlusion.

Blood leaves the brain via a variety of channels, the most important of which are the internal jugular veins. There is considerable mixing of the blood from the two sides; approximately one-third of the blood in each internal jugular vein comes from the contralateral side of the brain.

Measurement

The Kety-Schmidt technique

The classical technique for the measurement of cerebral blood flow is that developed by Kety (Kety and Schmidt, 1948). With this technique the subject inhales a constant, low concentration of nitrous oxide until the cerebral arterial and venous N_2O tensions have become equal. The amount of gas taken up by the brain during this equilibration period is then estimated from the concentrations of nitrous oxide in sequential samples of arterial and cerebral venous blood, and equated to the product of the venous N_2O tension at equilibrium, multiplied by the blood/gas partition coefficient for nitrous oxide (*see* below).

With the usual technique, the subject inhales 15 per cent nitrous oxide for 10 minutes. Arterial and jugular venous samples are taken intermittently during this period and analysed for nitrous oxide. As would be expected, the arterial concentration reaches a plateau more rapidly than does the venous concentration (*Figure 5.4*); but at the end of 10 minutes, the two are almost identical. The brain is then saturated with nitrous oxide, and the amount dissolved in 100 g of tissue equals $\lambda\, C_{v10}$, where λ is the blood/brain partition coefficient for nitrous oxide (the ratio of its solubility — ml 100 g^{-1} — in brain tissue/its solubility —

ml ml^{-1} — in blood), and C_{v10} is the concentration (ml ml^{-1}) of nitrous oxide in cerebral venous blood at the end of the 10 minute equilibration period. The amount of nitrous oxide taken up during the equilibration period is also, of course, given by the shaded area between the curves of *Figure 5.4* times the cerebral blood flow, so that the latter quantity can readily be calculated.

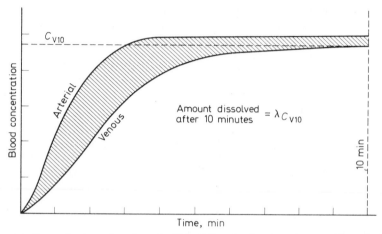

Figure 5.4. Determination of total cerebral blood flow by the Kety nitrous oxide technique (for explanation see text)

It is now more customary to use a radioactive gas such as ^{85}Kr, rather than nitrous oxide. Estimation of such a radioisotope is considerably easier than is the case with nitrous oxide and it is possible to use very low concentrations, and so avoid any possibility that the indicator gas has a pharmacological action on the cardiovascular system.

With the Kety technique cerebral venous blood is normally obtained from one jugular bulb, and this is assumed to contain blood which is representative of the cerebral venous drainage as a whole. Fortunately, it appears that there is normally little difference between blood from the two sides of the brain, and little contamination from extra-cerebral sources.

The other assumption on which the Kety technique depends is that the cerebral tissues are completely saturated with nitrous oxide at the end of 10 minutes. This condition is not completely satisfied even with a normal circulation (*see Figure 5.4*); and the discrepancy is likely to be greater when cerebral blood flow is reduced. To avoid errors from this source, some workers extend the equilibration period up to 20 or 25 minutes; others extrapolate the venous concentration until it becomes identical to the arterial concentration (Lassen and Munck, 1955). Cerebral blood flow calculated in this way is some 10 per cent lower than when the equilibration process is truncated after 10 minutes.

Measurement of local cerebral blood flow

The Kety technique measures mean blood flow through the whole cerebral circulation; it gives no indication of the way in which this total flow is partitioned between different areas. More recently, techniques have been developed for the estimation of blood flow in relatively discrete areas of the brain (Høedt-Rasmussen, 1965). With these techniques cerebral blood flow is calculated from the rate at which a radioactive isotope is cleared from a given region of the brain. The indicator used is commonly a radioactive inert gas such as ^{133}Xe. This is a gamma-emitter and may, therefore, be measured by externally-placed scintillation counters which, with suitable collimation, may be 'focused' onto relatively small regions of tissue.

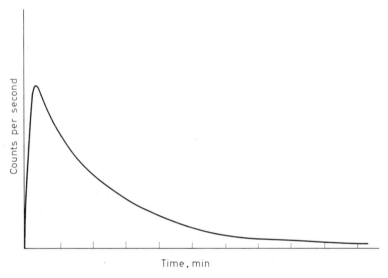

Figure 5.5. Cerebral radioactivity, measured with external scintillation counter, following injection of a bolus of radioactive ^{133}Xe into carotid artery (diagrammatic).

The variation of cerebral radioactivity with time, following the injection into the internal carotid artery of a bolus of radioactive xenon dissolved in saline is shown in *Figure 5.5*. The concentration of isotope rises rapidly to a peak and then decays away at a rate which depends on the rate of cerebral blood flow. Recirculation occurs to only a minor extent because the majority of injected gas is removed from the pulmonary capillary blood during a single passage through the lungs.

Cerebral blood flow is calculated as follows: provided there is no recirculation, that is an arterial concentration of zero, the rate at which isotope is removed from a given region of brain is $\dot{Q}C_v$, where

$\dot{Q}$ is the local blood flow, and

C_v is the concentration of isotope in blood draining the region under consideration.

The amount (M) of isotope dissolved in the brain at any instant is proportional to the cerebral gas tension, which is assumed to be equal to the venous tension. M is hence equal to λC_v, where λ is the blood/brain partition coefficient.

It is then possible to set up the differential equation:

$$-dM/dt = \dot{Q}C_v = \dot{Q}M/\lambda$$

This has the solution $M = Mo \; e^{-Q\lambda t}$ (Thompson, 1946), where Mo is the amount of gas in the brain at time $t = 0$.

The decay constant $(\dot{Q}/\lambda)$ may be determined in the usual way by plotting the relationship between log M against t. This gives a straight line with gradient $-\dot{Q}/\lambda$. If λ is known, therefore, cerebral blood flow may be calculated.

In fact, the decay curve usually has at least two components, that is it is of the form $M = Mo_1 \; e^{-k_1 t} - Mo_2 \; e^{-k_2 t}$. Therefore a plot of log M against time has *two* straight segments, corresponding to the two components of the exponential. It is generally assumed that the decay constant k_1 and k_2, refer to blood flow in the grey and white matter respectively. However, radioactivity from the exposed cerebral cortex of animals, following the injection of the beta emitter [85]Kr, shows that, even in this case, the decay curve may be analysed into two components, despite the fact that beta particles can penetrate through less than 1 mm brain tissue, and therefore presumably come solely from the cerebral grey matter (Harper, 1965). Due to this difficulty there is at present some uncertainty about the interpretation of blood flow measurements by the radioactive clearance technique, although most workers, perhaps rather too readily, accept their validity. Lassen (personal communication) points out that, in all tissues where the comparison has been made, blood flow measurements with electromagnetic flow meters agree closely with flows calculated from the first decay constant of the radioactivity clearance curve (*see also* page 147).

Normal values

The overall cerebral blood flow, measured by the nitrous oxide technique is approximately 50 ml min^{-1} 100 g^{-1} of brain tissue (Wade and Bishop, 1962). Since the weight of the normal brain is approximately 1.5 kg, the total blood flow is about 750 ml min^{-1}, that is, one-eighth of the total cardiac output at rest. The mean cerebral arterio-venous oxygen content difference is 6.3 ml 100ml^{-1} (Wade and Bishop, 1962), although the reported range is disturbingly large (3–10 ml 100 ml^{-1}). There is some evidence that cerebral blood flow may decrease with age. Even in health it may be reduced by 20 per cent at the age of 70 (Fazekas, Alman and Bessman, 1952).

An a-v difference of 6 ml 100 ml^{-1} corresponds to a cerebral oxygen consumption of approximately 3 ml min^{-1} 100 g^{-1} of tissue or 45 ml min^{-1} for the whole brain. Cerebral metabolism therefore accounts for roughly 20 per cent of the body's resting oxygen consumption.

Using the radioactive isotope clearance technique Høedt-Rasmussen (1965) found a mean flow of 77.7 ml min^{-1} 100 g^{-1} of cortical grey matter, and 20.3 ml min^{-1} 100 g^{-1} of white matter. The mean blood flow, determined by combining these values in the correct proportions, is 48 ml min^{-1} 100 g^{-1} of brain tissue, a figure which agrees well with results obtained by the Kety-Schmidt technique.

Factors affecting cerebral blood flow

Driving pressure

As in the case with other tissues, cerebral blood flow depends on the ratio of driving pressure to vascular resistance. In contrast, however, to the situation in other tissues, cerebral vascular resistance is influenced to a considerable extent by changes of extravascular pressure, that is, by intracranial pressure — the pressure between the skull and the brain. This pressure is transmitted via the cerebrospinal fluid to the blood vessels in the subarachnoid space and to the cerebral ventricles; and under normal conditions it closely parallels cerebral venous pressure. In man, cerebral blood flow is said not to be significantly reduced until intracranial pressure has risen to approximately 30 mm Hg (Kety, Shenkin and Schmidt, 1948).

The driving pressure across the cerebral vascular bed is normally relatively constant, because arterial pressure is stabilized by baroreceptor reflexes (*see* page 96). Even when the driving pressure does vary, however, the cerebral circulation is capable of a considerable degree of autoregulation (*see* page 92); cerebral blood flow does not fall until arterial pressure has decreased to 50–70 mm Hg (Lassen, 1959). Below this level, vasodilatation is insufficient to compensate for the reduced driving pressure, and consciousness may be lost when arterial pressure falls tò 35 mm Hg (Finnerty, Witkin and Fazekas, 1954). The degree to which cerebral autoregulatory ability may be impaired by disease, e.g. arteriosclerosis, is unknown.

Sympathetic innervation

Despite the fact that the cerebral vessels receive a profuse sympathetic innervation from the stellate and superior cervical ganglia, this appears to be of little functional importance. Stellate ganglion block has little effect on human cerebral blood flow (Scheinberg and Jayne, 1950). Recent histological studies (Falck, Nielson and Owman, 1968) have shown that the cerebral adrenergic nerve endings are distributed mainly to the larger cerebral vessels, which lie outside the brain tissue proper, rather than to the true resistance vessels.

Oxygen and carbon dioxide tensions

The chief factor which affects the cerebral vascular resistance is the P_{CO_2} and P_{O_2} of the arterial blood. A rise of Pa_{CO_2} causes cerebral vasodilatation, as does a fall of Pa_{O_2}. The former is, however, by far the more potent stimulus. Raising Pa_{CO_2} to 52 mm Hg increases cerebral blood flow by 70 per cent (Kety and Schmidt, 1948); hyperventilation to a Pa_{CO_2} of 26 mm Hg reduces it to about two-thirds of normal (Kety and Schmidt, 1946).

P_{CO_2} A composite curve of the relationship between cerebral blood flow and Pa_{CO_2} has been constructed by Paterson (1965) (*Figure 5.6*). An increase of Pa_{CO_2} has a greater effect on blood flow than does a decrease of similar magnitude. When P_{CO_2} falls below 20 mm Hg, there is little further decrease of flow, nor any further increase when the tension is increased above about 100 mm Hg.

Considerable uncertainty exists about whether the changes of blood flow induced by changes of P_{CO_2} are a response to carbon dioxide *per se* or to the simultaneously-occurring changes of hydrogen ion concentration. Recent work (French, Vale and Brock, 1968) however, suggests that the cerebral vessels

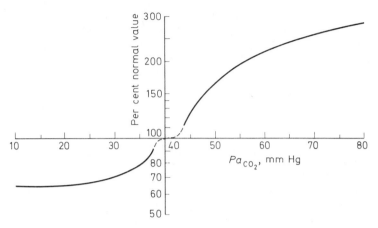

Figure 5.6. Relationship between total cerebral blood flow and Pa$_{CO_2}$ *(redrawn from Paterson, 1965)*

respond mainly to changes of hydrogen ion concentration in the extravascular fluid (which in turn depends on the intravascular P_{CO_2}), and only slightly to changes of intravascular $[H^+]$.

P_{O_2} The inhalation of hypoxic gas mixtures causes an increase of cerebral blood flow; inhalation of pure oxygen causes a small decrease. Kety and Schmidt (1948) found that the inhalation of 10 per cent oxygen increased mean cerebral blood flow by 35 per cent; the inhalation of 100 per cent oxygen reduced it by 13 per cent. The response of the cerebral circulation to differing oxygen tensions has been intensively investigated by McDowall (1966), who took pains to maintain Pa_{CO_2} constant while varying Pa_{O_2}. This precaution is necessary because changes of Pa_{CO_2} may alter pulmonary ventilation, and the resulting changes of Pa_{CO_2} may themselves affect cerebral blood flow.

The relationship, at constant P_{CO_2} between cerebral blood flow and Pa_{O_2} is shown in *Figure 5.7a.* Hypoxia has little effect on blood flow until Pa_{O_2} falls to 50–60 mm Hg; below this level, however, vascular resistance decreases rapidly with decreasing oxygen tension. The relationship between cerebral blood flow and cerebral venous P_{O_2} is shown in *Figure 5.7b;* flow begins to increase when the venous oxygen tension falls to approximately 40 mm Hg.

The inhalation of oxygen at pressures in excess of one atmosphere causes a moderate reduction of cerebral blood flow. Lambertsen et al. (1953) found that the inhalation of 100 per cent oxygen at 3.5 atmospheres reduced cerebral flow by 25 per cent. This decrease appears to be independent of any associated hypocapnia; and it occurs even when Pa_{CO_2} is maintained constant (Harper, Jacobson and McDowall, 1965).

Paradoxical response of damaged cerebral vessels to vasoactive agents

The brain and cerebral circulation are enclosed in a rigid box, the cranium, therefore changes of vascular calibre in one area must cause reciprocal changes in other areas.

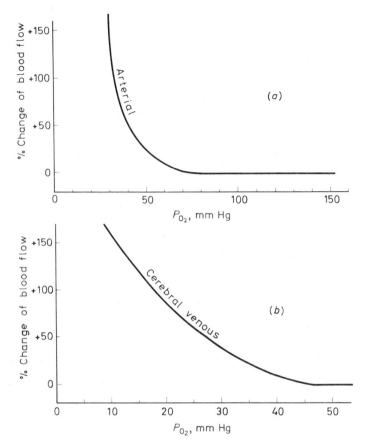

Figure 5.7. Relationship, at constant $Paco_2$, *between total cerebral blood flow and (a) arterial* Po_2, *(b) cerebral venous* Po_2 *(redrawn from McDowall, 1966)*

In the vicinity of regions of brain damage there may be local vascular paralysis, with the result that blood flow is excessive in relation to the region's oxygen requirements; venous blood from these regions is less desaturated than normal and appears red (luxury perfusion). The paralysed vessels in such a region of brain damage do not exhibit autoregulation and therefore cannot respond normally to hypertension or hypotension. An increase of vascular volume in a normal area of the brain may compress the paralysed vessels and cause a decrease of cerebral perfusion of the damaged regions. This is the phenomenon of intra-cerebral 'steal'. Conversely, vasoconstriction of the normal vessels may direct blood to the damaged area -- inverse steal. Lassen calls this the 'Robin Hood syndrome' because the damaged regions of the cerebral circulation improve their perfusion at the expense of the normal and previously rightly-perfused regions of brain.

Halothane causes cerebral vasodilatation, but may cause a decrease of blood flow by the steal phenomenon in areas of brain damage, with deleterious consequences to the patient. The same comment applies to respiratory acidosis (*see* page 191).

THE HEART

Anatomy

The myocardial blood supply is from the two coronary arteries which arise at the aortic root from the coronary sinuses. The right artery supplies mainly the right ventricle; the left supplies mainly the left ventricle; there is usually, however, a greater or lesser degree of overlap between the two sides. In man, the right coronary artery is predominant in 50 per cent of subjects, the left in 20 per cent, and the two are of equal importance in the remainder (Ross, Mosher and Shaw, 1961). Anastomoses between the two vessels are functionally very inadequate (Linder, 1966).

The majority of myocardial venous drainage is to the right atrium via the coronary sinus. Some blood returns to this chamber via the anterior cardiac veins, which usually enter separately from the coronary sinus. There is also some venous drainage directly into the ventricular cavities on both sides of the heart. In the left ventricle this forms one source of 'pulmonary venous admixture' because the blood in these vessels is relatively desaturated with oxygen, therefore its passage into the left ventricle dilutes the arterial blood returning from the lungs and lowers its oxygen tension, thus causing an oxygen tension difference between the alveolar gas and the arterial blood — an $(A - a)$ Po_2 difference.

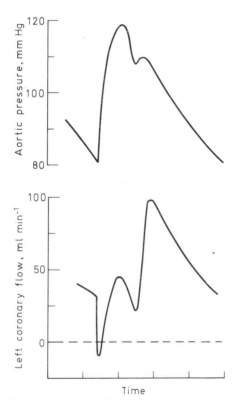

Figure 5.8. *Variation of coronary blood flow during cardiac cycle (semi-diagrammatic)*

The amount of blood returning to the left ventricle in this way is small, and constitutes only about 1 per cent of the total cardiac output (Ravin, Epstein and Malm, 1965). Its physiological influence is, however, somewhat enhanced by the marked desaturation of coronary venous blood (*see* page 133). If a coronary venous oxygen content of 9 ml 100 ml^{-1} is assumed, it may be calculated (Kelman and Nunn, 1968) that the return of 1 per cent of the total cardiac output to the interior of the left ventricle would cause an $(A - a) P_{O_2}$ difference of about 7 mm Hg.

With these anatomical communications between the interior of the heart and the myocardial microcirculation, the possibility exists that oxygenated blood may pass from the interior of the left ventricle into the myocardial capillaries during systole. It has been shown experimentally that isotopically-labelled blood does indeed penetrate for some distance into the endocardium, but the relevance of this finding to normal man, and particularly to patients with myocardial ischaemia is uncertain.

The myocardial circulation is peculiar also in that the vessels are rhythmically compressed during each ventricular systole. This not only alters the overall haemodynamic resistance of the coronary vascular bed, but also moves blood physically from one part of the myocardial circulation to another. Studies in animals with chronically implanted electromagnetic flowmeters (Granata et al., 1965) have shown that coronary blood flow is momentarily reversed during early systole (*Figure 5.8*); and that maximum flow occurs during diastole when the ventricular muscle is relaxed and the intraventricular pressure is minimal. Approximately 70 per cent of the total flow occurs during this phase of the cardiac cycle.

In ventricular fibrillation rhythmic compression of the coronary vessels does not occur; flow is, therefore, considerably increased initially, although it gradually returns to normal as a result of autoregulatory constriction (*see* page 92) of the coronary vessels.

Measurement

The standard method for the measurement of human coronary blood flow is a modification of Kety's nitrous oxide technique (*see* page 136). Applied to the coronary circulation, this requires simultaneous measurement of the nitrous oxide concentrations in arterial and coronary venous blood. The latter may be obtained via a modified cardiac catheter. Coronary sinus catheterization is, however, a difficult technique which is succcessful in only about 40 per cent of patients, even in the most experienced hands (Wade and Bishop, 1962). Krasnow et al. (1963) have measured myocardial blood flow by a modification of the nitrous oxide technique using ^{131}I-labelled antipyrine.

The blood in the coronary sinus is derived mainly from the left ventricle, therefore myocardial blood flow as estimated by this technique is actually left ventricular flow. But it is probable that, expressed per unit weight, the blood flows of the two ventricles are not greatly dissimilar.

Myocardial blood flow may also be estimated with radioactive gases by techniques similar to those used for the cerebral circulation (*see* page 136). Radioactive [85]Kr dissolved in saline can be injected into the aorta in the region of the coronary ostia, and its subsequent rate of removal from the myocardium estimated by serial blood samples from the coronary sinus. It is also possible to use a gamma-emitting isotope such as ^{133}Xe, and to measure its myocardial concentration by an external precordial counter. This technique has been used in man by Ross et al. (1964), and in lower animals by McBride and Ledingham (1968).

Normal values

The average myocardial blood flow, measured by the nitrous oxide technique, is approximately 80 ml min^{-1} 100 g^{-1} of tissue (Wade and Bishop, 1962). Assuming an average cardiac weight of 300 g, this gives a total coronary flow of 250 ml min^{-1}, or approximately 1/20 of the total resting cardiac output. Resting myocardial oxygen consumption is approximately 10 per cent of the total body consumption; so that coronary venous blood is therefore markedly desaturated in oxygen (*see* page 143).

Coronary blood flow is, of course, considerably increased during exercise, although precise figures for man are not easy to obtain. A figure of 400 ml min^{-1} 100 g^{-1} has been suggested by Folkow and Neil (1971).

Factors affecting coronary blood flow

Investigation of the factors which affect coronary blood flow is complicated by the fact that this depends not only on external factors, such as blood gas tensions and arterial blood pressure, but also on the amount of work which the heart is performing under the conditions of measurement. In addition, the rhythmic contraction and relaxation of the myocardium limits the time available for blood flow, which in consequence depends on the ratio of systole to diastole, and thus on heart rate. Tachycardia is accompanied by a decrease of the duration of diastole in comparison to that of systole (*see Table 7.2,* page 173).

Arterial pressure

As is the case with other vascular beds, flow through the coronary circulation is increased by an increase of arterial pressure. Flow is, however, not directly proportional to mean blood pressure because the coronary vessels are capable of a certain amount of autoregulation. This phenomenon is, however, less marked than it is in the cerebral circulation.

In shock (*see* Chapter 9) arterial blood pressure is usually considerably reduced. Severe arterial hypotension may be accompanied by a reduction of coronary blood flow sufficient to cause myocardial damage; in less severe cases, however, the reduction of myocardial perfusion may not be sufficient to cause damage because it is accompanied by a simultaneous decrease of cardiac work. During spinal anaesthesia, arterial hypotension may be accompanied by a considerable reduction of myocardial energy requirements; there may then be a marked reduction of coronary perfusion with no evidence of myocardial damage (*see* page 104).

Oxygen and carbon dioxide tensions

Coronary flow depends on arterial Po_2 and Pco_2. Flow is increased by hypoxia and hypercapnia; the former is, however, by far the more important stimulus. Some workers, in fact, deny that hypercapnia has any effect on coronary vascular resistance. A decrease of arterial pH has little effect on coronary perfusion, although it may be accompanied by arterial hypotension (Eckenhoff, Hafkenschiel and Landmesser, 1947).

In the whole body an increase of $Paco_2$ is accompanied by an increase of cardiac output (*see* page 191), therefore hypercapnia usually causes an increase of myocardial blood flow induced by the increased cardiac work. Vance, McBride and Ledingham (1967) found a roughly linear relationship between coronary perfusion and Pco_2.

Heart rate

Diastole is seriously curtailed by tachycardia. It might therefore be expected that, since the majority of coronary blood flow occurs during diastole, coronary perfusion would be reduced at high heart rates. Paradoxically, however, there is evidence that coronary flow may actually be *increased* by tachycardia, presumably due to the increased work which the heart performs under these circumstances. In experimental animals total coronary flow appears to increase in proportion to heart rate; coronary stroke flow remains constant (Gregg, 1963).

Autonomic activity

The effects of changes of sympathetic tone on the coronary circulation are difficult to assess. It appears, however, that increased sympathetic activity usually increases coronary blood flow, both in the heart–lung preparation and in the intact animal. The extent to which these changes are directly due to sympathetically-induced vasodilatation is, however, uncertain. Even if blood pressure remains constant, sympathetic stimulation causes an increase of heart rate accompanied by an increase of cardiac work; increased perfusion under these circumstances may be due to locally-produced vasodilator metabolites rather than to enhanced sympathetic activity *per se*. Feigl (1967) showed in dogs that sympathetic stimulation after administration of a beta-blocking drug causes a very small increase of coronary vascular resistance.

Vagal stimulation has little effect on coronary flow in the intact animal; it may, however, cause vasodilatation in the isolated heart–lung preparation (*see also* Feigl, 1967).

Adrenaline (and to a lesser extent noradrenaline) causes an increase of myocardial blood flow due, at least in part, to increased cardiac work. Acetylcholine is also said to increase flow, but the mechanism is obscure. The beneficial effects of nitroglycerine in *angina pectoris* are probably due mainly to peripheral vasodilatation (decrease of afterload, *see* page 116) rather than to coronary vasodilatation.

THE KIDNEY

Anatomy

The renal glomeruli are supplied by afferent arterioles. These arise at right angles from the interlobular arteries, which arise from the arcuate arteries lying at the corticomedullary junction, and then running outwards through the renal cortex. As an arteriole enters a glomerulus it divides into several smaller branches which give rise to the glomerular capillaries. These then recombine to form the efferent glomerular arteriole, which immediately divides again to form the peritubular capillary plexus. This drains ultimately into the interlobular veins. The cells of the walls of the afferent renal arterioles are in places modified to form the juxtaglomerular apparatus which secretes renin (*see* page 130).

The *vasa recta* arise from the efferent arterioles of juxtamedullary glomeruli, and pass down into the renal medulla in close apposition to the loops of Henle. After making a $180°$ turn they return towards the cortex to drain directly into the interlobular veins.

Changes of smooth muscle tone in either the afferent or efferent glomerular arterioles alter blood flow through the glomerular capillaries. Constriction of the efferent vessels reduces blood flow and, at the same time, increases the proportion of plasma filtered by the glomerulus (the filtration fraction); afferent arteriolar constriction reduces both blood flow and the filtration fraction.

The afferent arterioles of the renal vasculature are well supplied by sympathetic nerves from the lower thoracic and upper lumbar segments of the spinal cord. The vessels are very sensitive to sympathetic stimulation and to circulating catecholamines. The renal vascular bed is therefore one of the first to become shut down when sympatho-adrenal activity is increased during physiological stress. It was suggested by Trueta et al. (1947) that, under these circumstances, blood is shunted from the renal cortex to the renal medulla. This mechanism is not, however, now thought to be of importance in man, although it does seem to occur in the rabbit, the species on which the original studies were made (*see also* page 148).

The glomerular capillaries have especially permeable, wide pores (0.1 μm in diameter). They are, however, surrounded by a well-defined basement membrane, and by the cells of the visceral layer of Bowman's capsule. It has been suggested that it is the spaces between the latter cells which constitute the true filtration membrane.

Measurement

Para-aminohippuric acid (PAH) clearance

Renal blood flow is conveniently measured by the Fick principle (*see* page 256). Flow is assumed to equal the quotient of the rate at which a given substance is removed from the blood by the kidney, divided by its arteriovenous concentration difference. In symbols:

$$\dot{Q} = U_c/(C_a - C_v),$$

where $\dot{Q}$ is the renal flow;

> U_c is the rate at which the substance is excreted ('cleared') by the kidney; and
>
> C_a and C_v are, respectively, its arterial and venous concentrations.

Certain substances are particularly convenient for this measurement because they are almost completely removed from the blood during a single passage through the kidney. The renal venous concentration is then almost zero so that the above equation may be written $\dot{Q} = U_c/C_a$, or to use the more usual abbreviations:

$$\dot{Q} = uv/P$$

where $\dot{Q}$ is the renal plasma flow;

> u is the concentration of PAH in the urine;
>
> v is the urinary flow rate; and
>
> P is the concentration of PAH in the plasma.

Suitable substances for measuring renal blood (actually plasma) flow by this technique are diodrast and para-aminohippuric acid (PAH). Bergström et al. (1959) showed that PAH extraction exceeds 90 per cent in the normal subject. This figure is not significantly diminished by physiological stress, such as the administration of adrenaline or pitressin (Epstein, 1964), although PAH excretion may, of course, be seriously impaired in the presence of renal disease.

It is generally assumed that PAH clearance remains relatively normal under most forms of general anaesthesia (*see* page 202). The small quantity of PAH which remains in the renal venous blood probably represents blood flow to non-functional areas of the kidney, such as perirenal fat. Therefore, although the estimated blood flow may be slightly too low if the venous PAH concentration is assumed to be zero, the calculated flow probably represents the perfusion of functioning renal tissue, and is therefore a physiologically valid measurement.

Normally, this technique requires the system to be in a steady state, that is, the concentrations of PAH in blood and urine must be constant. Provided this is so, however, a low urine flow does not invalidate the technique, although it may somewhat limit its accuracy. An abrupt decrease of urine flow may be accompanied by a 'transitory and apparently false' decrease of all renal clearances (Smith, 1951). The explanation for this finding is obscure.

Radioisotope clearance techniques

It is also possible to estimate renal blood flow by measuring the rate of removal of radioactive inert gases by a technique similar to that used in the brain (*see* page 136). Radioactive ^{133}Xe dissolved in saline may be injected down a renal artery catheter, and its concentration in the kidney monitored by an external counter (Ladefoged et al., 1965).

As is the case with the cerebral circulation, the decay curve can be resolved into several components with different decay constants. Under favourable conditions, four such components have been identified, which have been ascribed, respectively, to the cortex, the outer medulla, the inner medulla, and the perirenal fat. This technique has been validated in the dog by autoradiography (Rosen et al., 1967).

Normal values

The kidneys receive approximately one-fifth of the resting cardiac output, although they are responsible for only 7 per cent of the body's oxygen consumption (Wade and Bishop, 1962). The renal arterio-venous oxygen content difference is, therefore, very low, the mean value quoted by Wade and Bishop being approximately 1.3 ml 100 ml^{-1}. As is the case with the cerebral circulation, renal blood flow appears to decline with advancing age. Davies and Shock (1950) found that it fell from 680 ml min^{-1} m^{-2} in the fourth decade to 275 ml min^{-1} m^{-2} in the 9th decade. The average weight of the two kidneys in man is about 300 g, so that the renal blood flow is around 350 ml 100 g^{-1}.

Renal medullary blood flow

In the normal kidney most of the blood flow goes to the cortex; only about 1 per cent perfuses the medulla. The mean medullary blood flow found by Kramer, Thurau and Deetjen (1960) was approximately 20 ml min^{-1} 100 g^{-1}, compared with a flow of 400 ml min^{-1} 100 g^{-1} for the whole kidney. Daniel, Peabody and Prichard (1951) showed radiographically that blood took some 20 seconds to pass through the canine renal medulla. The medullary circulation time is probably comparable in man.

Despite its small amount, the blood flow of the renal medulla is of considerable physiological importance. It is in this region of the kidney that the urine is concentrated, and it is thought that the *vasa recta* are involved in this process. At present it is uncertain whether the *vasa recta* act simply as countercurrent exchangers to maintain medullary hyperosmolarity or, as suggested by Lever (1965), as countercurrent multipliers which actually generate medullary hyperosmolarity. Full understanding of the complex interactions between blood flow in the *vasa recta* and urine flow in the loops of Henle will depend on further knowledge of the factors which affect medullary blood flow, and of how this changes during diuresis and antidiuresis, and in response to sympathetic stimulation.

The Trueta shunt

As suggested on page 146, some workers believe that, during physiological stress, blood is diverted from the renal cortex to the medulla. This conclusion was, however, based on injection studies which are now known to be unreliable. Insull, Tillotson and Hayman (1950) injected Prussian blue into the kidney and showed that, with an injection pressure of 50 cm H$_2$O, it filled the entire kidney, whereas with an injection pressure of 25 cm H$_2$O it filled only the juxtamedullary glomeruli and *vasa recta*. It does appear, however, that cortical and medullary vessels may be independently controlled and that, in some species at any rate, sympathetic stimulation may cause cortical ischaemia while leaving medullary flow unchanged. This might produce an apparent diversion of blood flow from the cortex to the medulla, even when there is no true increase of medullary flow.

Factors affecting renal blood flow

Haemorrhage

During haemorrhage, renal blood flow is considerably reduced by intense sympathetic activity. This diverts the diminished cardiac output away from the kidney to tissues more immediately essential for the body's survival (*see* page 217). If the haemorrhage is sufficiently severe renal blood flow virtually ceases, and this, of course, may have serious consequences for the body as a whole (*see* Chapter 9).

Oxygen and carbon dioxide tensions

P_{CO_2} Renal blood flow is little affected by moderate changes of arterial carbon dioxide tension. Severe respiratory acidosis may, however, cause a marked *decrease* of renal perfusion (Selkurt, 1963). This response is abolished by renal denervation, therefore the increased vascular resistance appears to be due to increased sympathetic activity. Stone et al. (1958) found a large increase of renal vascular resistance during diffusion oxygenation, and they attributed this response to carbon dioxide retention.

P_{CO_2} Moderate hypoxia causes a small increase of renal blood flow. Berger, Gladstone and Horwitz (1949) reduced arterial P_{O_2} in normal subjects to 50 mm Hg and found that there was a small (13 per cent) increase of PAH clearance, with no significant rise of arterial blood pressure. Similar results have been obtained in dogs. Severe hypoxia causes considerable renal vasoconstriction and a corresponding decrease of renal blood flow.

Hyperoxia is accompanied by a decrease of renal blood flow. Norman, Irvin and Smith (1968) found that, in dogs, flow decreased by approximately 12 per cent when the inspired oxygen tension was raised from normal levels to 760 mm Hg; and by a further 15 per cent when oxygen was breathed at 2 atmospheres. In both cases the acid-base state of the blood was maintained constant.

SPLANCHNIC REGION

Anatomy

The liver receives a dual blood supply from the hepatic artery and portal vein (*Figure 5.9*). The former is its main oxygen supply, because hepatic arterial blood is fully oxygenated, whereas portal venous blood has already supplied the intestines and is, therefore, partially desaturated. The relative flows through the two systems are not accurately known, but extrapolation from animal experiments suggests that the hepatic artery contributes approximately one-quarter of the total hepatic blood flow. Grindlay, Herrick and Mann (1941) measured flows in the hepatic artery, portal vein and hepatic vein of dogs and found that the values were respectively 100, 350 and 450 ml min^{-1}.

The hepatic arterial and portal venous streams mingle at the periphery of the

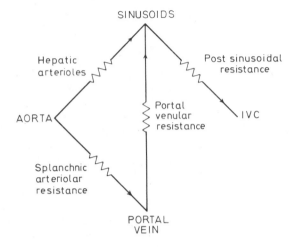

Figure 5.9. Diagram of hepatic circulation

hepatic lobules, and then flow through the hepatic sinusoids to the hepatic vein. The resistance of the small branches of the hepatic artery appears to be sufficient to reduce the pressure sufficiently to prevent reflux of hepatic arterial blood into the portal vein.

The hydrostatic pressure in the portal vein is low (6–12 mm Hg), therefore the pressure in the hepatic sinusoids must be lower still. To compensate, the effective colloid osmotic pressure of the plasma proteins is reduced by the high protein-permeability of the lining of these sinusoids (*see* page 83). Hepatic lymph contains about 6 per cent protein.

In common with other venous reservoirs, the portal system contains blood which can be discharged into the general circulation in a physiological emergency. The portal vessels have a well-developed muscular coat, which enables them to alter their capacity actively in response to nervous and hormonal stimuli. Dilatation of the intestinal resistance vessels in the presence of a constant hepatic vascular resistance causes storage of blood in the portal veins; constriction of the intestinal vessels, as in shock, has the reverse effect.

Measurement

Hepatic blood flow is usually measured by the Fick technique with a substance, such as bromsulphthalein (BSP), which is removed from the blood by the hepatic cells. It is not possible to measure the rate of hepatic excretion of BSP directly (as it is with the renal excretion of PAH), therefore the substance is infused into the blood stream at a constant rate until a steady state is attained. The rate of hepatic excretion is then assumed to equal the rate of infusion.

BSP is not completely cleared by the liver, therefore it is necessary to measure its concentration in the hepatic venous blood as well as in the arterial (or, more usually, systemic venous) blood. The necessity to catheterize the hepatic vein prevents this technique from being used in other than special centres.

The BSP method is based on the assumption that BSP is removed from the blood solely by the liver. The method assumes, in particular, that BSP is not removed by the intestine, so that its concentration in the portal vein is the same as in the hepatic artery. Extrahepatic removal of BSP seems, in fact, to be minimal and causes an overestimation of hepatic blood flow by only 1–2 per cent. A more important source of error is the intrahepatic storage of BSP which may occur following a change of plasma concentration; this error may be minimized by making measurements only when the plasma concentration is reasonably constant. Comparison of the BSP technique with direct determinations of hepatic blood flow in experimental animals gives agreement within 10 per cent (Drapanas, Kluge and Schenk, 1960).

It is possible to use other indicators. Indocyanine green is useful because its extrahepatic removal is virtually zero; 97 per cent is recoverable from the bile. It is also possible to use foreign particulate matter which is removed from the blood by the hepatic reticulo-endothelial cells. A variety of such substances has been used, for example radioactive gold colloid or heat-denatured albumen labelled with ^{131}I.

Normal values

Splanchnic blood flow measured by BSP clearance is approximately 1.5 l min^{-1} although there is considerable individual variation (Wade and Bishop, 1962). The mean arterio-venous oxygen content difference is 4.1 ml 100 ml^{-1} giving a calculated oxygen consumption of approximately 60 ml min^{-1}, 25 per cent of the resting oxygen consumption of the body.

Factors affecting splanchnic blood flow

Very little is known of the factors which affect splanchnic blood flow. McGinn, Mendel and Perry (1967) investigated the effects of changes of arterial pH and Pco$_2$ in rats, and found that there was a roughly linear relationship between splanchnic blood flow and Paco$_2$ If Paco$_2$ was maintained constant, however, changes of pH had little effect. During halothane anaesthesia in man hypercarbia causes an increase of splanchnic blood flow (Epstein et al., 1966).

SKIN

The cutaneous circulation is arranged so that, when necessary, a large amount of heat can be dissipated very rapidly. The skin contains large arterio-venous anastomoses which provide a low-resistance pathway, through which blood can flow rapidly when the body needs to lose heat. These anastomoses are found particularly in the fingers, toes and ears. Cutaneous blood flow is regulated chiefly to subserve the requirements of body temperature regulation.

Anatomy

Arteries reach the skin by running peripherally from the underlying muscles. This arrangement has the advantage that, during muscular exercise, blood from the active tissues can pass directly to the skin where heat may be rapidly dissipated. Blood returns either via superficial cutaneous veins or by the *venae comitantes* of the cutaneous arteries. This countercurrent arrangement of arteries and veins helps to conserve body heat because warm blood flowing peripherally in the arteries loses heat to the cold blood on its way back from the skin. Blood temperatures as low as $30°C$ have been recorded in the radial artery at a time when rectal temperature is normal (Milnor, 1974). (It is usual to correct measured pH and blood gas tensions to the core temperature of the subject, as measured by his oral or rectal temperature. The fact that blood samples may have a temperature considerably below the core temperature does not, however, lead to inaccuracy, because cooling in the artery presumably occurs anaerobically, that is, without the blood being able to take up or give off oxygen or carbon dioxide.)

When the limb is warm most of the blood returns to the heart via the cutaneous veins. The countercurrent mechanism is then not operative, and heat conservation does not occur.

Measurement

Venous occlusion plethysmography

Measurement of cutaneous blood flow is difficult. The most widely used method is based on the technique of venous occlusion plethysmography (*see* for example, Greenfield, 1960). A segment of the limb under investigation is placed in a rigid box (plethysmograph), and the venous return from the limb suddenly occluded. The rate of change of volume of the limb is then equal to the rate of arterial inflow; and may be assessed by means of a suitable volume recorder.

Of course, if this technique is applied to a complete limb, it measures *total* blood flow to both skin and muscle; however, if it is applied to the hand alone, the measured blood flow is almost entirely cutaneous, because the hand contains almost no muscle, and osseous blood flow is small.

Cutaneous blood flow is critically dependent on the temperature of the body and of its environment (*see* next page). The necessity of controlling these variables makes it difficult to obtain accurate results with the venous occlusion technique unless the greatest care is taken to maintain the environment of the limb — that is, the inside of the plethysmograph — at a constant temperature.

Radioisotope clearance

It is also possible to measure skin blood flow by a modification of the radioactive clearance technique, originally proposed by Kety (1949). This technique is based on the fact that the rate of disappearance of local radioactivity, following an injection of a radioisotope into the skin, is proportional to the cutaneous blood flow. A convenient isotope for this purpose is ^{22}Na (Barron and Veall, 1968). The chief snag with this technique is that it does not necessarily reflect changes of blood flow through arterio-venous anastomoses, because the blood in these channels does not come into close proximity to the injected material. The method is nevertheless useful, even though it is only semiquantitative; and is particularly valuable for the assessment of blood flow through skin pedicles; it is said that flow must be reduced to between 5 and 10 per cent of normal before viability of the pedicle is impaired.

Deduction from venous oxygen content

Provided the oxygen consumption of the skin remains constant, changes in the oxygen content of blood from cutaneous veins must indicate changes of skin blood flow. It is possible to combine this technique with analysis of blood from the underlying muscles — obtained via a percutaneously-introduced catheter, a technique originally developed by Mottram (1955) — and so obtain independent information about changes of skin and muscle blood flow.

Normal values

The mean value of cutaneous blood flow given by Wade and Bishop (1962) is 500 ml min^{-1} with an arterio-venous oxygen content difference of only 1.0 ml 100 ml^{-1}. There is, however, considerable variation from region to region; flow is greatest in the finger tips and earlobes, and least in the skin of the forearm and pretibial regions. In a cold environment there is marked cutaneous vasoconstriction, reducing the skin blood flow to as low as 20 ml min^{-1}; this vasoconstriction greatly increases the thermal insulation provided by the skin and subcutaneous tissues, and so minimizes heat loss from the body surface.

Factors affecting cutaneous blood flow

The increase of cutaneous blood flow on changing from a cold to a hot environment is very great. Scott, Bazett and Mackie (1940) found that such a change of environment caused blood flow through the fingers to increase from 1 ml min^{-1} 100 g^{-1} tissue to 80 ml min^{-1} 100 g^{-1}.

The stimulus to thermal dilatation of the cutaneous vessels may be either an increase of blood temperature acting directly on the temperature-regulating centre(s) in the hypothalamus, or an increase of afferent impulses from the skin reaching the temperature-regulating centre indirectly via the spinal cord and medulla. The application of radiant heat to the legs causes an increase of forearm blood flow in less time than it takes for the warmed blood to reach the postulated cerebral temperature-regulating centre.

It is thought that sweat gland activity is accompanied by local release of the proteolytic enzyme kallikrein; this enzyme then catalyses the formation of the vasodilator polypeptide kallidin (Webster and Pierce, 1963).

Local cutaneous reactions

The reactions of the cutaneous blood vessels to local stimulation was described 50 years ago by Sir Thomas Lewis (1927). Light stroking of the skin causes a 'white reaction', which is due to localized vasoconstriction, and is independent of the nerve supply. More intense stimulation causes the 'triple response' which consists of: localized vasodilatation (the 'red response'), oedema (the 'wheal'), and a surrounding area of reddening (the 'flush'), the localized response is probably a direct effect of trauma causing localized release of vasodilator chemicals, whereas the flush is due to an axon reflex, i.e. is neurally mediated and therefore abolished by local anaesthesia. The red reaction and wheal persist after neural degeneration.

Exposure of the skin to cold causes vasoconstriction, due partly to a direct effect on the blood vessels and partly to a reflex increase in sympathetic activity. The decrease of flow under these circumstances is accentuated by the increase of blood viscosity (*see* page 11). However, after about 10 minutes, the constricted vessels dilate — the phenomenon of cold vasodilatation — perhaps as a result of smooth muscle paralysis from the cold. This vasodilatation may considerably increase cutaneous heat loss, and so hasten a fatal outcome in cold immersion situations (Keatinge, 1972).

SKELETAL MUSCLE

The blood flow requirements of the skeletal muscles vary enormously from moment to moment. Muscular exercise causes a very marked increase of blood flow to the muscles, and also an increase of the percentage of the total cardiac output going to this region of the body (*Figure 5.3,* page 133); *see also* Chapter 7.

On a weight basis the resting oxygen consumption of skeletal muscle is very small; the large mass of this tissue, however, means that its total oxygen requirement is relatively large, accounting for 20–30 per cent of the body's resting expenditure.

Measurement

It is possible to measure blood flow to the forearm or calf by venous occlusion plethysmography (*see* below), or to infer changes of blood flow from changes of the oxygen content of blood from the deep veins, which drain predominantly the muscles (Mottram, 1955).

Venous occlusion plethysmography

Venous occlusion plethysmography gives a measure of the total blood flow to a limb. It is possible to correct for osseous blood flow (which in any case is not thought to be large), but in the forearm cutaneous flow may account for as much as 60 per cent of the total (Cooper, Edholm and Mottram, 1955), so that this technique really measures blood flow to *skin and muscle combined.* The cutaneous component may be considerably reduced, but not abolished, by iontophoresis of adrenaline into the skin (Edholm, Fox and MacPherson, 1956).

The mercury-in-rubber strain gauge (Whitney, 1953) may conveniently be used instead of a classical closed-box plethysmograph. It consists of a thin rubber tube filled with mercury, which is placed round the circumference of the forearm or calf. Changes of volume are then reflected in changes of limb circumference, measured as resistance changes of the mercury column.

Radioisotope clearance

It is also possible to assess skeletal muscle blood flow by measurement of the rate of clearance of an injected radioactive isotope. A suitable indicator for this purpose is ^{131}I dissolved in isotonic saline. As with other isotope clearance techniques, the decay curve may show more than one exponential component (*see* page 138), and there is controversy about the significance of each separate component.

Factors affecting resting muscle blood flow

Spontaneous hyperventilation causes a slight or moderate increase of forearm blood flow (Clarke, 1952), the muscle vessels being dilated and the skin vessels constricted. It should be remembered, however, that voluntary hyperventilation is unpleasant to many people, and may therefore stimulate sympathetic cholinergic vasodilator fibres (*see* page 90), thus causing muscular vasodilation.

Hypercapnia causes vasodilatation of muscular vessels by a direct effect, which is however, opposed by sympathetically-mediated vasoconstriction. An increase of Pa_{CO_2} therefore has an inconstant effect on forearm blood flow. During general anaesthesia the direct vasodilator effect is usually predominant and limb blood flow is generally increased (*see* page 203). The effects of acute hypoxia are similar to those of hypocapnia.

Bird and Telfer (1965) investigated the effects of hyperbaric oxygenation on forearm blood flow. They found that the inhalation of oxygen at 2 atmospheres reduced resting blood flow by 28.5 per cent. This finding may account in part for the relative inefficacy of hyperbaric oxygen in the treatment of peripheral vascular disease.

The regulation of muscle blood flow during exercise is considered in Chapter 7.

RECOMMENDED FURTHER READING

Anon. (1974). 'Mental Activity and Cerebral Blood-flow.' *Lancet* i, 440

Alexander, S. C. and Lassen, N. A. (1970). 'Cerebral Circulatory Responses to Acute Brain Disease: Implications for Anaesthetic Practice.' *Anesthesiology* 32, 60

Bonica, J. L., Akamatsu, T. J., Berges, P. U., Morikawa, K. and Kennedy, W. F. (1971). 'Circulatory Effects of Peridural Block. II. Effects of Epinethrine.' *Anesthesiology* 34, 514

Bonica, J. J., Berges, P. U. and Morikawa, K. (1970). 'Circulatory Effects of Peridural Block. I. Effects of Level of Analgesia and Dose of Lidocaine'. *Anesthiology* 33, 619

156 *Tissue Blood Flow*

Bonica, J. J., Kennedy, W. F., Akamatsu, T. L. and Gerbershagen, H. U. (1972). 'Circulatory Effects of Peridural Block. III. Effects of Acute Blood Loss.' *Anesthesiology* **36**, 219

Bradley, S. E. (1963). 'The Hepatic Circulation.' In *Handbook of Physiology, Circulation,* Vol. II, p. 1387. Washington; American Physiological Society

Brauer, R. W. (1963). 'Liver Circulation and Function.' *Physiol. Rev.* **43**, 115

Bromage, P. R. (1967). 'Physiology and Pharmacology of Epidural Analgesia.' *Anesthesiology* **28**, 592

Cooperman, L. H. (1972). 'Effects of Anaesthetics on the Splanchnic Circulation.' *Br. J. Anaesth.* **44**, 967

Cooper, K. E., Edholm, O. G. and Mottram, R. F. (1955). 'The Blood Flow in Skin and Muscle of the Human Forearm.' *J. Physiol.* **128**, 258

Grayson, J. and Mendel, D. (1965). *Physiology of the Splanchnic Circulation.* London; Edward Arnold

Heistad, D. D. and Abboud, F. M. (1974). 'Factors that Influence Blood Flow in Skeletal Muscle and Skin.' *Anesthesiology* **41**, 139

Hill, D. W. (1973). *Electronic Techniques in Anesthesia and Surgery,* 2nd edn, ch. 4. London; Butterworths

Kramer, K., Lochner, W. and Wetterer, E. (1963). 'Methods of Measuring Blood Flow.' In *Handbook of Physiology, Circulation,* Vol. II, p. 1277. Washington; American Physiological Society

Lassen, N. A. (1959). 'Cerebral Blood Flow and Oxygen Consumption in Man.' *Physiol. Rev.* **39**, 193

McDowall, D. G. (1969). 'Regional Blood Flow Measurement in Clinical Practice.' *Br. J. Anaesth.* **41**, 761

Mueller, H. S. (1972). 'Coronary Circulation.' In Ayres, S. M. and Gregory, J. J., *Cardiology: A Clinicophysiologic Approach,* p. 129. London; Butterworths

Rowe, G. G. (1974). 'Responses of the Coronary Circulation to Physiologic Changes and Pharmacologic Agents.' *Anesthesiology* **41**, 182

Selkurt, E. E. (1963). 'The Renal Circulation' In *Handbook of Physiology, Circulation,* Vol. II, p. 1457 Washington; American Physiological Society

Smith, A. L. and Wollman, H. (1972). 'Cerebral Blood Flow and Metabolism: Effects of Anesthetic Drugs and Techniques.' *Anesthesiology* **36**, 378

Strunin, L. (1975). 'Organ Perfusion during Controlled Hypotension.' *Br. J. Anaesth.* **47**, 793

Wade, O. L. and Bishop, J. M. (1962). *Cardiac Output and Regional Blood Flow.* Oxford; Blackwell

Willenkin, R. L. and Green, N. M. (1964). 'Circulatory Effects of Spinal and Epidural Anesthesia.' In Fabian, L. W., *Anesthesia and the Circulation,* p. 109. Philadelphia; F. A. Davis

Wollman, H. (1970). 'The Humpty Dumpty Phenomenon.' *Anesthesiology* **33**, 379

Veall, N. (1968). 'Diagnostic Uses of Radioisotopes. 8. Blood Flow.' *Hosp. Med.* **2**, 460

Woodcock, J. P. (1975). *Theory and Practice of Blood Flow Measurement.* London; Butterworths

Zelis, R. (1975). *The Peripheral Circulations.* New York; Grune and Stratton

Chapter 6 The Pulmonary Circulation

There are marked differences between the pulmonary and systemic circulations, related mainly to the different physiological roles of these two regions of the cardiovascular system. The pulmonary circulation is a low-pressure system, whereas the systemic circulation is a high-pressure system. The mean pressure in the pulmonary artery is approximately 17 mm Hg, compared with a mean systemic arterial pressure of 90 mm Hg. This pressure difference is reflected in the lower pressures in the pulmonary capillaries compared with those in the systemic capillaries (8 mm Hg as compared with 20–25 mm Hg), an important factor in the prevention of pulmonary oedema.

The other main difference between the pulmonary and systemic circulations is the fact that the pulmonary circulation is functionally homogeneous; the blood flow requirements of different regions of the lung do not vary greatly from moment to moment as is the case with many of the organs of the systemic circulation. The latter may be considered to consist of a number of vascular beds, connected in parallel between arterial and venous reservoirs in which the pressures are maintained relatively constant by homeostatic mechanisms, so that the flow through a given bed may readily be altered by adjustment of the tissue vessels (see page 89). In the pulmonary circulation, the need to divert blood from one region of the lung to another is slight because pulmonary blood flow is concerned primarily with oxygenating the mixed-venous blood, rather than with the nutritional requirements of the pulmonary tissues. The pulmonary circulation therefore consists of a relatively homogeneous vascular network lying between the pulmonary arterial and venous reservoirs.

Teleologically a possible reason for the low pressure in the pulmonary artery is the small vertical distance between the heart and the extremities of the lung. In contrast, in the systemic circulation there must be a considerable head of arterial pressure at the level of the heart on account of the large vertical distance between the heart and the brain (see page 4). (In the giraffe arterial blood pressure at heart level is approximately 300 mm Hg, therefore the arterial pressure in its cerebral circulation does not differ greatly from that in man.)

ANATOMY

In keeping with the low pressures in the pulmonary circulation, the walls of the pulmonary vessels are thinner than those of the systemic circulation. The walls of the right ventricle and pulmonary artery are only about one-third as thick as those of the left ventricle and aorta respectively. Harris and Heath (1962) calculate that the tension in the wall of the pulmonary artery is approximately 30 N m^{-1}, compared with 200 N m^{-1} in the aorta.

The pulmonary circulation is so arranged that the entire cardiac output, with the exception of 1–2 per cent which passes through the bronchial circulation (*see* below) flows through the pulmonary capillaries. The pulmonary vascular resistance is not required to vary widely under different physiological conditions as is the resistance in systemic organs such as the gut or skeletal muscles; therefore, the pulmonary arterioles (which may be defined as vessels of less than 100 μm diameter) possess no muscular tissue, and vary in diameter passively with changes of transmural pressure.

Changes of pulmonary vascular resistance are mainly passive; active changes in response to nervous stimulation or circulating hormones are functionally of little importance, although experimentally it is known that pulmonary vasoconstriction may be induced by hypothalamic stimulation (Anderson and Brown, 1967). Also, changes of local physiological gas tensions may induce variations of pulmonary vascular resistance with a consequent redistribution of pulmonary blood flow; such responses are important in minimizing inequalities of the ventilation/perfusion ratio throughout the lung fields (*see* page 163).

Bronchial venous drainage and pulmonary venous admixtures

The supporting tissues of the lung receive oxygenated blood from the systemic circulation via the bronchial arteries. The bronchial veins, which contain deoxygenated blood, empty mainly into the small pulmonary veins. This venous admixture causes a slight lowering of oxygen tension in the blood returning to the left side of the heart, and is one cause of the oxygen tension difference which always exists between the mixed-arterial blood and the so-called 'ideal' alveolar gas (*see* Nunn, 1969). Under normal circumstances the percentage of the cardiac output which returns via the bronchial circulation is only 1–2 per cent of the total (Ravin, Epstein and Malm, 1965); this proportion may, however, be considerably increased in disease, for example Fallot's tetralogy.

Assuming a bronchial arterio-venous oxygen content difference of 3 ml dl^{-1}, it may be calculated that, under normal circumstances a 2 per cent shunt of bronchial blood causes an alveolar-arterial oxygen tension difference of less than 4 mm Hg (*see* series II tables, Kelman and Nunn, 1968).

PRESSURES

Hydrostatic pressures in the right ventricle and pulmonary artery may be measured via a percutaneously-introduced cardiac catheter. The pressure in the left atrium may be measured either by direct puncture, or estimated by measurement of the 'pulmonary wedge pressure'. The introduction of the Swan–Ganz balloon catheter (Swan et al., 1970) has greatly simplified this measurement which is now made routinely in some intensive care units.

Pulmonary wedge pressure

To measure the pulmonary wedge pressure, a catheter is advanced through the right heart until it becomes impacted in a terminal branch of the pulmonary artery. The catheter tip is then presumed to be occluding the artery. Flow is then blocked, and since the branches of the pulmonary artery are end-arteries, it is a reasonable assumption that the wedged catheter samples the pressure, not in the pulmonary artery, but in the pulmonary veins or left atrium. A blood sample withdrawn through the catheter has the high oxygen saturation which is typical of pulmonary venous blood. There is, in fact, a good correlation between pulmonary wedge pressure and left atrial pressure (Luchsinger, Seipp and Patel, 1962), although the former is slightly the higher, suggesting that wedge pressure probably estimates the pulmonary venous pressure just distal to the pulmonary capillaries, rather than true left atrial pressure.

Pressures in the right ventricle and pulmonary arteries have waveforms similar to those in the systemic circulation, but only about one-sixth as high (*Figure 6.1*). The volumes of blood ejected by the two ventricles are almost identical, therefore the compliance of the pulmonary artery and its large branches must be correspondingly greater than that of the systemic arterial reservoir. This greater compliance depends mainly on the relative thinness of the walls of the pulmonary vessels.

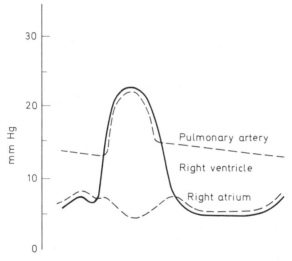

Figure 6.1. Pressure waveforms in right atrium, right ventricle, and pulmonary artery (semi-diagrammatic)

Right ventricular systole is preceded by contraction of the right atrium, which forces blood into the ventricle and raises the intraventricular pressure from approximately zero to several mm Hg above the surrounding intrathoracic pressure. This small pressure rise is followed by a much greater rise due to ventricular systole. When ventricular pressure exceeds the pulmonary arterial pressure—about 10 mm Hg at the end of diastole—blood is ejected out of the ventricle into the pulmonary artery. Peak right ventricle pressure is approximately 22 mm Hg; as systole subsides the intraventricular pressure falls rapidly to approximately 1 mm Hg, but the pulmonary arterial pressure is maintained by closure of the pulmonary valves. Pulmonary arterial pressure declines slowly during diastole to reach its lowest value of 10 mm Hg just before the start of the next systole. Mean pulmonary artery pressure is approximately 15 mm Hg.

With the technique of float catheterization of the right heart (Bradley, 1964), a fine, percutaneously-introduced catheter may be advanced through the heart without the necessity for X-ray control. The position of the catheter's tip is judged by observation of the pressure waveform. The change from the relatively steady atrial pressure to the large pressure swings which occur when the catheter passes through the tricuspid valve is easily observed, as is the change from a diastolic pressure of zero in the right ventricle to one of approximately 17 mm Hg as the catheter passes into the pulmonary artery.

Mean left atrial pressure is approximately 4 mm Hg, although quite large variations occur from subject to subject. Pulsation is greater than in the right atrium, partly because of the greater force of left ventricular systole, partly as a result of transmission of pressure oscillations through the pulmonary vascular bed, and partly due to the fact that the compliance of the left atrium and pulmonary veins is less than the compliance of the right atrium and systemic veins.

PULMONARY VASCULAR RESISTANCE

The whole of the cardiac output passes through the pulmonary circulation. The pressure difference between the pulmonary artery and left atrium is, however, considerably less than that between the aorta and the right atrium. Therefore the calculated pulmonary vascular resistance is much less than the systemic resistance (*see* page 18).

Although the pulmonary vasculature is well equipped with adrenergic nerve fibres, and can respond to circulating hormones and to changes of P_{O_2} and P_{CO_2}, pulmonary vascular resistance appears to depend more on passive changes of vascular calibre than on active vasoconstriction or vasodilatation.

An increase of cardiac output is accompanied by little increase of pulmonary arterial pressure until the flow has increased 3 or 4 times (West and Dollery, 1965). The pulmonary vasculature is so distensible that a small increase of intravascular pressure causes considerable vascular dilatation, therefore the vessels are able to transmit the increased flow with but little increase of pressure difference between the pulmonary artery and left atrium. If cardiac output increases by more than 4 times its resting value, however, the distensibility of the pulmonary vessels is no longer sufficient to accommodate the increased flow; pulmonary arterial pressure then rises even in patients without cardiopulmonary disease (Fowler, 1969).

Response of the pulmonary circulation to changes of physiological gas tensions

It is well recognized that uneven distribution of alveolar ventilation in relation to perfusion causes inefficiency of cardiopulmonary function. Relatively over-ventilated areas of lung produce an increase of physiological dead space; relatively over-perfused areas cause an apparent shunt of mixed-venous blood past the functioning lung tissue, with a consequent lowering of arterial P_{O_2} (Nunn, 1969). It would, therefore, be advantageous for the body to possess mechanisms which maintain the ventilation/perfusion ratio in individual alveoli or areas of lung close to the physiologically optimal value. In experimental animals, at any rate, this does in fact appear to be the case.

Alveolar Po_2 and Pco_2 in over-ventilated regions of lung are pulled towards the gas tensions of inspired air, whereas the gas tensions in relatively over-perfused areas are nearer to those of mixed-venous blood. Von Euler and Liljestrand (1946) showed that, in the cat, both hypoxia and hypercapnia cause an increase of pulmonary vascular resistance, presumably due to active vasoconstriction. This response would clearly tend to decrease blood flow through over-perfused regions where Pco_2 is relatively high and Po_2 relatively low.

Unfortunately, the difficulties of demonstrating such a response in intact man are considerable, chiefly because the pressure difference across the pulmonary vascular bed is so small. Not only is pulmonary arterial pressure considerably less than aortic pressure, but left atrial pressure is rather greater than right atrial pressure. The pressure difference between the pulmonary artery and left atrium is only 5 or 6 mm Hg, therefore halving pulmonary vascular resistance at constant flow causes a pressure change of only 2 or 3 mm Hg which is comparable to the error in the measurement of either of these quantities.

Hypoxia

In man, the inhalation of hypoxic gas mixtures causes an increase of pulmonary artery pressure roughly proportional to the reduction of arterial oxyhaemoglobin saturation (Fritts et al., 1960); left atrial pressure remains constant. This increase of pressure difference across the lungs is greater than can be accounted for by any simultaneous increase of pulmonary blood flow, and it therefore seems that hypoxia induces a generalized increase of pulmonary vascular resistance. In addition, unilateral hypoxia, induced by the administration of an hypoxic gas mixture to one lung, causes a redistribution of pulmonary blood flow towards the normally oxygenated lung (Himmelstein et al., 1958).

The anatomical site of the change of pulmonary vascular resistance is presumably the muscular pulmonary arteries, that is the vessels of between 100 μm and 1000 μm diameter which precede the pulmonary arterioles. The response can be elicited in the isolated perfused lung, therefore it does not appear to depend on an extrinsic nerve supply; nor is the hypoxic response of the human pulmonary circulation altered by extensive sympathectomy (Fishman, Fritts and Cournand, 1960). The reason that hypoxia causes vasoconstriction in the pulmonary circulation but vasodilatation elsewhere in the body is not known with certainty. However, Lloyd (1967) showed that isolated strips of pulmonary artery were relaxed by hypoxia; and it has therefore been suggested that in the intact animal, hypoxia acts via release of a vasoconstrictor substance. Amongst other substances, noradrenaline and histamine have been suggested for this role. Sykes et al. (1973) have shown that general anaesthesia can reverse hypoxically-induced pulmonary vasoconstriction.

Permanent residents at high altitudes tend to have pulmonary hypertension at rest, and show an exaggerated increase of pulmonary artery pressure during moderate exercise (Banchero et al., 1966). They also have abnormal muscularization of their pulmonary arterioles similar to that found in chronic *cor pulmonale* (Arias-Stella and Saldaña, 1963).

It is not clear whether the effects of inhaling hypoxic gas mixtures are due primarily to a diminished oxygen tension in the alveolar gas, in the pulmonary capillaries or in the mixed-venous blood. That mixed-venous oxygen tension appears to play a part is suggested by the fact that pulmonary vascular resistance is raised in carbon monoxide poisoning, a condition in which arterial P_{O_2} is normal but mixed-venous P_{O_2} is very low (Bergofsky et al., 1963).

Alternatively it is known that gases can diffuse across the very small distance which separates the alveoli and the muscular pulmonary arterioles; and Duke (1957) showed that perfusion of the lungs with hypoxic blood did *not* cause vasoconstriction if the alveolar P_{O_2} was normal. Also, the desaturation of the pulmonary arterial blood which is characteristic of exercise (*see* page 173) does not cause pulmonary vasoconstriction.

Hyperoxia

Most studies of the effects of increased oxygen pressure on pulmonary vascular resistance have been on patients with pulmonary hypertension, in whom the reactivity of the pulmonary vessels is far from normal. There is, however, some evidence from normal subjects which suggests that an increased inspired oxygen concentration may cause a decrease of pulmonary vascular resistance. Harris and Heath (1962) conclude that 'there is a continuous scale relating inspired oxygen concentration to pulmonary vascular resistance which extends from extreme hypoxia to extreme hyperoxia'. In dogs, however, Bain, Lancaster and Adams (1965) showed that pulmonary perfusion with blood of high P_{O_2} caused an increase, rather than a decrease, of pulmonary vascular resistance.

Hypercapnia

In the anaesthetized, artificially-ventilated dog an increase of inspired carbon dioxide concentration at constant minute volume causes pulmonary vasoconstriction (Bergofsky, Lehr and Fishman, 1962). This response is due primarily to change of pH because doubling the Pa_{CO_2} at constant pH has little or no effect. In addition, unilateral hypercapnia in man causes a redistribution of pulmonary blood flow towards the normal side. However, in cats, Viles and Shepherd (1968) found that carbon dioxide could induce pulmonary vasodilatation.

PULMONARY BLOOD FLOW

As a result of the elegant radioisotope studies carried out by West and his colleagues in the 1960s, it is now well recognized that blood flow is not uniform throughout the lung, but increases from above downwards (in the upright posture). The reason for this non-uniformity of pulmonary blood flow is that the pulmonary arterial pressure is fairly low, and thus comparable in magnitude with pressure differences due to gravity (*see* page 3).

(Of course, pressure differences due to gravity affect both the arterial and the venous sides of the circulation, and at first sight therefore it might seem that they would be without effect on blood flow. This indeed would be the case if the pulmonary vessels were rigid tubes; but they are not, and blood flow therefore depends not only on the driving pressure difference, but also on the transmural pressure. In the pulmonary apices the intravascular pressure is below the surrounding alveolar pressure, and the blood flow is minimal; whereas in the bases of the lung the intravascular pressure is high, so that the vessels are widely dilated and the resistance to blood flow is small.)

The consequences of this uneven pulmonary blood flow on gas exchange are discussed in detail by Nunn (1969).

It has been pointed out by West (1966) that the effect of the alveolar pressure on pulmonary blood flow is rather more complicated than might appear at first sight. There are several models of this situation; in the simplest the lung is divided into three zones: in the upper zone (zone I) the intravascular pressure is below the surrounding alveolar pressure, and the blood flow is virtually zero. In the lowest zone (zone III) both the pulmonary arterial and venous pressures exceed the surrounding alveolar pressure, so that the vessels are widely open and the blood flow depends on the arterio-venous pressure. In the middle zone (zone II) the situation is more complicated because the alveolar pressure lies somewhere between the arterial and venous pressures; and under these circumstances the blood flow depends not on the arterio-venous pressure difference, but on the difference between the pulmonary artery pressure and alveolar pressure. This being the case, it is likely that an increase of alveolar pressure as during intermittent positive-pressure ventilation (*see* page 193) may cause a diversion of blood flow from zone II to zone III, with a consequent increase in the effective size of zone I, and an increase of alveolar deadspace.

Pulsatile blood flow in pulmonary capillaries

The nitrous oxide technique for measurement of cardiac output (*see* page 266) has been modified to demonstrate pulsatile blood flow in the pulmonary capillaries (Lee and Dubois, 1955). The subject sits in an airtight box—a whole-body plethysmograph—and after attainment of a steady state takes a deep inhalation of nitrous oxide, and then holds his breath with open glottis. As nitrous oxide is taken up by the pulmonary capillaries, the amount of gas in the box falls, and this fall is reflected in a decrease of pressure in the box (Boyle's law). This technique has shown that the rate of uptake of nitrous oxide in the lungs is not constant, but appears to vary phasically with the heart beat; this fluctuation is usually interpreted as evidence that pulmonary capillary blood flow is pulsatile, although other interpretations are possible.

RECOMMENDED FURTHER READING

Aviado, D. M. (1965). *The Lung Circulation*. New York; Pergamon

Bergman, N. A. (1971). 'The Pulmonary Circulation.' In Evans, T. C. and Nunn, J. F., *General Anaesthesia*, 3rd edn, p. 262. London; Butterworths

Daly, I. de B.. and Hebb, C. O. (1967). *Pulmonary and Bronchial Vascular Systems.* Baltimore; Williams and Wilkins

Fishman, A. P. (1963). 'Dynamics of the Pulmonary Circulation.' In *Handbook of Physiology, Circulation*, Vol. II, p. 1667. Washington; American Physiological Society

Gillis, C. N. (1973). 'Metabolism of Vasoactive Hormones by Lung.' *Anesthesiology* **39**, 626

Green, J. F. (1975). 'The Pulmonary Circulation.' In Zelis, R., *The Peripheral Circulations*. New York; Grune and Stratton

Harris, P. and Heath, D. (1962). *The Human Pulmonary Circulation*. Edinburgh; Livingstone

Laver, M. B., Hallowell, P. and Goldblatt, A. (1970). 'Pulmonary Dysfunction Secondary to Heart Disease: Aspects Relevant to Anaesthesia and Surgery.' *Anesthesiology* 33, 161

Lee, G. de J. (1969). 'Blood Flow in the Lungs.' In Morgan Jones, A. (Ed.), *Modern Trends in Cardiology*, 2nd edn. London; Butterworths

Leigh, J. M. (1974). 'The Pulmonary Circulation.' In Scurr, C. and Feldman, S., *Scientific Foundations of Anaesthesia*. London; Heinemann

Milnor, W. R. (1972). 'Pulmonary Hemodynamics.' In Bergel, D. H., *Cardiovascular Fluid Dynamics*, p. 299. London; Academic Press

Permutt, S., Bromberger-Barnea, B. and Bane, H. N. (1962). 'Alveolar Pressure, Pulmonary Venous Pressure, and Vascular Waterfall.' *Med. thorac.* 19, 239.

Price, H. L., Cooperman, L. H., Warden, J. C., Morris, J. L. and Smith, T. C. (1969). 'Pulmonary Hemodynamics during General Anesthesia in Man.' *Anesthesiology* 30, 629.

Smith, N. T. and Hoffman, J. I. E. (1969). 'Evaluation of the Circulation—Pulmonary and Otherwise—in Man.' *Anaesthesiology* 30, 589.

Sykes, M. K., Davies, D. M. Chakrabarti and Loh, L. (1973). The Effects of Halothane, Trichloroethylene and Ether on the Hypoxic Pressor Response and Pulmonary Vascular Resistance in the Isolated Perfused Cat Lung.' *Br. J. Anaesth.* 45, 655

West, J. B. (1963). 'Distribution of Gas and Blood in the Normal Lungs.' *Br. Med. Bull.* 19, 53

Chapter 7 Cardiovascular Response to Exercise

The body's response to physical exercise has always interested physiologists because the stress of exercise activates various homeostatic mechanisms, and so helps understanding of their organization and function. In recent years the concept of 'testing under load' has become an accepted part of clinical practice, with formal exercise-testing playing an increasing role in the investigation of patients with cardiovascular or respiratory disease. In disease the body's (impaired) regulatory mechanisms may be sufficient to maintain homeostasis at rest, but are totally unable to cope with the additional demands of exercise.

Muscular contraction depends on the chemical energy which is liberated when adenosine triphosphate (ATP) is broken down to ADP. But the body's stores of ATP (and of its other source of high-energy phosphate, creatine phosphate) are sufficient for only a few seconds' exercise. ATP has therefore to be regenerated by the intramuscular breakdown of carbohydrate and fatty acids; and, although some of this energy may be derived from local glycogen stores, a sizeable proportion has to be provided from glucose and fatty acids which reach the muscle via the blood stream.

Muscular exercise thus requires a sufficient blood flow to the active muscles to provide adequate amounts of essential substrates, including oxygen.

(It is true, of course, that ATP can be regenerated also from the aerobic breakdown of glycogen to lactic acid—see page 220; but this mechanism is of strictly limited capacity, and is used mainly for short bursts of very intense exercise. In any case it produces large amounts of lactic acid which may have deleterious effects on other regions of the body.)

The large increase of muscle blood flow which occurs during exercise is accompanied by a similar increase of cardiac output, possibly to as much as six times its resting value, and by a decrease of blood flow to less active tissues such as the gut, kidneys and skin (but see below). The redistribution of cardiac output which occurs during exercise of moderate intensity is shown diagrammatically in *Figure 7.1*.

Any physical activity generates waste heat, and muscular contraction is no exception. In the short term this heat is stored as a rise of body temperature, and as an increase in the size of its central (homeothermic) core; but beyond a certain point it must be dissipated from the body, and this requires an increase of skin blood flow which imposes an additional strain on the body's cardiovascular system.

Although the general outline of the body's cardiovascular response to exercise is undisputed, many of the details are unclear, particularly the mechanism which causes muscular vasodilatation, and the increase of sympathetic stimulation to the heart and other tissues.

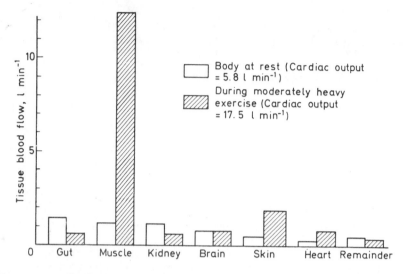

Figure 7.1. Redistribution of cardiac output during moderate exercise (figures from Wade and Bishop, 1962)

Unless otherwise stated the present account of the body's cardiovascular response to exercise refers to exercise in an upright posture, and in a thermally-neutral environment. The cardiovascular response to exercise in a hot environment is discussed in detail by Rowell (1974) (*see* Recommended Further Reading).

QUANTITATION OF EXERCISE

It is common experience that the body's cardiovascular responses to physical exercise vary according to the intensity of the exercise; and it is therefore desirable to have a means of quantifying exercise intensity. Comparisons can then more readily be made between the responses of different individuals.

During exercise on a bicycle ergometer, and to a lesser extent on a treadmill, it is easy to make a subject work at a prescribed rate simply by adjusting the load appropriately. The subject's work rate can then be expressed in terms of watts (or the older units kilo pond metres min^{-1} [kpm min^{-1}], 100 W $\simeq$ 600 kpm min^{-1}). The difficulty is that a work load which is difficult for a normal individual, and perhaps impossible for a patient with mitral stenosis, may be too easy for a trained athlete. But it is possible to get round this difficulty by adjusting the intensity of the exercise so that the subject exercises at a given *proportion of his total exercise capacity*; and under these circumstances it seems that the cardiovascular, respiratory and metabolic responses of a wide range of individuals are quantitatively similar, despite differences in their physical capabilities.

Maximal oxygen consumption ($\dot{V}_{O_2}$ max)

Provided that a subject is deriving his energy requirements from aerobic metabolism it is possible to find out how hard he is working simply by measuring his oxygen consumption ($\dot{V}_{O_2}$). If this is done then it is found that $\dot{V}_{O_2}$ increases roughly in proportion to the exercise intensity, provided this is below a certain level; but beyond this point further increases of exercise intensity do *not* result in an increased oxygen consumption, rather, in an increased production of energy from anaerobic metabolism (*see* page 220). The maximal uptake which a subject can achieve over a period of several minutes is known as his $\dot{V}_{O_2 max}$, or maximal aerobic capacity (Taylor, Buskirk and Henschel, 1955).

Provided that the subject is using more than 50 per cent of his total muscle mass, and provided that certain methodological errors are avoided, then it has been found that $\dot{V}_{O_2} max$ is highly reproducible from day-to-day, and that this is little affected by a variety of acute physiological stresses such as acute haemorrhage (Rowell, Taylor and Wang, 1964) and acute starvation (Henschel, Taylor and Keys, 1954). (It is, however, affected by changes in the subject's level of physical fitness as brought about by prolonged bed-rest or physical training—Saltin et al., 1968).

It has been found that $\dot{V}_{O_2} max$ varies markedly with the subject's habitual physical activity, from 30–45 ml kg^{-1} in sedentary men to as high as 85 ml kg^{-1} in top-grade endurance athletes (Ekblom and Hermansen, 1968). In general, it declines with age; and it is, of course, severely reduced in chronic heart disease.

There is some dispute about the physiological basis for the observed plateau of oxygen uptake which occurs above a certain work load. Kaijser (1970) suggests that the limitation is the muscles' ability to utilize oxygen; but most workers believe that the limitation is the rate at which oxygen can be delivered to the exercising tissues by the cardiovascular system. This concept is supported by the fact that oxygen breathing increases a subject's $\dot{V}_{O_2} max$, roughly in proportion to the increase in arterial oxygen content.

As already mentioned the cardiovascular response of an individual is related more to his *relative* work load (actual $\dot{V}_{O_2}$/maximal $\dot{V}_{O_2}$) than to his actual work load (*see also* below).

TISSUE BLOOD FLOW

During exercise blood flow to the exercising muscles is very considerably increased above its resting level; at the same time blood flow to non-exercising parts of the body, such as the skin, gut, kidney and non-exercising muscles, is decreased.

This redistribution of blood flow permits the achievement of a very high overall oxygen extraction from the blood—of the order of 85 per cent during intense exercise (Asmussen and Nielsen, 1952). If blood flow to non-exercising parts of the body were not restricted then such a high total oxygen extraction would not, of course, be possible, because deoxygenated blood from the exercising muscles would be diluted by relatively well-oxygenated blood from the body's non-active tissues.

Muscles

In general, skeletal muscle fibres are of two types: fast-twitch 'phasic' fibres and slow-twitch 'tonic' fibres. The former are adapted for rapid short-duration movements, while the latter—which contain large numbers of mitochondria as is necessary for prolonged aerobic metabolism—are able to maintain long-sustained contractions, such as those concerned in the maintenance of posture. It has been shown, in animals, that the resting blood flow is much greater in muscles which are composed predominantly of tonic fibres than in those which are composed mainly of phasic fibres. Also, capillary density and maximal blood flow are similarly greater in the postural muscles (Folkow and Halicka, 1968). In man phasic fibres are in the majority in most muscles.

A typical value for resting muscle blood flow is 2–5 ml min^{-1} 100 g^{-1} which, with an assumed total muscle mass of 30 kg, gives a resting blood flow of about 1–1.5 l min^{-1}. Elimination of the resting sympathetic vasoconstrictor tone causes only a relatively slight increase of muscle blood flow (roughly double), which indicates that the blood vessels in skeletal muscle have a large amount of inherent tone (*see* page 89).

During hard exercise, muscle blood flow may increase to as much as 50–75 ml min^{-1} 100 g^{-1}, i.e. total muscle blood flow during activities such as down-hill skiing, which involve the simultaneous use of most of the body's large muscles, may be as high as 20 or 25 l min^{-1}, or even higher in top-grade athletes. This considerable vasodilatation is due almost entirely to the local accumulation of vasodilator metabolites; it is not affected by sympathectomy.

It is said that muscular vasodilatation affects predominantly the precapillary resistance vessels, leaving the post-capillary vessels relatively undilated. This would be expected to cause an increase of intracapillary pressure, with loss of fluid from the circulation; and may account for the decrease of plasma volume which occurs even during a relatively short period of exercise, that is before the onset of sweating.

In contrast to this marked vasodilatation in the active muscles the vascular resistance of non-active muscles is increased, probably as a result of increased sympathetic activity (Bevegård and Shephard, 1967).

The vasodilator chemical(s)

The nature of the chemical—or most likely chemicals, because there is almost certainly more than one—which cause muscular vasodilatation during exercise is disputed. Muscle metabolism causes the breakdown of large molecules into smaller, more osmotically-active molecules; and it is thought that this local hyperosmolarity may cause muscular vasodilatation. Indeed, Mellander et al. (1967), have shown that there is a strong negative correlation between the osmolarity of the venous blood from an exercising muscle and its vascular resistance. Also, close intra-arterial injection of hyperosmolar fluids cause muscular vasodilatation.

Other candidates for the role of local muscular vasodilator are: potassium ions, hypoxia (which may potentiate the vasodilator action of potassium ions), increased hydrogen ion concentration, adenosine compounds, and a local increase of temperature.

Mechanical hindrance to muscle blood flow

It has been pointed out, elsewhere, how intermittent muscular contraction aids venous return by acting as a 'muscle pump' (*see* page 123); but muscular contraction may also impede local blood flow, particularly during isometric contractions (*see* later). Anaerobic metabolism in the relatively ischaemic muscles may then produce large local concentrations of lactic acid and other metabolites, and ischaemic pain.

The $\dot{V}_{O_2}$max determined during exercise on a bicycle ergometer is less than that measured on a treadmill, perhaps because high intramuscular pressures in the legs impede muscle blood flow (Åstrand and Saltin, 1961).

During less intense exercise, muscle metabolism can occur at a relatively constant rate, despite the phasically varying blood flow, by virtue of oxygen stored by intramuscular myoglobin.

Sympathetic vasodilator fibres

As already mentioned, muscle blood flow during well-established exercise is increased little or not at all by sympathectomy, being determined almost solely by the local accumulation of vasodilator metabolites. But the sympathetic nervous system *does* play a part in determining muscle blood flow, particularly just before and at the start of exercise.

The precise role of the sympathetic vasodilator fibres in man is uncertain; but they are thought to cause generalized muscular vasodilatation immediately before a period of exercise, the response being set in train by activity of higher nervous centres (*see* page 95). This increased blood flow is probably mainly through thoroughfare channels, rather than through the true exchange vessels (the capillaries); but then, when muscular activity starts, the precapillary sphincters open and the increased flow is immediately redistributed to the capillaries.

Splanchnic circulation

Blood flow to the splanchnic region decreases during exercise, roughly in proportion to its intensity. This is the case both in sedentary individuals and in

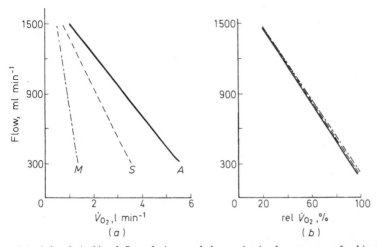

Figure 7.2. Splanchnic blood flow during graded exercise in three groups of subjects: M, patients with mitral stenosis; S, sedentary individuals; A, athletes (redrawn from Rowell, 1969)

athletes (Rowell, Taylor and Wang, 1964), and in patients with severely reduced exercise tolerances (Blackmon et al., 1967) (*Figure 7.2a*).

Despite the greatly differing exercise tolerances of the three groups just mentioned, Rowell has shown that if the blood flow is plotted against the subjects' *relative* oxygen consumption (actual $\dot{V}_{O_2}$/maximal $\dot{V}_{O_2}$) rather than against their *actual* consumption, then the three lines superimpose (*Figure 7.2b*). This is in keeping with the finding of Häggendal, Hartley and Saltin (1970), that the plasma concentration of noradrenaline (and therefore presumably sympathetic efferent activity) during exercise is increased roughly in proportion to the relative intensity of the work.

Kidneys

Renal blood flow is decreased during exercise, again roughly in proportion to the relative work load (Grimby, 1965).

Skin

Cutaneous blood flow is decreased during short-term exercise (Christensen and Nielsen, 1942), but may be increased during longer-term exercise as the need to lose heat from the body surface takes precedence over the need to divert blood flow to the exercising muscles (*see* later).

CARDIAC OUTPUT

The increase of muscle blood flow which can be achieved by redistribution from other regions of the circulation—as just described—is small in comparison with the muscles' metabolic needs. Obviously cardiac output must increase also. And it does: cardiac outputs of as high as 42 l min^{-1} have been measured in man during very intense exercise (Ekblom and Hermansen, 1968).

Athletes have considerably higher maximal cardiac outputs than less fit individuals, although at any given oxygen uptake their outputs are roughly the same (*Figure 7.3a*).

During exercise at up to about 70 per cent of maximum aerobic capacity the increase of cardiac output is roughly proportional to the subject's oxygen uptake (Åstrand et al., 1964). Above this level the increase is proportionately less, and there is increasing anaerobic metabolism in the muscles with a resulting lactic acidosis in the peripheral blood. Most workers consider that an inability to increase the cardiac output beyond a certain point is the chief limiting factor in determining a subject's maximal aerobic capacity (*see* earlier).

Heart rate and stroke volume (*Table 7.1*)

Most of the increase of cardiac output seems to be due to an increase of heart rate, rather than to an increase of stroke volume (*Figure 7.3c* and *d*); and, as with cardiac output, there is a roughly linear relationship between heart rate and

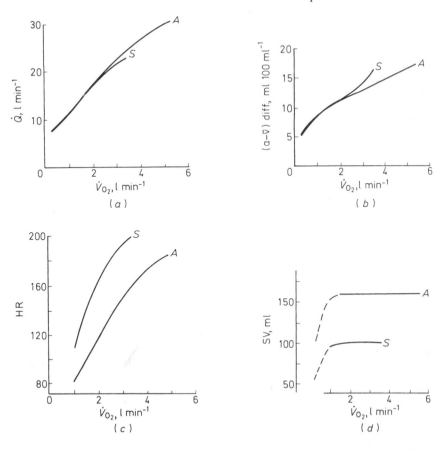

Figure 7.3. Relationship between oxygen consumption ($\dot{V}o_2$), cardiac output ($\dot{Q}$), (a–$\bar{v}$) O_2 diff., heart rate, and stroke volume during graded exercise in sedentary individuals (S) and athletes (A) (redrawn from Rowell, 1969)

Table 7.1   CARDIOVASCULAR ADJUSTMENTS TO EXERCISE IN
UPRIGHT MAN

	At rest (standing)	During exercise
Oxygen uptake	0.4 l min^{-1}	3–3.5 l min^{-1}
Cardiac output	5 l min^{-1}	25 l min^{-1}
Heart rate	70 min^{-1}	180 min^{-1}
End-diastolic volume	145 ml	180 ml
End-systolic volume	75 ml	40 ml
Stroke volume	70 ml	140 ml
(a–$\bar{v}$)O_2 difference	80 ml l^{-1}	140 ml l^{-1}
Cycle time	0.86 s	0.33 s
Ventricular systole	0.31 s	0.20 s
Ventricular diastole	0.55 s	0.13 s

(Figures modified from Folkow and Neil, 1971)

oxygen uptake over a wide range of exercise intensities. Above 70 per cent of the subject's maximal aerobic capacity the heart rate increases less rapidly, until at very high work rates it reaches a maximum of about 200 beats min^{-1} in young individuals, and rather less in older people.

The maximal heart rate of a trained athlete is slightly less than that of a sedentary individual. But the main difference between the two is in their heart rates at submaximal work loads: not only does the athlete have a lower resting pulse rate, but his exercising pulse rate at any given work load is less than that of a sedentary individual. Cardiac output in the athlete is maintained by a higher stroke volume.

Stroke volume increases little with increasing exercise intensity except in mild exercise. On assuming an upright posture there is a small fall of stroke volume due to venous pooling in the legs; but this fall is reversed by low-intensity exercise presumably because the 'muscle-pump' (*see* page 123) promotes venous return, and therefore cardiac filling. Athletes have higher stroke volumes, not only at rest but also during exercise of all grades of intensity (*Figure 7.3b*).

Cause of increased cardiac output

As explained elsewhere (*see* Chapter 4) there are two general mechanisms by which cardiac output can be increased: the Starling mechanism and the effect of inotropic influences on the myocardium. From the above paragraphs it would seem that the former is of relatively little importance except during mild exercise in the upright posture, when it undoubtedly helps to maintain the stroke volume. Starling himself said in 1920, on the importance of his law in this context: '. . . it [an increase of end-diastolic volume] becomes imperceptible in the intact animal, and is not revealed, for instance, by any radiographic study of the heart during exercise'.

Most X-ray evidence in man suggests that the diastolic volume of the heart during exercise is little or not at all increased above its resting value.

There thus seems little doubt that the main cause of the increased cardiac output of exercise is increased sympathetic (and decreased parasympathetic) activity to the heart. But there is no really satisfactory explanation for the cause of this alteration of autonomic activity. To some extent it may be a result of higher nervous activity, as with the body's 'anticipatory response' to exercise; but it has also been shown that there is an additional increase of heart rate which is manifest even during the *first few seconds of exercise* (Asmussen and Nielsen, 1951). This suggests that the mechanism is a neuronal one; but at the present time it is not at all clear whether it is predominantly a reflex which originates in the active muscles (as is certainly the case with the increased pulmonary ventilation of exercise), or whether it is due to 'irradiation' of neuronal activity from the descending motor pathways to the cardiovascular centres as suggested by Goodwin, McCloskey and Mitchell (1972).

The chief difference between a fit individual and a less fit one, therefore, seems to be the greater stroke volume of the former, and this difference is well seen in the decrease of stroke volume which occurs after a relatively short period of enforced bed-rest. Saltin et al. (1968) showed that 21 days' bed-rest caused a fall of $\dot{V}_{O_2}$max of almost 28 per cent, and that the decrease was due mainly to a fall of cardiac stroke volume. Conversely, the same workers showed that physical training caused an increase of $\dot{V}_{O_2}$max which was due partly to an increase of stroke volume, and partly to an increased (a–v̄) oxygen difference. Hartley et al. (1969) showed that in older subjects the increase in $\dot{V}_{O_2}$max was due almost entirely to an increase of stroke volume.

OXYGEN DELIVERY TO THE EXERCISING MUSCLES (*Table 7.2*)

It has been calculated (Rowell, 1974) that the maximal increase in muscle blood flow which could be achieved simply by redistribution of an unchanged cardiac output would be about 3 l min^{-1}. With a normal arterial oxygen content this represents an oxygen flux to the muscles of about 600 ml min^{-1}. It is known (Wade and Bishop, 1962) that even patients who have a fixed cardiac output because of valvular heart disease can double their oxygen consumption by this mechanism.

Table 7.2 DEPENDENCE OF $\dot{V}_{O_2}$max ON HEART RATE, STROKE VOLUME AND (a–v̄) OXYGEN CONTENT DIFFERENCE IN THREE GROUPS OF SUBJECTS WITH VERY DIFFERENT EXERCISE CAPACITIES (FROM ROWELL, 1969)

	$\dot{V}_{O_2}$max (l min^{-1})		Heart rate (min^{-1})		Stroke vol. (ml)		(a–v̄)O_2 diff. (ml 100 ml^{-1})
Athletes	5.2	=	190	x	160	x	17
Sedentary	3.2	=	200	x	100	x	16
Mitral stenosis	1.6	=	190	x	50	x	17

Normally however, redistribution of cardiac output is a relatively unimportant factor in determining muscular blood flow during moderate or severe exercise, the most important factors being: increase of cardiac output and increase of the (a–v̄) oxygen content difference. This is shown diagrammatically in *Figure 7.4* which illustrates the well-known physiological principle, first adumbrated by Barcroft, that 'every adaptation is an integration'; that is, the body responds to stress, not by a single mechanism, but by integration of several mechanisms—in the present case by increases of heart rate, stroke volume, (a–v̄) oxygen content difference, and acidosis which helps oxygen unloading in the tissues (*see* below).

Oxygen extraction from the blood by the working muscles seems to be very nearly complete. Saltin et al. (1968), for example, measured the oxygen content of the femoral venous blood and found that it was only 1.4 ml 100 ml^{-1} with a P_{O_2} of 12 mm Hg and a pH of 7.09. In this situation oxygen unloading from haemoglobin is undoubtedly aided by the shift of the dissociation curve which occurs as a result of local acidosis (from increased production of CO_2 and lactic acid), and from a local rise of temperature.

It may be calculated (Kelman and Nunn, 1968) from the above figures, that, even ignoring the effect of temperature, the Bohr shift raises the local venous P_{O_2} by approximately 7 mm Hg, i.e. by 70 per cent.

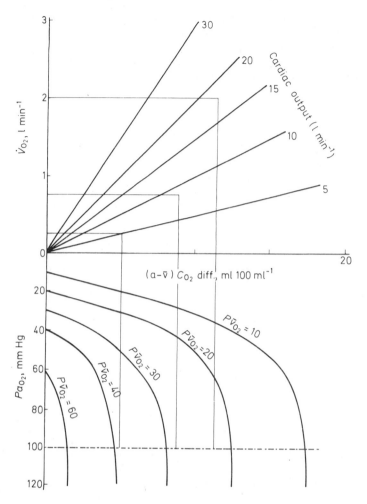

Figure 7.4. 'Two-quadrant' diagram of tissue oxygenation during three levels of exercise (rectangular lines). Arterial oxygen capacity assumed to be 20 ml 100 ml⁻¹

ARTERIAL BLOOD PRESSURE

It is usually said that mild or moderate exercise is accompanied by an increase of systolic blood pressure, and by a smaller increase or by a small decrease of diastolic pressure. But there is a complication: accurate recording of arterial pressure during exercise requires an indwelling arterial cannula; and this may give inaccurate results when blood flow is rapid. The reason is that the kinetic energy of the flowing blood as it impinges against the end of the cannula produces an artificially high pressure reading which reflects *both* the kinetic and the pressure energy of the blood (*see* page 23). Marx et al. (1967), for example, measured aortic pressure during exercise, and found lower values by using a catheter with side-holes than by using one with a single end-hole.

For this reason it is probable that in the past arterial pressure during exercise has been somewhat overestimated. Indeed, it is possible that the mean blood pressure during some forms of intense exercise may fall slightly as the output of the heart is unable to keep pace with widespread vasodilatation which occurs in the exercising muscles.

Åstrand et al. (1965) measured intra-arterial blood pressure during graded arm and leg exercise; and they found that, at a given percentage of the subject's $Vo_{2\,max}$, the blood pressure was much higher during arm exercise than during leg exercise. This suggests that arm exercise—such as shovelling snow, cranking a car—may throw a particularly heavy strain on the cardiovascular system, and should therefore be avoided in patients who have impaired myocardial circulation. (A similar increase of blood pressure occurs with isometric exercise, and may throw a similar strain on the heart—*see* below.)

CARDIOVASCULAR RESPONSE TO PROLONGED EXERCISE

Prolonged exercise at any given sub-maximal work load is characterized by a gradual increase of heart rate, a phenomenon sometimes referred to as 'cardiovascular drift'. Saltin and Stenberg (1964), for example, investigated the effects of severe prolonged exercise at 75 per cent of $Vo_{2\,max}$; and they found that it was characterized by a small increase of cardiac output (and of whole body oxygen consumption) with a 15 per cent increase of heart rate, and a rather smaller decrease of stroke volume.

There is dispute about the cause of this cardiovascular drift, but it seems to be related in some way to the body's need to dissipate increasing amounts of heat as exercise is prolonged (*see* earlier). This need could affect the cardiovascular system in at least two ways: dilatation of the cutaneous resistance vessels would tend to lower the arterial blood pressure, and might therefore cause a compensatory increase of cardiac sympathetic activity; alternatively, dilatation of the cutaneous capacitance vessels might reduce the central blood volume (*see* page 120), thereby reducing the cardiac stroke volume, and so causing a compensatory increase of heart rate. In this connection it is noteworthy that Ekelund and Holmgren (1964) did indeed find a fall of right ventricular end-diastolic volume during prolonged exercise.

ISOMETRIC EXERCISE

The way in which muscular contraction tends to impede muscle blood flow during ordinary (isotonic or dynamic) exercise has already been mentioned; this is even more the case during isometric, or static, exercise, where there is an unremitting impediment to muscle blood flow. Lind and his colleagues (Humphreys and Lind, 1963; Lind and McNicol, 1967) showed that forearm blood flow during sustained hand-grips increased with increasing tension up to about 30 per cent of the subject's maximal voluntary contraction (MVC), but that above this level it decreased again. During contractions greater than about 70 per cent of MVC blood flow was virtually zero.

The reason for this finding is, of course, that muscular contraction impedes blood flow, despite the marked vasodilatation which accompanies all forms of muscular activity; and this effect is more marked at higher muscle tensions. (In keeping with this idea is the fact that muscle blood flow immediately after a period of isometric exercise is considerably greater than it is during the exercise.)

These changes in muscle blood flow are accompanied by marked, and progressive, increases of arterial blood pressure due partly to an increase of cardiac output and partly to an increase of peripheral resistance. For example, Lind and McNicol (1967) found that at the end of a period of sustained hand-grip at 30 per cent of MVC the *mean* arterial blood pressure was 160 mm Hg, and the systolic pressure was over 220 mm Hg. The cause of this increase of blood pressure is uncertain, but teleologically its purpose is obviously to try and maintain perfusion to the contracted, and therefore ischaemic, muscles.

It was found by the original investigators of the body's cardiovascular response to isometric exercise, and it has been recently confirmed (McCloskey and Streatfield, 1975), that the response is related not to the mass of muscle involved, but to the strength of the contraction in relation to the muscles' maximal contractile ability. This has important clinical implications because it means that a severe strain can be imposed on the cardiovascular system by the isometric contraction of quite a small group of muscles, for example, the small muscles of the hand.

It is perhaps worth mentioning also that isometric exercise has very little effect on a person's general cardiovascular fitness, that is on his ability to carry out long-term dynamic exercise. Isometric exercise must therefore be considered to be generally undesirable; and it is not a recommended form of physical training, except perhaps for such sports as wrestling and weight-lifting (*see* Recommended Further Reading).

RECOMMENDED FURTHER READING

Anon. (1975). 'Let me carry your Suitcase.' *Lancet* ii, 754

Åstrand, P. O. and Rodahl, K. (1970). *Textbook of Work Physiology.* New York; McGraw-Hill

Bevegard, B. S. and Shepherd, J. T. (1967). 'Regulation of the Circulation during Exercise in Man.' *Physiol. Rev.* **47**, 178

Campbell, E. J. M. (1967). 'Exercise Tolerance.' *Sci. Basis med. Ann. Rev.* p. 128

Carlsten, A. and Grimby, G. (1966). *The Circulatory Response to Muscular Exercise in Man.* Springfield, Ill.; Charles C. Thomas

Chapman, C. B. (1967). 'Physiology of Muscular Exercise.' *American Heart Association Monograph*, No. 15

Cotes, J. E. and Davies, C. T. M. (1969). 'Factors underlying the Capacity for Exercise: A Study in Physiological Anthropometry.' *Proc. roy. Soc. Med.* **62**, 10

Donald, K. W., Lind, A. R. McNicol, G. W., Humphreys, P. W., Taylor, S. H. and Staunton, H. P. (1967). 'Cardiovascular Responses to Sustained (Static) Contractions.' *Circ. Res.* **20** (Suppl. 1), 15

Guyton, A. C., Jones, C. E. and Coleman, T. G. (1973). *Cardiac Output and its Regulation,* 2nd edn, ch. 25. Philadelphia; W. B. Saunders

Folkow, B. and Neil, E. (1971). *Circulation,* ch. 22. Oxford University Press

Gollnick, P. D. and King, D. W. (1969). 'Energy Release in the Muscle Cell.' *Med. and Sci. in Sports* **1**, 23

Jones, N. L. (1967). 'Exercise Testing.' *Br. J. Dis. Chest* **61**, 169

Kjellmer, I. (1965). 'Studies on Exercise Hyperaemia.' *Acta Physiol. scand.* **64** (Suppl. 244), 1.

Lind, A. R. (1970). 'Cardiovascular Responses to Static Exercise (Isometrics, Anyone?).' *Circulation* **41**, 173

Rowell, L. B. (1969). 'Circulation.' *Med. and Sci. in Sports* **1**, 15

Rowell, L. B. (1974). 'Human Cardiovascular Adjustments to Exercise and Thermal Stress.' *Physiol. Rev.* **54**, 75

Rushmer, R. F. (1971). *Cardiovascular Dynamics,* 3rd edn, ch. 7. Philadelphia; Saunders

Rushmer, R. F., Smith, O. A., Jr. and Lasker, E. P. (1960). 'Neural Mechanisms of Cardiac Control during Exertion.' *Physiol. Rev.* **40** (Suppl. 4), 27

Simonson, E. (1971). *Physiology of Work Capacity and Fatigue.* Springfield, Ill.; Charles C. Thomas

Vatner, S. F. (1975). 'Effects of Exercise on Distribution of Regional Blood Flows and Resistances.' In Zelis, R., *The Peripheral Circulations.* New York; Grune and Stratton

Wade, O. L. and Bishop, J. M. (1962). *Cardiac Output and Regional Blood Flow.* Oxford; Blackwell

Chapter 8   The Circulation and General Anaesthesia

General anaesthesia represents a more or less severe departure from the body's normal physiological state and may be accompanied by marked departures from normality of several important cardiovascular parameters. The causation of these abnormalities is complex and depends on the interaction of many individual factors, which may act either in opposition or in concord. It has been aptly remarked that general anaesthetics have general actions on the body (Price, 1961): they act not only on the central nervous system, but have also a number of actions on other bodily systems. Some of the most important of these 'side effects' are on the heart and circulation.

All the commonly-used general anaesthetic agents, with the possible exception of nitrous oxide, have a depressant action on the myocardium and peripheral vascular bed (Moffitt and Sessler, 1964). Although the extent of this depression varies with the agent under consideration, there is, in general, a close correlation between the potency of a given agent as an anaesthetic and its depressant effects on the cardiovascular system.

The situation is complicated, however, by the fact that the direct cardiovascular depression is antagonized, to an extent which varies with the agent under consideration, by homeostatic mechanisms such as increased sympathetic stimulation to the heart and blood vessels, and increased adrenal catecholamine secretion. During light anaesthesia with ether, and particularly with cyclopropane, cardiac output may be normal or even above normal because, under these circumstances, there is a marked increase of sympathetic activity; during light halothane anaesthesia, however, cardiac output may be severely reduced, because the administration of this agent is accompanied by little compensatory sympathetic activity. With deepening anaesthesia, the body's homeostatic mechanisms may become obtunded, and cardiac output may then be decreased even with agents such as ether or cyclopropane.

Para-anaesthetic agents

The function of the cardiovascular system is affected also by drugs which are given as adjuvants to the main anaesthetic agent. Potent analgesics such as morphine and phenoperidine may cause circulatory depression, or may potentiate the cardiovascular effects of general anaesthetic agents. Cardiac output during cyclopropane anaesthesia in unpremedicated patients is often above normal, whereas after the administration of morphine it is usually reduced (Li and Etsten, 1957). Conversely the administration of large doses of morphine

(2 mg kg^{-1}) with controlled ventilation with oxygen causes an increase of cardiac output and peripheral vasodilatation (Wong et al., 1973).

Muscle relaxants also have effects on the cardiovascular system; and these effects must be taken into account when considering cardiovascular regulation during general anaesthesia (*see* later).

Blood gas tensions

In addition to the effects of anaesthetic and para-anaesthetic agents, it is necessary to consider also the effect on the cardiovascular system of abnormalities of arterial blood gas tensions. With modern anaesthetic techniques serious reductions of arterial oxygen tension are less likely to occur than formerly; but abnormalities of arterial P_{CO_2} and pH are of almost universal occurrence. During spontaneous ventilation there is often a significant respiratory acidosis, even in the absence of airway obstruction; and during artificial ventilation Pa_{CO_2} is almost always below normal, because of excessive alveolar ventilation in the presence of reduced whole body carbon dioxide production.

Surgical stimulation

Finally, the cardiovascular response to surgical stimulation must be considered. Traction on peritoneal ligaments may cause cardiovascular depression and a severe reduction of cardiac output. Conversely, painful stimuli, particularly those from superficial tissues, may, during light anaesthesia, cause increased sympathetic stimulation and increased cardiac output.

CATECHOLAMINE RELEASE AND SYMPATHETIC ACTIVITY DURING GENERAL ANAESTHESIA

It has been known for more than half a century that the administration of certain anaesthetic agents, both to man and experimental animals, is accompanied by increased sympathetic activity and increased catecholamine secretion by the adrenal medullae. The extent of this increased sympathetic activity varies greatly with the agent under consideration. Ether and cyclopropane, for example, are accompanied by marked sympatho-adrenal activity, whereas the reverse is the case with halothane. An increase of Pa_{CO_2} may also cause increased sympathetic activity.

It is uncertain whether the sympathetic overactivity which accompanies general anaesthesia with certain agents is due to direct stimulation of the autonomic-nervous system or to the body's response to circulatory depression. The administration of ether to a headless animal, however, is said to cause increased sympathetic activity which suggests that part at least of the response is due to direct stimulation. The same interpretation may be placed on the fact that cyclopropane abolishes the depressor response normally initiated by carotid sinus stimulation.

Ether

Elliott (1912) showed, in animals, that ether anaesthesia was accompanied by a diminution of the pressor activity of adrenal medullary extracts, and that this depletion could be prevented by splanchnic nerve section. Price (1957) showed in man during laparotomy under ether anaesthesia, that adrenaline entered the circulation at a rate of approximately 0.5 μg min^{-1} and noradrenaline at approximately 4 μg min^{-1}. The ratio of adrenaline to noradrenaline secreted by the human adrenal is approximately 4 : 1 (von Euler, 1954), therefore the majority of the sympathetic amines found by Price was presumably derived from sympathetically-innervated tissues other than the adrenal medullae. It is recognized clinically that the administration of ether may cause peripheral gangrene in patients who have sympathectomized (and therefore catecholamine-sensitized) extremities (Felder et al., 1951). This is presumably a result of vasoconstriction induced by circulating catecholamines.

More recently Millar and Biscoe (1965, 1966) have shown that there is increased pre- and postganglionic sympathetic activity during ether anaesthesia in the rabbit.

Cyclopropane

Cyclopropane also causes depletion of adrenal medullary catecholamines (Elmes and Jefferson, 1942). In 1959 Price and his colleagues demonstrated that cyclopropane anaesthesia in man is accompanied by an increased plasma catecholamine concentration roughly proportional to the alveolar cyclopropane concentration of anaesthetic agent. Increased sympathetic activity has also been directly demonstrated by Millar and Biscoe (Millar and Biscoe, 1965; Biscoe and Millar, 1966b).

Although the rate of disappearance of exogenous noradrenaline is less than normal during cyclopropane anaesthesia, this decrease is not sufficient to account for the greatly increased plasma noradrenaline levels which have been found experimentally under these circumstances. Indeed Ngai, Diaz and Ozer (1969) showed that the uptake and retention of intravenously-injected tritiated noradrenaline during cyclopropane anaesthesia was normal.

It has also been shown by Price and Price (1962) that the action of adrenaline on strips of isolated rabbit aorta is enhanced by cyclopropane, suggesting that part of its hypertensive action is due to a direct action on vascular smooth muscle.

Halothane

In contrast to what happens with ether and cyclopropane, halothane anaesthesia appears to abolish the normal sympatho-adrenal response to arterial hypotension and respiratory acidosis. Administration of this agent is not accompanied by elevation of plasma catecholamine levels even during profound hypotension (Price et al., 1959). Indeed it is the lack of adrenal medullary response during halothane anaesthesia which makes this a valuable agent for use in patients with phaeochromocytomas (Etsten and Shimosato, 1965).

This is not to say, however, that sympathetic activity is completely in abeyance during halothane anaesthesia. It has been shown that ganglion blockade enhances the circulatory depression which normally accompanies halothane anaesthesia (Severinghaus and Cullen, 1958). In addition, Millar and Biscoe (1965, 1966) have demonstrated sympathetic activity in both pre- and postganglionic sympathetic neurones during halothane anaesthesia, although the clinical significance of this finding is uncertain because some at least of their experimental animals were profoundly hypotensive at the time of measurement.

It has also been suggested that the apparent lack of sympathetic activity during halothane anaesthesia is partly due to the fact that this agent antagonizes the peripheral actions of noradrenaline on both smooth and cardiac muscle.

Despite the fact that halothane is usually thought to cause ganglion blockade (Raventós, 1961), Biscoe and Millar (1966b) found that, in this respect, it did not appear to be more potent than cyclopropane or ether. It appears therefore that part at least of the marked circulatory depression which accompanies halothane anaesthesia is due to its depressant action on the heart and (perhaps) vascular smooth muscle. Black and McArdle (1962) found that halothane decreased vascular responsiveness to intravenously-infused noradrenaline. Also, it has recently been demonstrated by Millar et al. (1969) that, in the cat, halothane may reduce preganglionic sympathetic activity (as compared with the increase previously found by these workers).

Is sympathetic overactivity beneficial?

The sympathetic overactivity which is induced by some agents is probably advantageous since it counteracts their primary depressant action on the cardiovascular system, and maintains the circulation in a relatively normal state. Excessive sympathetic activity may, however, be accompanied by ventricular dysrhythmias (*see* page 196). The high therapeutic index (lethal dose: anaesthetic dose) possessed by cyclopropane is probably due to the sympathetic stimulation which it causes and to the way in which it enhances the response of peripheral tissues to sympathetic activity. It should be noted, however, that, although arterial blood pressure may be normal during cyclopropane anaesthesia, it is so only at the expense of arteriolar constriction: despite a relatively normal blood pressure, cardiac output is often decreased to a greater or lesser extent, particularly at higher anaesthetic concentrations.

Effect of general anaesthesia on the baroreceptor reflex

In the past decade various workers, in particular Millar, have investigated the effect on various anaesthetic agents on the baroreceptor reflexes. For obvious reasons, these techniques must be limited to lower animals; but the results are of interest, although their application to intact man must clearly be made with caution.

Anaesthetic agents appear, in general, to sensitize the baroreceptor nerve endings. At a given arterial pressure the action potential frequency in the afferent fibres from the carotid sinus is increased by inhalation of various anaesthetics. This effect has been demonstrated with ether, trichlorethylene and chloroform (Robertson, Swan and Whitteridge, 1956), cyclopropane (Price and Widdicombe, 1962), and halothane (Biscoe and Millar, 1964).

Other things being equal, such sensitization would be expected to cause marked cardiovascular depression with bradycardia and hypotension. However, electrical stimulation of afferent baroreceptor nerves and simultaneous recording of preganglionic efferent sympathetic activity reveals a progressive depression of central transmission during administration of increasing concentrations of cyclopropane, ether and halothane (Biscoe and Millar, 1966a), the effect being most marked with cyclopropane, less so with halothane, and minimal or non-existent with nitrous oxide. By removing the inhibitory effects of afferent baroreceptor impulses such depression of central transmission might be expected to cause increased efferent sympathetic activity, as is in fact the case with some anaesthetic agents (*see* above).

CARDIAC FUNCTION DURING ANAESTHESIA

The difficulties involved in measuring myocardial contractility—that is the inherent ability of the myocardium to convert chemical into mechanical energy—have been considered elsewhere (*see* page 47). However, despite these difficulties there is little doubt that most commonly-used agents cause myocardial depression, whether this is measured with the isolated heart-lung preparation (*see* below), or by more sophisticated techniques such as determination of the myocardial force-velocity curve (*see* page 45). In many cases, however, the primary depressant action of the anaesthetic agent is counteracted partially or completely by the sympatho-adrenal overactivity which accompanies some forms of general anaesthesia.

Whether a given degree of myocardial depression results in a decrease of cardiac output depends on the simultaneous state of the peripheral circulation. As shown by Prys-Roberts and Gersh (Prys-Roberts et al., 1972b; Gersh et al., 1972) halothane causes myocardial depression, but at normal levels of Pco_2 little or no peripheral vasodilatation. The weakened heart is therefore required to eject blood against a normal peripheral resistance; and, as a result, the cardiac output, and to some extent the arterial pressure, falls. (This is particularly likely to occur in hypertensive patients in whom the systemic vascular resistance is abnormally high—*see* page 243). Reduction of $Paco_2$ causes an increase of systemic vascular resistance, and the greater load which this imposes on the halothane-weakened heart causes a further reduction of cardiac output. Myocardial contractility is little affected by hypocapnia (Foëx and Prys-Roberts, 1975).

Conversely, hypercapnia causes peripheral vasodilatation, with an increased cardiac output due mainly to the decreased load presented to the heart (Prys-Roberts et al., 1968).

Brown and Crout (1971), using the isolated cat papillary muscle, investigated the effect of various anaesthetic agents on myocardial contractility. The different agents all depressed myocardial contractility in a qualitatively similar manner; but the degree of myocardial depression with equipotent anaesthetic doses of the different agents was not the same, the order being halothane > methoxyflurane > cyclopropane > diethyl ether. Administration of propranolol had no effect, a finding which suggests that the observed differences were not due to β-adrenergic stimulation, as some workers have suggested.

The heart-lung preparation is useful for demonstrating primary myocardial depression, because the heart is completely denervated and isolated from the effects of circulating hormones produced in other regions of the body. All the commonly-used general anaesthetic agents cause depression of the heart-lung preparation, that is, a decrease of cardiac output at a given right atrial pressure (Price and Helrich, 1955; Flacke and Alper, 1962).

Myocardial function during anaesthesia has also been investigated by use of the Walton–Brodie strain-gauge arch; but for the reasons given in Chapter 2 (*see* page 46) this technique is now used less commonly than in the past. It does, however, have the advantage that it may be used in man when the bridge may be temporarily sutured to the surface of the heart exposed at thoracotomy. With this technique, for example, Boniface, Brown and Kronen (1955) found a progressive decrease of ventricular contractile force with increasing depth of anaesthesia during the administration of ether, cyclopropane or chloroform. During light anaesthesia with agents such as ether or cyclopropane, which cause marked sympathetic activity, there was often an increase of contractile force, indicating that the compensatory sympathetic overactivity was greater than the primary myocardial depression (*see* above). Mahaffey et al. (1961) showed that the administration of halothane, in a concentration greater than 1.2 per cent progressively decreased myocardial contractile force in both dogs and patients. Even nitrous oxide may cause myocardial depression; Craythorne and Darby (1965) showed that the contractile force of the canine right ventricle was decreased by the administration of this agent, even in a concentration as low as 50-75 per cent.

Ventricular function curves

Determination of ventricular function curves (Sarnoff, 1955), that is, the relationship between ventricular stroke work and mean atrial pressure, gives information about cardiac function in the relatively intact animal. The results must, however, be interpreted with some care (*see* below). This technique is particularly valuable because it gives information about the individual function of the two ventricles. It has been used both in patients (Price et al., 1962) and in experimental animals.

Etsten and Li (1962) investigated the effects of ether and cyclopropane on ventricular function in closed-chest and otherwise unmedicated dogs. They found that light anaesthesia with both agents was accompanied by movement of the ventricular function curve upwards and to the left; that is, the ventricle was able to perform more work at a given atrial pressure than in the unanaesthetized state. These functional changes were similar to those induced by stimulation of the stellate ganglion.

Deep ether anaesthesia caused a marked depression of the left, but not of the right, ventricular function curve. This might be interpreted as evidence that ether depresses the left ventricle, but has little effect on the right ventricle. Other techniques, however, such as measurement of myocardial force by a Walton– Brodie strain-gauge arch, suggest that this agent depresses both ventricles equally.

The answer to this paradox lies in the fact that stroke work depends on the product of stroke volume and mean arterial pressure; a decrease of arterial pressure at constant stroke volume must cause a decrease of ventricular stroke work. During deep ether anaesthesia there is a decrease of systemic, but not of pulmonary vascular resistance; therefore ether anaesthesia is accompanied by a corresponding decrease of left ventricular stroke work. In contrast, pulmonary arterial pressure remains relatively constant, as does right ventricular stroke work. Etsten and Shimosato (1964) showed that, if the systemic arterial resistance was artficially restored to normal, the left ventricular function curve moved upwards and to the left until the curves of the two ventricles did not differ significantly.

Cyclopropane causes little depression of either ventricle, even at high concentrations (Etsten and Li, 1962). This appears to be due to the fact that, during this form of anaesthesia, systemic arterial blood pressure is normal or even raised, therefore there is not the apparent depression of left ventricular function which occurs at the same depth of anaesthesia with ether.

Shimosato, Li and Etsten (1963) showed that halothane depresses the function of both ventricles and, as with ether, the decrease of left ventricular stroke work is associated with a decrease of mean aortic pressure. During halothane anaesthesia, however, artificial restoration of arterial pressure does not completely restore ventricular function to normal.

CARDIAC OUTPUT DURING ANAESTHESIA

Regulation of cardiac output is a complex subject. As explained in Chapter 4, cardiac output depends on the interrelationship between the state of the peripheral circulation and the efficiency of the cardiac pump, although normally the peripheral circulation is the more important factor (Guyton, 1968). General anaesthesia affects both factors to an extent which depends on the depth of anaesthesia, the agent(s) being used, the level of $P\text{CO}_2$, and the adjuvant drugs.

A knowledge of the probable cardiac output is of considerable practical importance to the anaesthetist, if for no other reason than that a change of output affects the rate of uptake or elimination of gaseous anaesthetic agents (*see* page 207).

Changes of cardiac output must, however, be considered also in relation to the perfusion needs of the body as a whole. There is a natural tendency to assume that, if cardiac output is reduced, some tissues must be ischaemic and therefore deprived of essential nutrients. This is not necessarily the case, because what is important is not the absolute blood flow, but the relationship between a tissue's metabolic needs and the rate at which these are supplied by the blood. During some modes of general anaesthesia, for example, cardiac output may be considerably reduced below what would be appropriate for a conscious resting subject; but the body's oxygen consumption is reduced in proportion, and there is, therefore, no true perfusion defect. Under these circumstances the oxygen content of the mixed-venous blood is normal. Alternatively, under other circumstances, the fall of cardiac output may outstrip the reduction of whole body oxygen consumption, so that the oxygen content difference between arterial and mixed-venous blood is greater than normal, indicating that the patient is suffering from stagnant hypoxia.

Despite the marked falls of cardiac output which accompany some forms of general anaesthesia (Prys-Roberts et al., 1968), there is little evidence that the body is harmed by such departure from normality. To the physiologist, however, it would seem logical to place the onus on the anaesthetist to demonstrate conclusively that he is not harming his patient when he deliberately induces a more or less severe departure from the normal physiological state (*see also* Blenkarn et al., 1975). (It should also be remembered in this context, that respiratory alkalosis may cause considerable reductions of cerebral blood flow (*see* page 139), and there is some evidence that cerebral metabolism may be impaired during hyperventilation. Cohen et al. (1968) found that the pattern of cerebral metabolism during extreme hyperventilation ($P_{CO_2} < 20$ mm Hg) was similar to that found in the presence of indisputable cerebral hypoxia; *see also* page 140).

Studies on normal volunteers

Since the first edition of this book a group of investigators in California has made a series of very carefully controlled measurements of the cardiovascular effects of various inhalational anaesthetic agents. These findings are valuable in that they apply to a controlled situation: constant deep body temperature, constant arterial P_{CO_2}, no additional drugs, no surgical stimulation, and so on. But they must, of course, be extrapolated with care to actual clinical situations, where anaesthetics are perforce given in a less carefully-controlled manner, where premedication and/or surgical stimuli may modify the body's responses, and where the patient may be less fit than the young normal adults studied by the Californian workers.

Except where stated otherwise the following paragraphs refer to findings during the first hour of anaesthesia. These findings are summarized in

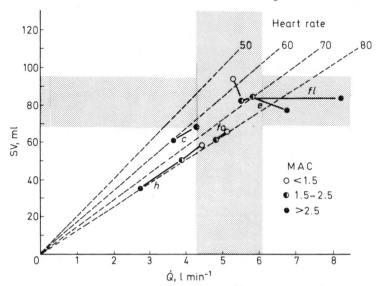

Figure 8.1. Relationship between cardiac output ($\dot{Q}$) and stroke volume during anaesthesia with halothane (h), cyclopropane (c), isoflurane (fo), diethyl ether (e), and fluroxene (fl). Shaded bands, range of values found in same subjects before induction of anaesthesia

Figures 8.1, 8.2 and *8.3*, which are based on the following papers: Cullen, Eger and Gregory (1969a, b), Cullen et al. (1970), Eger et al. (1970), Gregory et al. (1971), and Stevens et al. (1971). In preparing these Figures, experimentally-determined cardiac outputs and whole-body oxygen consumptions have been

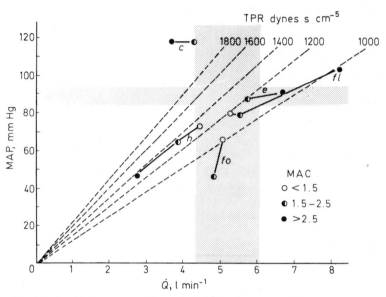

Figure 8.2. *Relationship between cardiac output ($\dot{Q}$) and mean arterial pressure (MAP) with different anaesthetic agents. (Symbols and shaded bands have same significance as in Figure 8.1)*

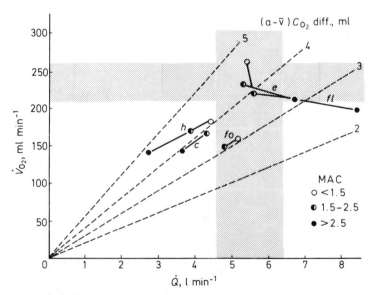

Figure 8.3. *Relationship between cardiac output ($\dot{Q}$) and whole body oxygen consumption ($\dot{V}_{O_2}$) with different anaesthetic agents. (Symbols and shaded bands have same significance as in Figure 8.1)*

normalized to a body weight of 70 kg. The shaded bands show the range of values found in the same subjects before induction of anaesthesia. The MAC values used were based on those found by Saidman et al. (1967), and are therefore to some extent arbitrary, although doubtless of the right order of magnitude.

Halothane caused a significant depression of cardiac output, even during light anaesthesia; and this depression became greater as anaesthesia was deepened. Cyclopropane caused no depression of cardiac output with light anaesthesia, but some depression at deeper levels. The ethers, diethyl ether and fluroxene, caused little change of cardiac output with light anaesthesia, and significant *increases* at deeper levels. Isoflurane caused minimal depression of cardiac output at any level of anaesthesia.

In the main these changes of cardiac output were due to changes of stroke volume, rather than to changes of heart rate, although there was tachycardia at the deeper levels of anaesthesia with ether, and particularly fluroxene.

Systemic vascular resistance was increased even at light levels of anaesthesia with cyclopropane, causing a marked increase in blood pressure. With halothane, ether, and fluroxene peripheral resistance remained roughly constant, and mean arterial pressure therefore varied as the cardiac output. With isoflurane the systemic vascular resistance was markedly reduced at deeper levels of anaesthesia, resulting in a decrease of arterial pressure of roughly the same magnitude as that found with halothane.

With isoflurane and cyclopropane whole-body oxygen consumption was reduced roughly in proportion to the decrease in cardiac output; with halothane the decrease in oxygen consumption was proportionately rather greater, with some widening of the $(a-\bar{v})$ oxygen content difference; and with ether and fluroxene the decrease was rather less, resulting in a decrease of the $(a-\bar{v})$ oxygen difference.

All agents caused an increase of skin blood flow at the lighter levels of anaesthesia. As anaesthesia was deepened, however, the flow returned to normal levels with fluroxene and halothane, but remained increased with cyclopropane and ether. No agent except isoflurane caused much alteration of muscle blood flow at light levels of anaesthesia; halothane however, caused a consistent decrease of muscle flow with increasing depth of anaesthesia.

In general, right atrial pressure was increased with all these agents, more so at the deeper levels of anaesthesia.

Except in the case of isoflurane it was found that prolongation of anaesthesia to beyond four hours resulted in an increase of cardiac output compared with its value after one hour's anaesthesia. This finding was particularly dramatic in the case of fluroxene, where cardiac output at the end of four hours' anaesthesia had roughly twice its control (conscious) value. There were accompanying decreases of right atrial pressure suggesting that the output changes were due to improved cardiac function. At the present time there seems to be no satisfactory explanation for this finding which, although perhaps not of great clinical importance, adds another dimension—that of duration of anaesthesia—to the problems of interpreting cardiac output measurements made during general anaesthesia.

The same workers (Smith et al., 1970) investigated the cardiovascular effects of adding 70 per cent nitrous oxide to a halothane/oxygen anaesthetic mixture, as is, of course, common clinical practice. The addition caused an increase of arterial blood pressure, with an increased peripheral resistance and decreased forearm blood flow; cardiac output was unchanged. There were signs of increased sympathetic activity with pupillary dilatation and increased plasma noradrenaline levels. In a control experiment in which 70 per cent nitrogen was added to the halothane/oxygen mixture the cardiovascular changes were minimal, a finding which suggests that nitrous oxide has a genuine pharmacological effect on the cardiovascular system.

It is not at all easy to be dogmatic about the clinical importance of these findings. Of the five agents investigated halothane caused by far the greatest decrease of cardiac output, together with an increase of the (a–v̄) oxygen content difference; and arterial blood pressure, particularly at the deeper levels of anaesthesia, were severely depressed. But, as Eger, Smith and Cullen (1971) point out, these changes were accompanied by no evidence of impaired cardiac metabolism (normal ECG), nor of whole body underperfusion (no metabolic acidosis). Indeed, they said: 'the greater reduction in myocardial work with halothane may make it the anaesthetic of choice for patients with impaired coronary perfusion'. Conversely, they also point out that 'the better maintenance of pressure and perfusion relative to consumption with the other agents suggests greater safety when organs other than the heart have limited perfusion'.

Perhaps the most interesting of these results are those obtained with isoforane. This agent caused a marked decrease of arterial blood pressure without causing a concomitant decrease of cardiac output, although there was probably some tissue underperfusion because a larger proportion of the total flow was directed to the skin and muscles than before induction of anaesthesia. There was also very little evidence of cardiac depression with this agent, as indicated by no increase of right atrial pressure nor change of ballistocardiogram amplitude; this finding is, of course, in marked contrast to what happens with halothane.

Earlier investigations

Ether

Clinical anaesthesia with ether produces no consistent change of cardiac output (Kubota, Schweiger and Vandam, 1962; Jones et al., 1962), although there is little evidence of cardiovascular depression, and some patients in these studies had outputs above the normal range. At deeper levels of anaesthesia, ether induces an increase of heart rate, perhaps due in part to vagal blockade, which is not, however, complete because atropine causes a further tachycardia to approximately 150 beats min^{-1}.

In man, central venous and pulmonary artery pressures are increased during ether anaesthesia (Johnson, 1951). This increase of pulmonary artery pressure is said to cause, on occasion, reversal of shunt blood flow through a patent interventricular septum.

Ether decreases limb blood flow, and increases limb vascular resistance, especially at deeper levels of anaesthesia. But although the arterial pressure is usually normal, or even above normal, during light ether anaesthesia there is often hypertension at deeper levels, indicating that (despite the increased circulating noradrenaline concentrations) the vasoconstriction is not generalized.

The studies of Price and Price (1962) showed that ether depresses the responsiveness of the vascular smooth muscle to noradrenaline.

Cyclopropane

Cyclopropane increases cardiac output at low concentrations and decreases it at higher concentrations (Jones et al., 1960). There is, in addition, an increase of total peripheral resistance, which accounts for the mild to moderate hypertension commonly found during this form of anaesthesia, particularly if there is CO_2 retention. At deeper levels of anaesthesia this increase of peripheral resistance prevents development of hypotension despite the decrease of cardiac output. Cardiac rate is normal except following the administration of atropine when, as with ether, there is marked tachycardia due to sympathetic overactivity.

Cyclopropane is similar to ether in that its administration is accompanied by an increase of right atrial and pulmonary arterial pressures.

Halothane

The values of cardiac output which have been found during halothane anaesthesia by different investigators vary considerably. Payne, Gardiner and Verner (1959) found no change during the administration of 2 per cent halothane, whereas Severinghaus and Cullen (1958) found an approximately 30 per cent reduction with an inspired halothane concentration of 1.5 per cent. These differences may be due in part to the method used to induce anaesthesia: cardiac output appears to be less when anaesthesia is induced with thiopentone than when it is induced with halothane alone. An even more important factor is, however, inconsistency of blood gas tensions (*see* page 191).

The general consensus of opinion seems to be that, at normal carbon dioxide tensions, cardiac output is reduced to a greater or lesser extent by halothane. Prys-Roberts et al. (1968) found that the mean output during 1 per cent halothane anaesthesia (after induction with thiopentone 150–250 mg) was $3.32 \, l \, min^{-1} \, 70 \, kg^{-1}$ body weight at a Pa_{CO_2} of 47.7 mm Hg (spontaneous ventilation) and $3.10 \, l \, min^{-1} \, 70 \, kg^{-1}$ body weight at a Pa_{CO_2} of 43.3 mm Hg (artificial ventilation, normal mean intrathoracic pressure).

The decrease of cardiac output which accompanies the administration of halothane is, however, not in itself sufficient to account for the marked systemic hypotension found during this form of anaesthesia. There is also a reduction of systemic vascular resistance (Deutsch et al., 1962).

With the passage of time, cardiac output tends to return towards normal, but the systemic resistance remains low as, to a lesser extent, does the arterial blood pressure. The cause of this gradual improvement of cardiac output is not clear. It does not appear to be due entirely to changes of plasma volume consequent on arterial hypotension, although it is known that there is, in general, an inverse relationship between plasma volume and intravascular pressure (Price, Helrich and Conner, 1956).

The decrease of systemic peripheral resistance during halothane anaesthesia is attributed by most workers to diminution of sympathetic tone to the resistance vessels. This decreased tone appears to be due partly, but not entirely, to ganglion blockade (Enderby, 1960). In addition, it has been suggested that halothane antagonizes the peripheral action of sympathomimetic amines (Burn, 1959). There is also evidence that it stimulates β-adrenergic receptors (Klide, 1966); such stimulation would induce vasodilatation in certain organs, thus lowering the total peripheral resistance.

Although there may be a reduction of total peripheral resistance during halothane anaesthesia, the response of patients to pressor drugs is disappointing. This is mainly due to the fact that vasoconstriction induced by these agents increases the load on a myocardium which is already depressed by halothane, so that there may be no increase, or even a decrease, of cardiac output (*see also* page 116). Although the administration of vasopressor agents may be accompanied by an improvement of arterial blood pressure, it may not be accompanied by a corresponding improvement of tissue perfusion (*see* Chapter 9).

Heart rate is generally slow during halothane anaesthesia, and is usually increased by the administration of atropine. This increase of rate may be accompanied by an increase of arterial pressure. It is not, however, nearly as marked as during anaesthesia with ether or cyclopropane. Occasionally, marked bradycardia may occur during light halothane anaesthesia; this appears to be due to sensitization of cardiac receptors to parasympathetic stimulation. Halothane may also stimulate parasympathetic activity by a central action (Price, Linde and Morse, 1963).

Short-acting barbiturates

It is well recognized clinically that intravenous injection of short-acting barbiturates may cause a marked fall of arterial blood pressure, particularly when the injection is made relatively rapidly. Prys-Roberts et al. (1971b) showed that a hypotensive response is particularly likely to occur in untreated hypertensive patients (*see* page 247). In a comparison between thiopentone and methohexitone in normal clinical dosage, Dundee and Moore (1961) showed that the fall in blood pressure on induction of anaesthesia was greater with thiopentone.

The main cause of arterial hypotension following intravenous barbiturates is almost certainly an acute reduction of cardiac output consequent on a reduction of myocardial contractile strength. The depressant effect of thiopentone on the isolated heart-lung preparation was shown by Prime and Gray (1952) and by Price and Helrich (1955). Its effect on intact humans has been investigated by many workers, e.g. Flickinge et al. (1961) who found a fall of cardiac output from $5.85 \, \mathrm{l \, min^{-1}}$ to $4.57 \, \mathrm{l \, min^{-1}}$ immediately after induction of anaesthesia with thiopentone (100–400 mg); arterial blood pressure was, however, relatively well maintained by a simultaneous (presumably reflex) increase of total peripheral resistance from 1375 dyne s $\mathrm{cm^{-5}}$ to 1630 dyne s $\mathrm{cm^{-5}}$. Rowlands et al. (1967) found a somewhat smaller reduction of cardiac output after administration of methohexitone ($1.2 \, \mathrm{mg \, kg^{-1}}$).

The effects of these drugs on the peripheral circulation are unclear, but it is likely that high circulating concentrations may cause peripheral vasodilatation by a direct effect on the resistance vessels and may so accentuate the hypotension (Sankawa, 1965). They also cause dilatation of the peripheral capacitance vessels (Watson, Seelye and Smith, 1962), but the decrease of 'venous return' (*see* page 117) caused by this mechanism is probably not significant in relation to the decrease of cardiac output, which is almost certainly due mainly to a reduced myocardial contractility.

There is little catecholamine secretion during thiopentone anaesthesia; thiopentone appears to resemble halothane in blocking normal sympathetic activity.

RESPIRATORY ACIDOSIS

It has been known for at least 50 years that anaesthesia with ether, chloroform or nitrous oxide may cause acidosis. It was not until 1925, however, that Koehler showed that the increased hydrogen ion concentration was due to carbon dioxide retention, rather than to accumulation of non-volatile acids. Since that time there have been many reports of respiratory acidosis during anaesthesia with most of the commonly-used agents. For example, Ivanov, Waddy and Jennings (1967) found that Pa_{CO_2} rose, on average, to 57 mm Hg during routine halothane anaesthesia, while in individual patients it could be as high as 70 mm Hg.

Effects of hypercapnia

The effects of carbon dioxide on the cardiovascular system are complex. Hypercapnia appears to cause direct depression of both cardiac muscle and

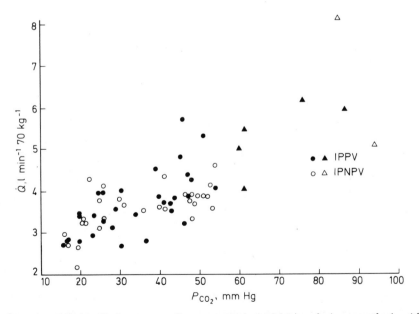

Figure 8.4. Relationship between cardiac output and arterial P_{CO_2} during anaesthesia with 70 per cent nitrous oxide in oxygen during intermittent positive pressure ventilation (IPPV) and intermittent positive-negative pressure ventilation (IPNPV)

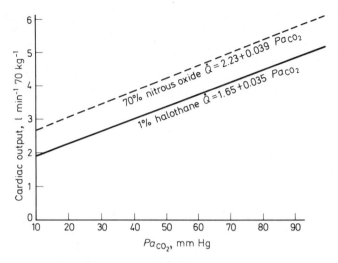

Figure 8.5. Regression lines relating cardiac output and Pa_{CO_2} during anaesthesia with 1 per cent halothane or 70 per cent nitrous oxide in oxygen

Table   8.1 SLOPE   OF   CARDIAC   INDEX/Pa_{CO_2} RELATIONSHIP   DURING ANAESTHESIA WITH DIFFERENT INHALATIONAL ANAESTHETICS (FIGURES FROM CULLEN AND EGER, 1974)

Anaesthetic agent	Cardiac index/Pa_{CO_2} (ml mm Hg^{-1})	Reference
None	95	Cullen and Eger (1974)
Halothane 1%	23	Prys-Roberts et al. (1967)
Isoflurane 1.8%	48	Cromwell et al. (1971)
Cyclopropane 25–30%	51	Cullen, Eger and Gregory (1969b)
Fluroxene 9%	65	Cullen et al. (1971)

vascular smooth muscle but, at the same time, it causes reflex stimulation of the sympatho-adrenal system, which compensates to a greater or lesser extent for the primary cardiovascular depression. The situation is, therefore, very analogous to the way in which the cardiovascular depression of some general anaesthetic agents may be diminished or abolished by a compensatory increase of sympathetic activity (*see* page 179).

Price and Helrich (1955) showed that an increase of Pa_{CO_2} depressed the isolated canine heart. A fall of 0.5 pH units (corresponding to an increase of hydrogen ion concentration of approximately 300 per cent) caused a 50 per cent reduction of myocardial contractile force. Bouckaert and Leusen (1951) showed that an increase of CO_2 tension increased sympathetic activity, and Tenney (1960) demonstrated that it increased the rate of catecholamine secretion from the adrenal medulla.

In conscious subjects elevation of arterial P_{CO_2} causes increased myocardial contractility and cardiac output, with a decrease of systemic vascular resistance (Cullen and Eger, 1974). During anaesthesia there is a roughly linear relationship between Pa_{CO_2} and cardiac output (*Figures 8.4* and *8.5*); but the slope of this relationship depends on the depth of anaesthesia, and the agent under consideration (*see Table 8.1*).

Conversely, during respiratory alkalosis sympathetic activity appears to be reduced. Moster et al. (1969) showed, in dogs, that the rate of spontaneous postganglionic sympathetic activity during nitrous oxide anaesthesia was reduced by hypocapnia, even though Pa_{O_2} and arterial blood pressure were unchanged.

ARTIFICIAL VENTILATION

Many workers have demonstrated a decrease of cardiac output during artificial ventilation, but they have often failed to distinguish adequately between the effects of changes of Pa_{CO_2} and of changes of intrathoracic pressure, both of which may occur simultaneously. An increase of intrathoracic pressure may, for the reasons considered in Chapter 4, page 117, impede the flow of blood back to the heart, and so reduce cardiac output. Fortunately, the body is able to compensate, at least partly, for this increased pressure, although there is little doubt that the use of an excessive inflation pressure or of an unphysiological inspiration:expiration ratio may reduce cardiac output during intermittent positive pressure ventilation (IPPV). This is especially the case in patients with hypovolaemia or ganglion blockade.

Artificial ventilation of the paralysed, anaesthetized patient is usually accompanied by respiratory alkalosis, because alveolar ventilation is excessive for the patient's reduced metabolic rate. Alveolar, and therefore arterial P_{CO_2}, is proportional to the quotient of the body's carbon dioxide production divided by its alveolar ventilation. Carbon dioxide production may be reduced during general anaesthesia because body temperature is sub-normal, or because the body's total energy requirements are reduced by muscular paralysis, or by a reduction of cardiac work. Mild hypothermia is especially liable to occur during long operations with open pleural or peritoneal cavities.

Respiratory alkalosis versus raised intrathoracic pressure

It is possible to investigate the effect of changes of Pa_{CO_2} during IPPV while maintaining intrathoracic pressure constant by the use of an appropriate degree of expiratory sub-atmospheric airway pressure.

Prys-Roberts et al. (1967) studied paralysed, artificially-ventilated patients anaesthetized with 70 per cent nitrous oxide. Mean intrathoracic pressure was maintained at the same level as during spontaneous ventilation, while Pa_{CO_2} was varied by changing the inspired carbon dioxide concentration. When no carbon dioxide was added to the inspired gas mixture the alveolar minute volume was sufficient to induce a moderate degree of hypocapnia. Under these conditions, the mean cardiac output was significantly reduced ($3.43 \ l \ min^{-1} \ 70 \ kg^{-1}$ body weight) below the value found when Pa_{CO_2} was normal ($3.86 \ l \ min^{-1} \ 70 \ kg^{-1}$).

At normal Pa_{CO_2}, however, there was no significant difference between cardiac output during intermittent positive pressure ventilation with a raised mean intrathoracic pressure ($4.09 \ l \ min^{-1} \ 70 \ kg^{-1}$ body weight) and with intermittent positive-negative pressure ventilation with a normal intrathoracic pressure ($3.86 \ l \ min^{-1} \ 70 \ kg^{-1}$). The maximum inflation pressure used by these workers was, however, limited to 30 cm H_2O, and the increase of mean intrathoracic pressure was only 4 cm H_2O.

Cardiac output was significantly greater during spontaneous ventilation (4.43 l min^{-1} 70 kg^{-1}) than during artificial ventilation with the same mean intrathoracic pressure and Pa_{CO_2} (4.09 l min^{-1} 70 kg^{-1}). This reduction of cardiac output was presumably due to decreased efficiency of the diaphragmatic pump (*see* page 123). During spontaneous ventilation, descent of the diaphragm is accompanied by an increase of abdominal pressure and a decrease of intrathoracic pressure. This pressure gradient helps to return blood to the heart. During artificial ventilation by intermittent airway pressure, however, diaphragmatic descent is accompanied by an increase of intrathoracic pressure, which tends to prevent the return of blood to the heart, thus leading to a reduction of cardiac output.

When Pa_{CO_2} was increased above normal there was a further increase of cardiac output with a roughly linear relationship between cardiac output and P_{CO_2} over a wide range of values of the latter variable (*Figure 8.4*). There is a similar linear relationship between cardiac output and Pa_{CO_2} during anaesthesia with 1 per cent halothane in oxygen (Prys-Roberts et al., 1968). (*Figure 8.5*).

The haemodynamic consequences of artificial ventilation have recently been reviewed by Conway (*see* Recommended Further Reading). In this article he points out that the inspiratory/expiratory ratio is of more importance in determining pulmonary blood flow than the shape of the pressure waveform (Adams et al., 1970).

Relationship between Pa_{O_2} and P_{CO_2}

Kelman and Prys-Roberts (1967) also found an interesting relationship between Pa_{O_2} and Pa_{CO_2} during halothane anaesthesia. When Pa_{CO_2} was raised there was an accompanying increase of Pa_{O_2} (*Figure 8.6*). A similar finding has been reported in anaesthetized dogs by Egli (1965). Although the precise explanation of this phenomenon is uncertain, Kelman et al. (1967) suggest that changes of mixed-venous oxygen content should theoretically cause changes of the alveolar-to-arterial (A—a) P_{O_2} difference, and therefore changes of Pa_{O_2}. An increase of cardiac output at constant whole-body oxygen consumption should be accompanied by an increase of mixed-venous oxygen content; the passage of this well-oxygenated blood through pulmonary shunts should then cause a decrease of the (A—a) P_{O_2} difference and a consequent increase of Pa_{O_2}. This mechanism, together with the linear relationship between Pa_{CO_2} and cardiac output described above, would account for the experimental findings shown in *Figure 8.5*.

This theory, of course, assumes that total body oxygen consumption is relatively independent of Pa_{CO_2}. Although there was considerable scatter of individual results, the mean calculated oxygen consumption found by Prys-Roberts et al. (1968)—*Figure 8.7*—was almost identical during hypocapnia, eucapnia and hypercapnia, suggesting that the proposed explanation is probably reasonable.

More recently a similar increase of Pa_{O_2} has been found to accompany the increase of cardiac output which occurs during laparoscopy (Kelman et al., 1972).

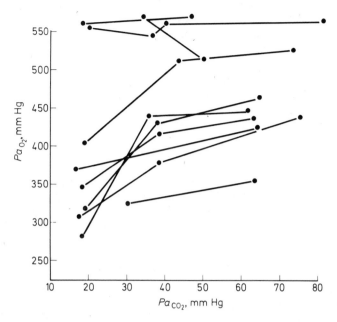

Figure 8.6. *Relationship between arterial Po₂ and Pco₂ in ten patients, anaesthetized with 1 per cent halothane in oxygen*

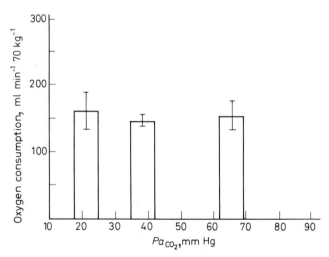

Figure 8.7. *Calculated oxygen consumption during hypocapnia, eucapnia and hypercapnia in ten patients anaesthetized with 1 per cent halothane in oxygen*

Valsalva manoeuvre

The effects of an increase of airway pressure on the cardiovascular system can conveniently be investigated by use of the Valsalva manoeuvre (Bernstein and Orkin, 1965). This technique not only gives information about the ability of the cardiovascular system to withstand an increase of intrathoracic pressure, but also about the integrity of various cardiovascular reflexes.

The essential features of the normal response (Hamilton, Woodbury and Harper, 1936) are, that the blood pressure does not fall appreciably during application of the positive airway pressure, being maintained by tachycardia and an increase of peripheral resistance; that the release of airway pressure is accompanied by a transient and rapid increase of arterial pressure as the heart ejects blood into a peripheral circulation which has momentarily an inappropriately high systemic vascular resistance; and that this transient hypertension is accompanied by a reflex bradycardia. A response which does not show these features is said to be 'blocked'.

Blackburn et al. (1973) found that the response in young patients was normal during halothane/nitrous oxide/oxygen anaesthesia even when the patients were given beta-blocking and ganglion-blocking drugs in a dosage sufficient to induce moderate arterial hypotension. The response was, however, blocked at deeper levels of anaesthesia. Scott, Slawson and Taylor (1969), on the other hand, found that it was consistently abnormal in anaesthetized patients who were old and/or 'ill'.

VENTRICULAR DYSRHYTHMIAS DURING GENERAL ANAESTHESIA

It has been known for many years that general anaesthesia with certain agents, chloroform in particular, may be accompanied by serious cardiac dysrhythmias, such as ventricular tachycardia or fibrillation. Understanding of the causation of such dysrhythmias is clearly of great importance to practising clinicians. Unfortunately, however, experimental investigation of this problem has proved unrewarding, and Price (1967) comments: 'This field suffers from two important disadvantages (1) results are not exactly duplicable from one day to the next, one investigator to another, between animals or even in the same animal as time passes; (2) the mechanisms involved are obscure and possibly numerous'. In other words, we just do not know what causes cardiac dysrhythmias during general anaesthesia.

Role of respiratory acidosis

It appears that, in the presence of a sensitizing agent, the development of cardiac dysrhythmias requires either injection of exogenous adrenaline or noradrenaline, or increased sympathetic nervous activity, or respiratory acidosis (the effects of which are probably also due to enhanced sympatho-adrenal activity—*see* page 192). Ventricular dysrhythmias which accompany respiratory acidosis in the experimental animal may be abolished by stellate ganglion block (Price et al., 1958).

The factors which influence the occurrence of ventricular dysrhythmias during human anaesthesia have been extensively studied during cyclopropane anaesthesia by Lurie et al. (1958), and by Black et al. (1959) who investigated the effects of halothane. In both cases spontaneous dysrhythmias rarely occurred in the absence of respiratory acidosis, while conversely there was a Pco_2 threshold, above which dysrhythmias always occurred. Dysrhythmias were, however, more difficult to induce in the presence of arterial hypotension. The dysrhythmic threshold to respiratory acidosis during halothane anaesthesia was a Pa_{CO_2} of 60–70 mm Hg, when arterial pressure was normal, and 85–140 mm Hg in the presence of pronounced arterial hypotension. During the administration of cyclopropane, which is commonly accompanied by an elevation of arterial pressure, the P_{CO_2} threshold was usually only slightly above 40 mm Hg.

Role of the vagi

Discussion of the pathogenesis of cardiac dysrhythmias during general anaesthesia is complicated also by uncertainty about the role played by the vagi. In the absence of sensitizing agents, neither the injection of adrenaline nor increased sympathetic activity causes cardiac irregularities unless the vagi are intact (Price, 1967); and if it is assumed, as Hoffman and Cranefield (1964) suggest, that abnormal rhythms arise from aberrant foci of spontaneous electrical activity distal to the S-A node, then it can be argued that parasympathetic activity is necessary to prevent the normal dominance of impulses generated by the normal pacemaker. During anaesthesia with a sensitizing agent, however, the abolition of parasympathetic activity by injection of atropine may actually induce dysrhythmias; under these circumstances the anaesthetic agent appears to take over whatever is the essential dysrhythmia-generating role of the parasympathetic system.

There is also evidence that ventricular dysrhythmias only appear when the heart rate is above a certain level (Vick, 1966). It may be, therefore, that the effect of vagal blockade is simply to increase heart rate above this critical level. It has been shown in dogs that adrenaline-induced dysrhythmias during cyclopropane anaesthesia may be converted to sinus rhythm by vagal stimulation.

Nature of Cardiac Sensitization

The sensitizing action of anaesthetic agents seems to be directly on the myocardium, because such sensitization has been demonstrated on the isolated heart-lung preparation (Fawex, 1951). Some agents are far more prone to induce dysrhythmias than others. Ether appears to be relatively innocuous; and the question therefore arises: in what way does ether differ from most other general anaesthetic agents? One marked difference which may be relevant is the fact that both chloroform and cyclopropane cause an increase of the ventricular refractory period, whereas ether has no such effect (Smith et al., 1962). Also it is known that chloroform increases the temporal dispersion of the recovery of myocardial excitability, and the consequent non-uniformity of excitability and conduction-velocity might be expected to favour the genesis of dysrhythmias.

In view of the putative role of sympatho-adrenal overactivity in the causation of ventricular dysrhythmias, many workers have recommended the prophylactic use of β-blockers such as propranolol. But although there appears to be little doubt of their effectiveness for this purpose (Johnstone, 1966), their mode of action is open to question because they appear to have local anaesthetic activity as well as being true β-blockers. Under most circumstances, dysrhythmias during general anaesthesia may be abolished by simpler and more physiological means, such as the prevention or correction of carbon dioxide retention or anaesthetic overdose.

REGIONAL BLOOD FLOW

The microcirculation

Studies by Baez, Zauder and Orkin (1962) on the microcirculation by the techniques described on page 82 have shown that light anaesthesia with ether, cyclopropane or halothane is accompanied by an increase of vasomotion (*see* page 92) of the precapillary sphincters, and by increased vascular sensitivity to topically-applied sympathomimetic amines. Deep anaesthesia with these agents is, however, accompanied by reduced vasomotion, by decreased vascular sensitivity to adrenaline, and, ultimately, by marked vascular dilatation. Methoxyfluorane depresses spontaneous vascular activity even during light anaesthesia.

Direct measurement of vascular calibre during light ether or cyclopropane anaesthesia shows that the arterioles, but not the venules, are constricted; with deepening anaesthesia, however, the arterioles return to normal, while the venules become dilated. In contrast, light halothane anaesthesia is accompanied by little change of arteriolar diameter, whereas deeper anaesthesia with this agent causes dilatation of both the pre- and post-capillary vessels.

In general, therefore, the microcirculatory response to general anaesthesia is in accord with what is known about the effect of different agents on sympathetic activity (*see* page 179). It is, however, difficult to be dogmatic about the functional significance of the observed changes. It could be argued that increased vasomotion of precapillary sphincters tends to divert blood from the true capillaries, and that if this response is excessive, capillary flow may become insufficient for the metabolic needs of the tissue. On the other hand, if the vessels become dilated, as they do during the deeper levels of anaesthesia, blood may stagnate in the capillaries, with equally deleterious effects on tissue nutrition. Under these circumstances the situation may be rather similar to the capillary stagnation which occurs during irreversible shock (*see* page 224).

The correlation between animal experiments and what happens in intact man is at best uncertain. The experimental findings described above should, therefore, be interpreted with caution.

A new technique

Amory, Steffenson and Forsyth (1971) used the technique of injecting radioactively-labelled microspheres into the circulation of rhesus monkeys to determine the blood flow to a wide variety of organs, both in absolute terms and as a percentage of the total cardiac output (*see* their *Tables 10* and *20*). As other workers have noted, Amory found a dose-related fall of arterial pressure during halothane anaesthesia, due in part to a fall of cardiac output, and also—in

Table 8.2 ORGAN BLOOD FLOW, AS PERCENTAGE OF PRE-ANAESTHETIC VALUES, IN MONKEYS ANAESTHETIZED WITH HALOTHANE: S—SPONTANEOUS; C—CONTROLLED VENTILATION. (FIGURES FROM AMORY, STEFFENSON AND FORSYTH, 1971.)

| | *End-tidal halothane concentration* | | | |
	0.8%, S	0.8%, C	1.2%, C	1.2%, S
Heart	51%	49%	37%	39%
Brain	64%	65%	89%	71%
Kidneys	106%	101%	92%	87%
Skin	86%	76%	38%	51%
Skel. muscle	34%	33%	25%	34%

Table 8.3 CARDIOVASCULAR VARIABLES IN MONKEYS ANAESTHETIZED WITH HALOTHANE, COMPARED WITH VALUES IN UNANAESTHETIZED CONTROLS: S—SPONTANEOUS; C—CONTROLLED VENTILATION. (FIGURES FROM AMORY, STEFFENSON AND FORSYTH, 1971.)

| | *End-tidal halothane concentration* | | |
	0.8%, S	0.8%, C	1.2%, C
Mean art. pressure	55%	55%	44%
Heart rate	82%	82%	78%
Cardiac output	82%	76%	68%
Total peripheral resistance	68%	72%	64%

contrast to the findings of Prys-Roberts and colleagues (1972)—to a fall of systemic vascular resistance, even with controlled ventilation.

Myocardial blood flow was decreased proportionately more than the decrease of cardiac output, but in direct proportion to the decrease in left ventricular work. Cerebral blood flow was decreased in proportion to the fall of arterial pressure at the lower halothane concentration; but proportionately less at the higher concentration. Interestingly, the fall of blood flow was most marked in the cerebral hemispheres and the diencephalon. Renal blood flow was well maintained with a decrease of local vascular resistance (a finding which is in marked contrast to that of Deutsch et al. (1966), who found a decrease of PAH clearance in healthy volunteers anaesthetized with 1.5 per cent halothane). Splanchnic flow was decreased in proportion to the fall of arterial pressure. Cutaneous blood flow was little changed at the lower halothane concentration, but decreased at the higher concentration; this finding might, however, have been a reflection of altered thermal balance. Blood flow to the skeletal muscles was markedly reduced at both levels of anaesthesia, with a large increase of local vascular resistance.

The myocardium

In general, myocardial blood flow is linked to the cardiac metabolic rate by the mechanisms described on page 143. The decrease of cardiac work which occurs during halothane anaesthesia, for example, is accompanied by a corresponding decrease of myocardial blood flow; and conversely, an increase of cardiac work, as occurs during exercise (*see* page 170), is accompanied by an increase of myocardial flow. It is necessary, however, to remember that what is true for the normal circulation does not necessarily apply in the presence of arterial disease. In hypertensive patients, for example, Prys-Roberts, Meloche and Foëx (1971a) showed that the hypotension which is characteristic of halothane anaesthesia may be accompanied by evidence of myocardial ischaemia, despite the greatly reduced cardiac work. Conversely, an increase of cardiac work as a result of peripheral vasoconstriction may give rise to myocardial ischaemia when the coronary vessels are unable to dilute sufficiently to permit a sufficient increase of coronary blood flow.

Myocardial blood flow during induction of anaesthesia has been studied in man by Pelligrini (1957) who found that flow was transiently reduced by the intravenous injection of thiopentone. This decrease was, however, accompanied by a parallel reduction of cardiac output, suggesting that it was due mainly to a reduction of cardiac work, and that there was no true myocardial ischaemia. It has been demonstrated in the isolated mammalian heart, that thiopentone may cause coronary vasoconstriction; and it is thus possible that, during the induction of human anaesthesia, the arterial concentration of thiopentone may rise sufficiently to cause coronary vasoconstriction and cardiac dysrhythmias.

The brain

Thiopentone

Thiopentone causes a reduction of cerebral oxygen consumption and, in the presence of a normal Pa_{CO_2}, this reduced metabolic rate is accompanied by a parallel reduction of cerebral blood flow (Pierce et al., 1962). The cerebral vessels however remain sensitive to carbon dioxide: hyperventilation causes a further reduction of flow, whereas respiratory acidosis restores it to normal levels, or even above.

Nitrous oxide and hyperventilation

During anaesthesia with nitrous oxide there is a slight reduction of cerebral perfusion when Pa_{CO_2} is normal, while there may be evidence of cerebral anaerobic metabolism when Pa_{CO_2} is reduced below 15 mm Hg (Alexander et al., 1965). Under these circumstances, however, there is a marked shift of the oxygen dissociation curve due to the Bohr effect, therefore the cerebral hypoxia is not necessarily due entirely, or even mainly, to cerebral ischaemia. If the normal cerebral venous oxygen content is taken to be 14 ml 100 l^{-1}, reduction of Pa_{CO_2} from 40 mm Hg to 15 mm Hg would reduce the cerebral venous oxygen tension from 35 mm Hg to 27 mm Hg, even if blood flow remained unchanged (Kelman and Nunn, 1968).

Halothane

During halothane anaesthesia there appears to be a reduction of cerebral vascular resistance, but there is dispute about whether this is due to accumulation of vasodilator metabolites, that is, to autoregulation (*see* page 92), or to a direct vasodilator action of halothane on the cerebral vessels (Smith, 1973). Most workers believe that, at normal CO_2 tensions, cerebral perfusion is increased by halothane anaesthesia, and this effect is even more marked in the presence of hypercapnia. McDowall (1967), for example, found that cerebral blood flow in dogs, anaesthetized with 2 per cent halothane in nitrous oxide and oxygen, was increased by approximately 35 per cent over the value found during anaesthesia with nitrous oxide and oxygen alone. This finding has been confirmed in man by Christensen, Høedt-Rasmussen and Lassen (1967). McDowall, Barker and Jennett (1966) found that the inhalation of 0.5 per cent halothane caused a rise of CSF pressure, presumably due mainly to cerebral vasodilatation.

Lowering *Pa*CO_2 during halothane anaesthesia causes cerebral vasoconstriction, but the arterial hypotension which accompanies the respiratory alkalosis seems to be the more important factor in reducing cerebral perfusion under these circumstances.

Hypercapnia must be avoided in cases of head injury lest the increase of cerebral blood flow may cause cerebral ischaemia in areas of cerebral damage—'intracerebral steal' (*see* page 141).

Cyclopropane

Cyclopropane tends to cause an increase of cerebral blood flow, especially when arterial pressure is raised. This is particularly the case in the presence of respiratory acidosis. Cyclopropane anaesthesia causes a reduction of *Pa*CO_2 (i.e. cerebral vasoconstriction) and usually a reduction of cerebral blood flow (Wollman et al., 1968).

Splanchnic region

Normocapnia

Splanchnic blood flow is reduced during most forms of general anaesthesia. At normal CO_2 tensions hepatic blood flow in man is reduced by anaesthesia with both cyclopropane (Price et al., 1965) and halothane (Epstein (R. M.) et al., 1966). In the case of cyclopropane the reduction of flow occurs despite the mild arterial hypertension which often accompanies this form of anaesthesia. With halothane the reduction of flow is due mainly to reduction of arterial pressure, although there is some evidence that halothane may cause splanchnic vasodilatation, thus limiting the decrease of blood flow which would otherwise occur. This decrease of hepatic perfusion which occurs with cyclopropane and halothane does not, however, appear to be sufficient to cause hepatic hypoxia (Price et al., 1966).

During nitrous oxide anaesthesia, splanchnic vascular resistance and blood flow are normal at normal CO_2 tensions (Epstein et al., 1961). Ether, however, appears to cause a decrease of hepatic vascular resistance and an increase of splanchnic blood flow (Galindo, 1965).

Hypercapnia

An increase of Pa_{CO_2} during halothane causes an increase of splanchnic blood flow, due to decrease of splanchnic vascular resistance (Epstein (R. M.) et al., 1966). With cyclopropane, however, respiratory acidosis tends to cause a reduction of splanchnic flow, presumably due to the increased sympathetic activity which occurs under these circumstances. A similar increase of splanchnic vascular resistance in response to respiratory acidosis has been reported during nitrous oxide anaesthesia (Cooperman, Warden and Price, 1968).

Kidney

Validity of the PAH clearance technique during general anaesthesia

In the past, doubt has been cast on the validity of estimates of renal blood flow based on measurements of PAH clearance during anaesthesia. It has recently been shown, however, that halothane does not reduce PAH extraction by the renal tubules (Deutsch et al., 1966); therefore it is probable that PAH clearance *does* give a satisfactory estimate of renal blood flow during most forms of general anaesthesia.

Cyclopropane

Most general anaesthetics reduce renal plasma flow, glomerular filtration rate and the rate of excretion of water and electrolytes by the kidney (Papper and Papper, 1964). Deutsch, Pierce and Vandam (1967) showed that the administration of 50 per cent cyclopropane in oxygen to unpremedicated human volunteers increased renal vascular resistance and reduced effective renal plasma flow by 42 per cent. Glomerular filtration rate was simultaneously reduced by 39 per cent. These changes were accompanied by intense antidiuresis, partially reversible by alcohol, a finding which suggests that it was due, not only to reduction of glomerular filtration, but also to an enhanced secretion of ADH. There was also an increased circulating renin concentration, presumably induced by the reduction of renal blood flow.

Ether

The effects of ether on renal haemodynamics are similar to those of cyclopropane, but less marked. This may be due to the fact that ether appears to cause local relaxation of renal vascular smooth muscle (Miles and de Wardener, 1952).

Halothane

Deutsch et al. (1966) investigated the effects of halothane anaesthesia (1.5 per cent in oxygen) on renal blood flow in human volunteers, and found that flow was reduced in proportion to the reduction of arterial pressure which normally accompanies halothane anaesthesia. They also found renal plasma flow to be reduced by 38 per cent under similar circumstances, accompanied by a marked reduction of GFR. Renal vascular resistance was slightly increased. Conversely, MacDonald (1969) investigated the effects of halothane anaesthesia (0.5 per cent) on renal cortical blood flow in dogs, and found that it caused little change when arterial pressure was normal, while in the presence of arterial hypotension flow was increased rather than decreased, presumably because halothane reverses the sympathetically-induced vasoconstriction which accompanies arterial hypotension.

Skin and skeletal muscles

There is considerable disagreement between different workers who have attempted to measure limb blood flow during various forms of general anaesthesia. This is presumably due to the many factors which control blood flow through this region of the circulation (*see* page 151), and in particular to the conflicting effects of anaesthetic agents and of CO_2 on the cutaneous blood vessels.

Skin

Cutaneous blood flow is increased by all the commonly used general anaesthetic agents (Eger, Smith and Cullen, 1971); but the mechanism, and particularly the role played by sympathetic ganglion-blockade is disputed (Akester and Brody, 1969). Obviously a wide variety of mechanisms could cause such vasodilatation: central abolition of sympathetic tone, autonomic ganglion-blockade, prevention of noradrenaline release from post-ganglionic sympathetic terminals, or a direct depressant action on the vascular smooth muscle. Perhaps the mechanism is not the same for all agents.

This cutaneous vasodilatation, of course, increases heat loss from the body, sometimes to an extent which is sufficient to cause a drop of core temperature of several degrees. The inhalation of halothane increases limb blood flow and, at the same time, reduces the responsiveness of the cutaneous vessels to intravenously-infused noradrenaline (Black and McArdle, 1962).

Skeletal muscle

Under similar circumstances there is often a marked *decrease* of blood flow through the skeletal muscles, so that the total vascular resistance of the forearm may be normal or increased. Thomson (1967) found that the resistance of the cutaneous vessels was decreased during the induction of anaesthesia with thiopentone, cyclopropane and halothane, while the resistance of the muscular vessels was increased with thiopentone and cyclopropane, but unchanged with halothane. It is said that nerve block does not abolish the increase of vascular resistance in the skeletal muscles which occurs during cyclopropane anaesthesia. This finding casts doubt on the obvious explanation that the vasoconstriction is due to increased sympathetic activity; it may, however, be due to an increased concentration of circulating catecholamines.

The pulmonary circulation

Very little is known about the response of the pulmonary vascular bed to general anaesthesia. This lack of knowledge is due mainly to the difficulties inherent in the investigation of this region of the circulation. It is known, however, that pulmonary artery pressure is raised during anaesthesia with both cyclopropane (Etsten et al., 1953), and with halothane (Wyant et al., 1958). In the case of cyclopropane this appears mainly due to increase of pulmonary vascular resistance plus a small increase of left atrial pressure; with halothane, however, the pulmonary resistance appears to be normal (Price et al., 1969). In the latter case the mild pulmonary hypertension is presumably due to increase of left atrial pressure consequent on the myocardial depression which inevitably accompanies halothane anaesthesia.

CARDIOVASCULAR EFFECTS OF SURGICAL STIMULATION

It is known that surgical stimulation may be accompanied by marked cardiovascular responses. Some of these changes may be due to abnormal postures necessary for adequate surgical exposure, or to interference with venous return by retractors or surgical packs; most, however, appear to be reflex in nature.

Studies of cardiovascular function during general anaesthesia may, therefore, give unreliable results when made during or immediately after surgery. Such investigations should preferably be made before the start of surgery, although clearly care must be taken to ensure that anaesthesia is not thereby excessively prolonged.

Depressor response

Many regions of the peritoneum are extremely sensitive to traction; stimulation of such regions causes marked cardiovascular depression. The regions from which this type of response may be elicited include the duodenum and coeliac axis, the hepato-duodenal ligament, the gall bladder, the greater omentum and the broad ligament of the ovary. The precise afferent pathways involved have not been determined with certainty; it appears, however, that impulses from the parietal peritoneum run via somatic nerves, while impulses from the visceral peritoneum probably reach the central nervous system via afferent nerves which run in the sympathetic chain to enter the thoracic region of the spinal cord.

In addition to these peritoneal responses, traction on the pulmonary hilum, traction on the external ocular muscles, or laryngoscopy (particularly if roughly performed) may also cause severe cardiovascular depression.

Traction on the mesentery may reduce cardiac output by as much as 50 per cent for a few seconds (Folkow et al., 1962). The response is particularly marked during light anaesthesia, although this is probably partly due to the fact that the cardiovascular system is so depressed by deeper levels of anaesthesia that further reflex depression cannot occur to any appreciable extent. It has been suggested that the increased incidence of myocardial infarction which occurs after surgery to the biliary tract may be due to arterial hypotension induced by peritoneal traction on the structures in the region of the *porta hepatis* (Mendelsohn and Monheit, 1956).

Because these cardiovascular depressor reflexes are mediated as much by decrease of resting sympathetic tone as by increase of parasympathetic activity, the administration of atropine has little effect in their prevention unless there is pronounced bradycardia (Price, 1967). The reflexes can, however, be abolished by blocking their afferent pathways by local anaesthesia.

Pressor response

In contrast to the cardiovascular depression which may accompany peritoneal traction, painful stimulation of superficial structures, such as the skin and tracheal mucosa, may cause tachycardia accompanied by an increase of cardiac output and arterial pressure. This response is accompanied by sympathetically-mediated constriction of blood vessels in the skin, gut and kidney, and by vasodilatation in skeletal muscles. This latter response is mediated by sympathetic cholinergic fibres (*see* page 90). The afferent fibres involved in this type of pressor response reach the central nervous system via the ordinary somatic nerves.

As is the case with the depressor reflexes, pressor responses are obtunded by deeper levels of anaesthesia (Johansson, 1962). It is known, however, that the response is still present during light surgical anaesthesia, and, under these circumstances, blood flow to the muscles of the calf and forearm may be considerably increased by superficial surgical stimulation (Shackman, Graber and Melrose, 1952).

CARDIOVASCULAR EFFECTS OF MUSCLE RELAXANTS

It is generally assumed that the cardiovascular actions of the commonly-used muscle relaxants are slight and clinically insignificant. But the literature on this subject is confused and there are conflicting opinions on almost every point. This is doubtless due in part to the difficulty of controlling such factors as intrathoracic pressure and Pa_{CO_2} during the administration of such drugs.

Succinylcholine

The cardiovascular effects of succinylcholine are not marked; indeed the human cardiovascular system has been said to be 'practically unchanged' by the administration of this drug (Halldin and Wåhlin, 1959). Such cardiovascular effects as may occur appear to be no longer detectable after 10 to 15 minutes. Graf, Ström and Wåhlin (1963) suggest that the cardiovascular effects of succinylcholine may occasionally be of clinical significance, particularly when it acts in conjunction with other drugs, or in the presence of severe departures from physiological normality.

It should be noted, also, that the increase of plasma potassium concentration which accompanies the administration of succinylcholine may at times be sufficient to cause cardiac arrest. This is particularly the case in burned patients (Roth and Wüthrich, 1969).

d-Tubocurarine (Smith and Whitcher, 1967)

Other than causing a transient fall of arterial blood pressure, d-tubocurarine has little or no effect on the human cardiovascular system. The cause of this hypotension is disputed—it may be due to myocardial depression, to ganglion blockade, to histamine release, or to chemically-induced peripheral vasodilatation. It is known that in dogs histamine may be released by small doses of tubocurarine; and Westgate, Gordon and Bergen (1962) showed that approximately 20 per cent of curarized patients had an elevated plasma histamine level. Curare causes little or no tachycardia.

Gallamine

In contrast to tubocurarine, gallamine causes in increase of heart rate and, probably, of the force of myocardial contraction. Kennedy and Farman (1968) found a mean increase of heart rate of 40 per cent after the administration of gallamine in a dose of 0.5–1.0 mg kg^{-1}. This tachycardia was accompanied by a 35 per cent increase of cardiac-output, and by a small rise of arterial pressure.

The effect of gallamine on the heart appears to be due to the fact that it blocks parasympathetic activity, while leaving the sympathetic system normally active. Some workers suggest that this antiparasympathetic activity is relatively specific to the heart (Paton, 1959); definite evidence on this point is, however, lacking.

Alcuronium

Alcuronium, in a dose of 0.15 mg kg^{-1} body weight, causes a small increase of heart rate, about 10 per cent accompanied by a small decrease of cardiac output (Kennedy and Kelman, 1970). Mean arterial blood pressure is unaffected.

Pancuronium

Pancuronium, in a dose of 0.07 mg kg^{-1} body weight, causes a fairly marked increase of heart rate, about 25 per cent, accompanied by a smaller increase of cardiac output and of mean arterial blood pressure—about 10 per cent (Kelman and Kennedy, 1970).

EFFECT OF CHANGES OF CARDIAC OUTPUT ON RATE OF UPTAKE OF ANAESTHETIC AGENTS

If the lungs were completely unperfused, the inhalation, at constant minute volume, of a steady inspired concentration of a gaseous anaesthetic agent would cause its alveolar concentration to rise exponentially towards the inspired concentration, with a time constant equal to alveolar ventilation divided by total lung volume (*Figure 8.8*). This is approximately what happens with an almost insoluble gas such as helium.

If the inspired gas is appreciably soluble in blood, however, the alveolar (and therefore arterial) concentration rises less rapidly, because gas is removed from

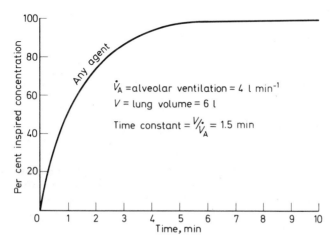

Figure 8.8. *Exponential rise of alveolar concentration of any gaseous anaesthetic agent in the absence of pulmonary blood flow*

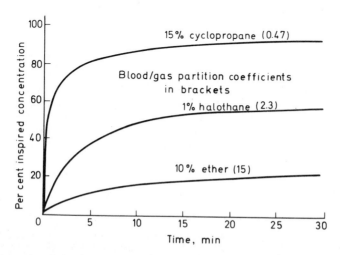

Figure 8.9. *Rise of alveolar concentration of cyclopropane, halothane and ether at constant inspired concentration, alveolar ventilation and cardiac output (redrawn from Eger, 1963).*

the alveoli by the pulmonary blood flow. The alveolar concentration is then determined by two factors: on the one hand, alveolar ventilation tends to wash gas into the lungs, on the other hand, blood flow through the pulmonary capillaries tends to remove gas from the alveoli. The alveolar concentration at any time is a balance between these two processes.

This being so, the rate of rise of alveolar concentration must be influenced by the rate of pulmonary capillary blood flow—the cardiac output—and by the blood solubility of the gas. A very soluble gas, such as ether (blood/gas partition coefficient = 15) is removed from the alveoli more rapidly than a less soluble gas, such as nitrous oxide or cyclopropane (partition coefficient = 0.47). Therefore the alveolar concentration, expressed as a percentage of the inspired concentration, rises less rapidly with ether than with cyclopropane (*Figure 8.9*). Halothane, with a blood/gas partition of 2.3, occupies an intermediate position.

The concentration effect

The rate of rise of alveolar anaesthetic concentration varies also with the inspired concentration. This is the concentration effect (*see* Eger, 1964), by which the higher the inspired concentration, the more rapid is the approximation of alveolar and inspired concentrations. If the inspired concentration were 100 per cent, alveolar concentration would rise at the same rate for all gases; however much gas had been taken up from the lungs, the alveolar concentration would remain unchanged. When the inspired concentration is less than 100 per cent, however, gas uptake reduces the alveolar concentration, thus slowing the rate of approach to equilibrium for any given agent; the lower the inspired concentration, the slower is the rate of rise of alveolar concentration.

Changes of cardiac output

The effect of changes of cardiac output on the rate of equilibration between the alveolar and inspired concentrations of halothane is shown in *Figure 8.10*. As would be expected, the concentration rises most rapidly when cardiac output is low. The effect of changes of cardiac output on anaesthetic uptake is minimal with an insoluble agent such as nitrous oxide or cyclopropane, but is very marked with a soluble agent such as ether. It is well recognized clinically that induction of anaesthesia with ether may be unexpectedly (unexpected to the unwary, that is) rapid in shocked patients, whereas in a similar patient the rate of induction with cyclopropane is relatively normal. Conversely, in patients with hyperdynamic cardiovascular systems the induction of anaesthesia with ether may be unexpectedly prolonged. After 20 minutes, the reduction of alveolar concentration caused by a 300 per cent increase of cardiac output is roughly 3 per cent in the case of nitrous oxide (blood/gas partition coefficient 0.47), 38 per cent in the case of halothane (partition coefficient 2.3) and 47 per cent in the case of ether (partition coefficient 15), all agents administered in clinical concentrations (Eger, 1963).

Of course, clinically a change of cardiac output is normally accompanied by a change of the distribution of total blood flow between the different body tissues (*see* Chapter 9). The effect of this factor on anaesthetic concentrations in the

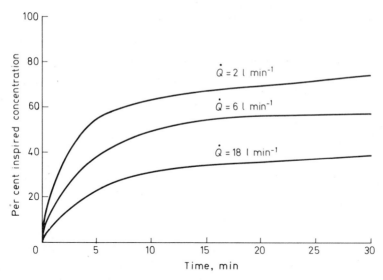

Figure 8.10. *Rise of alveolar concentration of halothane at constant alveolar ventilation, but various cardiac outputs (redrawn from Eger, 1963)*

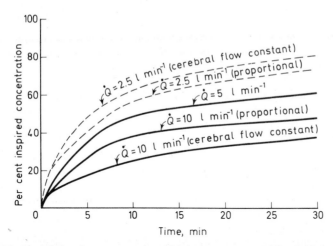

Figure 8.11. *Rise of alveolar concentration of halothane at constant inspired concentration and alveolar ventilation, but various cardiac outputs and cerebral flows (redrawn from Munson, Eger and Bowers, 1968)*

blood has recently been investigated by Munson, Eger and Bowers (1968) who compared the rate of rise of alveolar concentration in a five-compartment model of the circulation, on the assumptions that:

1. the relative perfusion of different organs remained the same as cardiac output was varied,
2. changes of cardiac output were accompanied by a constant cerebral blood flow and therefore by disproportionately greater changes of blood flow to other tissues (*Figure 8.11*).

The influence of changes of cardiac output on the rate of uptake of anaesthetic agent is greater when cerebral blood flow remains constant. This, of course, is the situation typically found in shock, when cardiac output is considerably reduced but cerebral perfusion is relatively well maintained (*see* Chapter 9).

Anaesthetic uptake at constant alveolar concentration

In practice, induction of general anaesthesia is usually achieved by maintaining a relatively constant alveolar, rather than a constant inspired, concentration of anaesthetic agent. It is therefore necessary to consider also the effect of cardiovascular changes on the rate of uptake of anaesthetic agents at constant alveolar concentration (Eger, 1964). In this case uptake is initially greater than with a constant inspired concentration; later it becomes less.

Changes of cardiac output make a marked difference to the initial rate of uptake, especially with soluble agents such as ether and methoxyfluorane. With ether, an increase of cardiac output from 4 to 8 l min^{-1} causes an increase of the initial rate of uptake from about 430 ml min^{-1} to 810 ml min^{-1}; an increase of output to 16 l min^{-1} increases the initial rate to approximately 1500 ml min^{-1}.

CARDIAC OUTPUT DURING EXTERNAL CARDIAC MASSAGE

The increasing involvement of anaesthetists in the resuscitation of critically ill patients makes a brief comment on cardiac output during external cardiac massage not out of place in a book aimed primarily at clinicians and particularly at anaesthetists.

Most evidence suggests that the cardiac output which can be achieved by external massage is considerably less than that produced by a spontaneously-beating heart. During cardiac massage blood flow through the heart is often limited by valvular incompetence due to dilatation of the atrio-ventricular valve-rings, particularly on the right side. Such incompetence may cause venous pulsation which may be wrongly interpreted as evidence of a satisfactory arterial pressure pulse (Gall, 1965).

Although the systolic blood pressure may be relatively normal during external massage, the diastolic and mean pressures are low, as is the cardiac output. Gall suggests that no technique of cardiac massage, internal or external, can produce an output greater than 50 per cent of normal. MacKenzie et al. (1964) measured cardiac output in three patients undergoing external massage and found a mean cardiac index of 0.92 l min^{-1} m^{-2} body surface, compared with 1.85 l min^{-1} m^{-2} after resumption of a spontaneous heart-beat. Del Guercio, Commaraswamy and State (1963) found a mean cardiac index during external massage of 0.61 l min^{-1} m^{-2} (about $\frac{1}{6}$ normal) with an average circulation time of 88.5 seconds.

Despite these rather depressing figures, there is no doubt that patients can survive external cardiac massage for periods up to 2 hours, and may recover consciousness during this procedure. The peripheral blood flow which is achieved is, however, seldom sufficient to prevent the occurrence of considerable metabolic acidosis, which may militate against the satisfactory resumption of a spontaneous heart-beat (*see* page 220).

RECOMMENDED FURTHER READING

Adams, A. P. (1975). 'Techniques of Vascular Control for Deliberate Hypotension during Anaesthesia.' *Br. J. Anaesth.* **47**, 777

Anon. (1971). 'Beta-blocking Drugs in Treatment of Cardiac Arrhythmias during Anaesthesia.' *Br. J. Anaesth.* **43**, 1

Baez, S. (1971). 'Anesthesia and the Microcirculation.' *Anesthesiology* **35**, 333

Black, G. W. (1971). 'Circulatory, Respiratory and Metabolic Effects of Inhalational Anaesthetics.' In Gray, T. C. and Nunn, J. F., *General Anaesthesia*, 3rd edn, p. 465. London; Butterworths

Buckley, J. J. (1964). 'Effects of Respiratory Acidosis upon the Circulation during Anaesthesia.' In Fabian, L., *Anesthesia and the Circulation*, p. 117. Philadelphia; F. A. Davis

Conway, C. M. (1975). 'Haemodynamic Effects of Pulmonary Ventilation.' *Br. J. Anaesth.* **47**, 761

Conway, C. M. and Ellis, D. B. (1969). 'The Haemodynamic Effects of Short-acting Barbiturates.' *Br. J. Anaesth.* **41**, 534

Cooperman, L. H. (1972). 'Effect of Anaesthetics on the Splanchnic Circulation.' *Br. J. Anaesth.* **44**, 967

Dowdy, E. G. (1964). 'Circulatory Effects of Neuromuscular Blocking Drugs.' In Fabian, L. W., *Anesthesia and the Circulation*, p. 97. Philadelphia; F. A. Davis

Etsten, B. E. and Li, T. H. (1962). 'Current Concepts of Myocardial Function during Anaesthesia.' *Br. J. Anaesth.* **34**, 884

Etsten, B. E. and Shimosato, S. (1964). 'Myocardial Contractility Performance of the Heart during Anaesthesia.' In Fabian, L. W., *Anesthesia and the Circulation*, p. 56. Philadelphia; F. A. Davis

Fabian, L. W. (1964). 'Circulatory Effects of Respiratory Alkalosis.' In Fabian, L. W., *Anesthesia and the Circulation*, p. 137. Philadelphia; F. A. Davis

Goldberg, A. H. (1968). 'Cardiovascular Function and Halothane. In Green, N. M., *Clinical Anesthesia: Halothane*, p. 24. Oxford; Blackwell

Katz, R. L. and Bigger, J. T. (1970). 'Cardiac Arrhythmias during Anesthesia and Operation.' *Anesthesiology* **33**, 193

Larson, C. P., Mazze, R. I., Cooperman, L. H. and Wollman, H. (1974). 'Effects of Anesthetics on Cerebral, Renal and Splanchnic Circulations: Recent Developments.' *Anesthesiology* **41**, 169

Merin, R. G. (1973). 'Inhalation Anesthetics and Myocardial Metabolism.' *Anesthesiology* **39**, 216

Millar, R. A. (1971). 'Some Effects of Inhalational Anesthetics on Neurocirculatory Control.' In Millar, R. A., *Pharmacological Topics in Anesthesia*. Boston; Little Brown

Munson, E. S., Eger, E. I., Bowers, D. L. (1973). 'Effects of Anesthetic-depressed Ventilation and Cardiac Output on Anesthetic Uptake: A Computer Nonlinear Simulation.' *Anesthesiology* **38**, 251

Price, H. (1960). 'General Anesthesia and Circulatory Homeostasis.' *Physiol. Rev.* **40**, 187

Price, H. L. (1966). 'The Significance of Catecholamine Release during Anaesthesia.' *Br. J. Anaesth.* **38**, 705

Price, H. L. (1967). *Circulation during Anaesthesia and Operation.* Springfield; Charles C. Thomas

Salanitre, E. (1975). 'The Role of Physiological Factors in Exchange of Anaesthetic Gas.' In Mushin, W. W., Severinghaus, J. W., Tiengs, M. and Gorini, S. *Physiological Basis of Anaesthesiology.* Piccin Medical Books

Shimosato, S. and Etsten, B. E. (1969). 'Effect of Anesthetic Drugs on the Heart: A Critical Review of Myocardial Contractility and its Relationship to Hemodynamics.' In Fabian, L. W., *Clinical Anesthesia: A Decade of Clinical Progress*, p. 17. Oxford; Blackwell

Siegel, J. H. (1969). 'The Myocardial Contractile State and its Role in the Response to Anesthesia and Surgery.' *Anesthesiology* **30**, 519

Smith, A. L. and Wollman, H. (1972). 'Cerebral Blood Flow and Metabolism: Effects of Anesthetic Drugs and Techniques.' *Anesthesiology* **36**, 378

Thyrum, P. T. (1972). 'Fluorinated Hydrocarbons and the Heart.' *Anesthesiology* **36**, 103

Zauder, H. L., Baez, S. and Orkin, L. R. (1964). 'Tissue Perfusion during Anesthesia.' In Fabian, L. W., *Anesthesia and the Circulation*, p. 79. Philadelphia; F. A. Davis

Chapter 9 Haemorrhage and Shock

The clinical syndrome known as shock is unfortunately all too familiar to clinicians and particularly to practising anaesthetists. Shock is not confined to the operating theatre and surgical ward; it also occurs in such acute medical conditions as coronary thrombosis and adrenal insufficiency.

The essential physiological defect in shock is almost always a reduction of cardiac output (*see* however, page 222). To a first approximation arterial blood pressure equals the product of cardiac ouput and total peripheral resistance (*see* page 75), therefore a reduction of cardiac output tends to be accompanied by a decrease of arterial blood pressure. Provided, however, that the reduction of pressure is not excessive, it is the deficiency of blood flow which is the more important physiological defect. Injudicious attempts to restore blood pressure to normal by the administration of potent vasopressor agents may be accompanied by a further decrease of cardiac output and by a paradoxical worsening of the patient's condition (*see* page 231).

The majority of cases of shock seen by the anaesthetist are at least partly due to hypovolaemia; therefore this chapter starts with a consideration of the problems of acute haemorrhage.

PRESSURE VERSUS FLOW

A clear understanding of the relationship between blood pressure and blood flow is essential before any discussion of haemorrhage and shock. Blood flow through any given vascular bed is proportional to the hydrostatic pressure difference between the arterial and venous ends of the bed, and inversely proportional to the resistance to flow. Since arterial pressure is normally much greater than venous pressure, it is usual to ignore the latter and to assume that blood flow is directly proportional to arterial pressure. When arterial pressure is low, or venous pressure is high, and particularly when both conditions occur simultaneously, as in shock due to myocardial damage (cardiogenic shock, *see* page 126), this simplification may not be entirely valid. Under most circumstances, however, the approximation is a reasonable one which considerably simplifies discussion about tissue perfusion.

The factors influencing the resistance to blood flow through a vascular network are considered in Chapter 1. If all the vessels comprising a given vascular bed decrease in diameter by 16 per cent, resistance to flow is doubled. If the vasoconstriction is of the same degree but limited to one segment only of a vascular bed, its effect on vascular resistance is correspondingly less.

The relationship, flow = pressure/resistance, applies both to the circulation as a whole and to blood flow through a single organ. For the circulation as a whole, the equation indicates that, neglecting venous pressure in comparison to arterial pressure, arterial pressure equals the product of cardiac output and total peripheral resistance. (This relationship applies strictly only to *mean* arterial pressure and *mean* blood flow. Arterial pressure and flow vary phasically throughout the cardiac cycle, but, because of inertia, pressure and flow are not always in phase. For most purposes this discrepancy may be neglected (*see also* page 231).)

In the case of a single organ or tissue, the equation indicates that blood flow is equal to arterial pressure (minus venous pressure) divided by the resistance of the vascular bed. If the resistances of the individual body tissues remained constant, therefore, an increase of arterial pressure would cause a generalized increase of tissue perfusion. However, under most conditions, resistance does *not* remain constant, therefore an increase of arterial pressure may not necessarily be accompanied by an increase of blood flow. It is necessary to consider also the way in which the increase of blood pressure is brought about.

An increase of cardiac output into a constant total peripheral resistance must, by the above relationship, be accompanied by an increase of arterial blood pressure; if the resistance of the various tissues remains constant, this increase of pressure must cause a generalized increase of blood flow. However, if cardiac output is constant, an increase of arterial blood pressure must be due to an increase of vascular resistance in some or all of the peripheral tissues; this vasoconstriction prevents the increase of flow which would otherwise occur as a result of the rise of arterial pressure. If cardiac output does not increase, the perfusion of an individual tissue may be unchanged, or even decreased, in the presence of an increase of arterial blood pressure.

The relationship between pressure and flow may also be considered in a somewhat different manner. This is to consider that the heart produces a certain total blood flow per unit time (the cardiac output) which is shared amongst the various organs in inverse proportion to their vascular resistances (*Figure 9.1a*). If cardiac output remains constant, an increase of blood flow to one tissue must inevitably by accompanied by a decrease of the flow available for the remaining tissues. A uniform overall increase of tissue resistance raises arterial pressure, but, unless it is accompanied by an increase of cardiac output, has no effect on tissue perfusion (*Figure 9.1b*).

An increase of resistance in some tissues, but not in others, increases the total peripheral resistance. It therefore increases arterial blood pressure, but, provided there is no increase of cardiac output, it must be accompanied by a decrease of blood flow to the vasoconstricted tissues and by an increase of flow to the passive tissues, that is, by a redistribution of a constant cardiac output (*Figure 9.1c*). The consequences of decreased blood flow to vasoconstricted tissues are considered on page 222 in the context of deteriorating shock.

An increase of cardiac output accompanied by a generalized decrease of tissue resistance results in a generalized increase of tissue perfusion, although arterial blood pressure may be unaltered or even diminished (*Figure 9.2*).

(Readers familiar with elementary electronics will find similarities between the way in which the heart may be considered either as a generator of pressure or as a generator of flow, and the way in which a transistor or thermionic valve may be considered either as a voltage generator or as a current generator. Without pushing the analogy too far, it may be remarked that arterial blood pressure is analogous to voltage, and blood flow to current.)

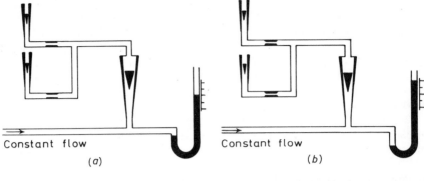

Constant flow

(a)

Constant flow

(b)

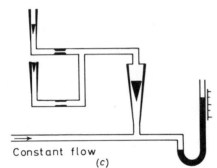

Constant flow

(c)

Figure 9.1. *Relationship between pressure and flow. (a) Normal situation. (b) Generalized increase of tissue resistance but total blood flow (cardiac output) unchanged—causes increase of blood pressure but no change of tissue blood flow. (c) Differential increase of tissue resistance but total blood flow (cardiac output) unchanged—causes increase of blood pressure and decrease of blood flow to constricted tissues with increase of flow to remaining tissues (from Kelman, G. R., 1969. 'Cardiac Output in Shock.' Int. Anaesth. Clin. 7, No. 4. Boston; Little, Brown and Company)*

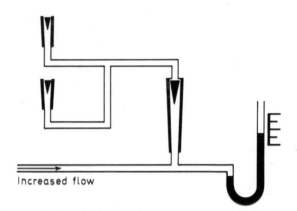

Increased flow

Figure 9.2. *Increase of total flow (cardiac output) in the presence of a generalized decrease of tissue resistance causes decrease of blood pressure and a generalized increase of tissue blood flow (from Kelman, G. R., 1969. 'Cardiac Output in Shock.' Int. Anaesth. Clin. 7, No. 4. Boston; Little, Brown and Company)*

Vasoconstrictor drugs

Treatment of shock with alphamimetic vasoconstrictor drugs (*see* page 229) causes intense vasoconstriction in tissues which are well supplied with alpha-adrenoceptive sites. This vasoconstriction causes an increase of total peripheral resistance, and therefore a rise of mean arterial pressure but, as there is usually no accompanying increase of cardiac output, there is diversion of blood away from the vasoconstricted tissues, with a reduction of blood flow to these regions.

The myocardial sympathetic receptors are predominantly β in type (*see* page 73), therefore the use of drugs which are predominantly alphamimetic has little effect on the efficiency of the cardiac pump, and does not restore a reduced cardiac output. Indeed, an increase of arterial blood pressure imposes an increased load on a heart already weakened by hypoxia or acidosis, and may thus cause a decrease, rather than an increase, of cardiac output (*see* page 228). Many workers therefore recommend the use of betamimetic or alphabetamimetic drugs for the treatment of shock rather than drugs such as noradrenaline, the action of which is predominantly on the alpha receptors. It must be remembered, however, that betamimetic drugs may decrease the efficiency of the heart and therefore cause a disproportionate increase of myocardial oxygen consumption.

HAEMORRHAGE

The differences between the clinical manifestations of acute and chronic haemorrhage are well known. In the former the defect is essentially of blood volume; in the latter it is of red cell mass. The body is far less tolerant of hypovolaemia than of anaemia: a 20 per cent reduction of blood volume may have serious consequences, whereas a similar reduction of red cell mass, with constant blood volume, causes but little physiological disturbance. Only the effects of acute haemorrhage are considered here.

Although the physiological disturbances which accompany acute haemorrhage are similar irrespective of whether the blood loss is external or internal, it should be remembered that internal haemorrhage into certain regions, such as the cranial cavity or pericardium, may interfere with the function of vital organs, and therefore have consequences out of proportion to the actual volume of blood lost. In a previously healthy young adult the acute loss of 20 per cent of the total blood volume results in moderate shock; the loss of 40–50 per cent results in severe shock and may be fatal.

Defence against hypovolaemia

Immediately following acute haemorrhage there is a period of hypovolaemia. If the initial haemorrhage is not too great, this initial phase is followed by gradual restoration of the blood volume to normal. If the loss exceeds a certain amount, however, it leads to a gradual deterioration of the body's physiological state and ultimately to death.

Transfer of interstitial fluid to the intravascular compartment

Acute hypovolaemia causes the rapid flow of interstitial fluid from the tissue spaces into the intravascular compartment. This occurs as a result of reduction of capillary pressure consequent on the arteriolar constriction and arterial hypotension which accompany haemorrhage. Even when the pressure in the large arteries is relatively normal, capillary pressure is reduced by the increased pressure drop along the constricted arterioles. After a massive acute haemorrhage a volume of fluid equivalent to 10–15 per cent of the initial blood volume may enter the bloodstream in 5 minutes.

The fluid which is drawn into the vascular compartment dilutes the haemoglobin and plasma proteins; therefore, although blood volume is restored partly or completely to normal, the oxygen-carrying power of the blood is severely reduced. Given normal hepatic function, the plasma protein concentration is restored to normal relatively rapidly by increased protein synthesis; restoration of the red cell mass, however, takes some weeks.

Increased sympatho-adrenal activity

The increased sympatho-adrenal activity which accompanies acute haemorrhage is considered on the next page.

Increased production of antidiuretic hormone and aldosterone

The body also reacts to a reduced blood volume by increased secretion of antidiuretic hormone (ADH) and of aldosterone (*see* page 128). These hormones promote the re-absorption of sodium and water from the renal tubules, although after a severe haemorrhage glomerular filtration may be so reduced that renal sodium loss is minimal anyway.

Haemodynamic consequences of hypovolaemia

Immediately after acute haemorrhage, there is a reduction of the circulating blood volume, and a consequent reduction of mean systemic pressure (*see* page 121). This causes a reduction of cardiac output with a consequent reduction of tissue blood flow and, usually, of arterial blood pressure. These reductions of pressure and flow cause compensatory responses throughout the cardiovascular system; and these responses tend to restore arterial pressure and cardiac output to normal.

Reflex response to hypovolaemia

The afferent neurones involved in these reflexes arise in the baroreceptors and chemoreceptors described in Chapter 3. The baroreceptors detect the reduction of mean arterial pressure, and also the reduction of pulse pressure; the chemoreceptors are stimulated by a reduction of their local blood flow, and by changes of Pa_{O_2} and Pa_{CO_2}. The reflex response of the body to this situation includes an increase of sympathetic tone to the veins, the heart, and to the systemic resistance vessels, and decreased vagal tone to the heart. In addition, there is increased stimulation of the adrenal medullae and enhanced secretion of adrenaline and noradrenaline from this organ.

Effect on mean systemic pressure

Two-thirds of the total blood volume is normally contained in the veins. These vessels are relatively distensible, therefore a moderate quantity of blood may be lost with but little decrease of venous pressure (and therefore of mean systemic pressure, *see* page 121). A more severe haemorrhage, however, causes a marked reduction of venous and mean systemic pressures, although the reduction is limited by compensatory sympathetic activity which reduces the capacity of the circulatory system (*see* page 121).

The increased respiratory movements which often accompany haemorrhage tend to drive blood back to the heart by increasing the efficiency of the respiratory pump; they therefore compensate partly for the reduction of mean systemic pressure.

Effect on resistance vessels

Increased sympathetic tone to resistance vessels causes vasoconstriction and an increase of total peripheral resistance. Arterial blood pressure is, therefore, relatively well maintained despite a marked reduction of cardiac output. It should be noted, however, that sympathetically-induced vasoconstriction is more marked in the precapillary than in the post-capillary resistance vessels. It is, therefore, accompanied by a reduction of capillary hydrostatic pressure, even when systemic arterial pressure is relatively normal. This reduction of capillary pressure permits the transfer of extracellular fluid into the vascular compartment (*see* page 84).

Vasoconstriction is particularly intense in tissues such as the skin, skeletal muscles, splanchnic area, and kidneys, which are of less immediate importance for the body's survival than such essential organs as the brain and heart. The coronary and cerebral resistance vessels show only minimal vasoconstriction in response to increased sympathetic activity (Green and Kepchar, 1959). Blood flow through these regions is therefore relatively well maintained even when skin, renal and splanchnic flow are virtually at a standstill.

Hypotension may, in fact, be accompanied by an actual reduction of vascular resistance in some tissues (autoregulation, *see* page 92), thus maintaining their perfusion despite the reduction of arterial pressure. There are, however, limits to this response, therefore a severe reduction of arterial blood pressure will probably be accompanied by some reduction of blood flow even through the brain where the blood vessels exhibit marked autoregulation. This is especially likely to be the case when the vessels are diseased.

This diversion of blood from the body's less vital organs is initially beneficial to the patient. But it may ultimately result in pathological changes in the ischaemic, hypoxic tissues, with the result that toxic substances are liberated into the general circulation, where they may damage organs which are not themselves hypoxic. This causes further deterioration of the patient's already severely disturbed homeostatic mechanisms, and may ultimately result in his death.

Effect on the heart

The effect of increased sympathetic tone to the heart is to increase both its rate and force of contraction; the increase of rate depends also on a decrease of parasympathetic tone. As a result, the efficiency of the cardiac pump is increased; it is able to pump an increased amount of blood at a given right atrial pressure, therefore cardiac output is restored partly to normal, despite a marked reduction of mean systemic pressure (*see* page 125).

Cholinergic sympathetic pathways

Emotional factors such as the sight of blood may cause fainting during an acute haemorrhagic episode. The sympathetic cholinergic fibres (*see* page 90) then cause widespread vasodilatation in the skeletal muscles with a consequent reduction of total peripheral resistance. There is, as a result, a marked fall of systemic arterial pressure, which then becomes insufficient to maintain cerebral perfusion in the upright position.

Tissue oxygenation during hypovolaemia

After a moderate haemorrhage the oxygen tension of the arterial blood is relatively normal as is its oxygen content before the onset of haemodilution. Indeed, the respiratory alkalosis which usually accompanies haemorrhage probably causes a small increase of arterial oxyhaemoglobin saturation, and therefore a slight, and clinically insignificant, increase of arterial oxygen content. However, in hypovolaemia, the blood flow to many organs is severely reduced although their oxygen consumption is unchanged, therefore such tissues have increased arterio-venous oxygen content differences and venous blood which is abnormally desaturated (stagnant hypoxia). This desaturation is usually reflected in changes of oxygen content and tension of the mixed-venous blood which, of course, is a weighted average of the venous drainage from all the peripheral tissues.

Since cardiac output is reduced while total body oxygen consumption is unchanged, or even increased, the mixed-venous blood after acute haemorrhage is abnormally desaturated. It should be noted, however, that, while an abnormally low mixed-venous oxygen tension inevitably means that the patient is suffering from hypoxia (whether hypoxic, anaemic or stagnant), a normal mixed-venous oxygen content cannot be taken as certain evidence that there is no hypoxia. In severe haemorrhage blood flow to some tissues virtually ceases and, although these tissues are indisputably hypoxic, this hypoxia does not influence the composition of the blood returning to the heart.

In the kidney the arterio-venous oxygen content difference remains constant even when its blood flow is reduced to 10 per cent of normal (Kramer, 1962). The majority of renal oxygen consumption is expended on the re-absorption of filtered sodium; therefore, when the tubular sodium load is reduced by decreased glomerular filtration, as occurs after haemorrhage, renal oxygen consumption is reduced proportionally.

The arterial hypoxaemia of severe haemorrhage

After severe haemorrhage there is commonly a reduction of arterial oxygen tension (Freeman, 1966). The precise cause of this hypoxaemia is uncertain; it does not appear to be due to alveolar underventilation because, except when the patient is *in extremis,* arterial P_{CO_2} is below normal, despite a marked increase of physiological dead space, presumably due to underperfusion of alveoli in the superior parts of the lung.

It should be noted, however, that, as a result of this increased dead space, the patient depends on a large respiratory minute volume to prevent CO_2 retention. If ventilation is depressed by morphine, or general anaesthesia, or by respiratory obstruction or chest injury, alveolar ventilation may be insufficient to eliminate metabolically-produced carbon dioxide and the patient then becomes acidotic and, if breathing air, hypoxic.

Since the arterial hypoxaemia of haemorrhage is not primarily due to alveolar hypoventilation, it is necessary to consider whether it is due to increased pulmonary physiological shunting. This does not, in fact, appear to be the case. Freeman and Nunn (1963) found in dogs subjected to severe haemorrhage that the calculated percentage physiological shunt was actually *reduced* from a control value of 5.5 per cent to 0.7–1.7 per cent. The mixed-venous blood, however, had a very low oxygen content, therefore the (A–a) P_{O_2} difference was not significantly different from normal.

Aerobic and anaerobic metabolism

Despite the increased oxygen extraction which occurs in the ischaemic, vasoconstricted tissues in shock, the amount of oxygen available to them may not be sufficient for their metabolic needs. There is then a decrease of tissue oxygen consumption which is a reflection of the fact that local metabolism has temporarily become anaerobic.

The details of tissue metabolism under aerobic and anaerobic conditions are discussed in standard textbooks on biochemistry (*see also* Nunn, 1969). Briefly, the pathways are as follows (*Figure 9.3*). The breakdown of glucose to carbon dioxide and water involves the conversion of phosphoglyceraldehyde to phosphoglyceric acid. This reaction is catalysed by DPN (diphosphopyridine nucleotide) which becomes reduced to DPNH in the process. DPNH is then re-oxidized to DPN by removal of hydrogen, and its transfer down a chain of flavoproteins and cytochromes, until ultimately it combines with molecular oxygen to form water.

In the absence of oxygen, oxidation of DPNH via the flavoprotein-cytochrome chain cannot occur. DPNH can, however, be oxidized to DPN by reacting with pyruvate, which in the process becomes reduced to lactate,

$$pyruvate + DPNH \rightleftharpoons lactate + DPN$$

Pyruvic acid is therefore diverted just before the point at which it normally enters the Krebs cycle, and becomes converted to lactic acid.* Ultimately, the breakdown of glucose stops altogether because accumulation of lactic acid

* The pK of lactic acid is approximately equal to 3.0.

prevents further conversion of pyruvate, and therefore further oxidation of DPNH.

In addition to possible deleterious consequences from the release of lactic acid into the general circulation, anaerobic metabolism produces considerably less energy than the complete breakdown of glucose to carbon dioxide and water. The complete aerobic breakdown of glucose produces 19 times as much energy (in the form of ATP) as does its anaerobic conversion to lactic acid.

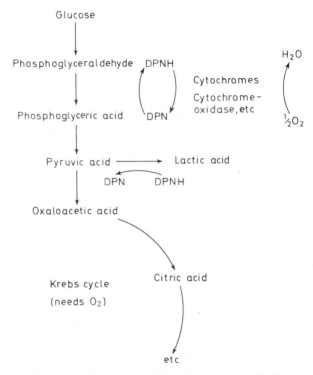

Figure 9.3. Aerobic and anaerobic carbohydrate metabolism

Lactic acidosis

When lactic acid enters the general circulation it induces a non-respiratory (metabolic) acidosis. This is, however, partly compensated by the respiratory alkalosis which usually accompanies haemorrhage; arterial pH is therefore partly restored to normal. The administration of large doses of analgesic narcotics such as morphine may however cause respiratory depression, and the resulting combination of respiratory and non-respiratory acidosis causes a marked reduction of arterial pH.

Cardiovascular effects of acidosis

Acidosis has deleterious effects on the cardiovascular system (*see,* for example, Wildenthal et al., 1968). It appears to have a primary depressant action on the myocardium, and also to reduce the responsiveness of the heart to sympathetic stimulation and sympathomimetic amines. There is little doubt that the acidosis which accompanies severe haemorrhage is a most important factor in the pathogenesis of so-called irreversible shock (*see* page 223), a condition in which cardiac output remains low despite adequate restoration of blood volume.

In addition, local tissue acidosis paralyses resistance vessels causing microcirculatory stasis. Initially, the post-capillary vessels are less affected than the precapillary vessels, with the result that the capillaries become overfilled with blood. Increased capillary pressure also causes increased loss of fluid into the tissue spaces. In 1923 Cannon asked 'where is the blood which is out of currency?'; part of the answer to his question would seem to be, in dilated tissue capillaries and the tissue spaces.

From animal experiments there is evidence that the mortality from acute haemorrhage depends on the size of the oxygen debt which develops as a result of anaerobic tissue metabolism (Crowell and Smith, 1964). These workers found that the probability of survival decreased rapidly when the oxygen debt exceeded a certain value, irrespective of the rate at which it developed. Dogs with a total debt of less than 100 ml kg^{-1} survived; those with a debt of more than 150 ml kg^{-1} died. The applicability of these figures to man is unknown; it is generally recognized, however, that severe metabolic acidosis is usually of poor prognostic significance in the shock syndrome.

Effect of acidosis on tissue oxygenation

Leaving out of consideration the effects of acidosis on tissue blood flow (*see* Chapter 5), its effects on the carriage of oxygen by the blood must be briefly considered. These are complex and depend on the circumstances. It is well known that acidosis shifts the oxyhaemoglobin dissociation curve downwards and to the right, with the result that pulmonary capillary blood is able to take up less oxygen than it would at normal *p*H. But in the tissues, for the same reason, the blood is able to give up oxygen more readily, that is, at a higher Po_2. It is therefore possible that under some circumstances acidosis may cause an increase of tissue venous oxygen tension despite the decreased arterial oxygen content; under other circumstances the pulmonary effect is dominant, and acidosis then results in a severe fall of arterial oxygen content, and in a lowered venous oxygen tension.

SHOCK

Guyton (*see* Recommended Further Reading) defines shock as 'a state of circulation in which tissues in widespread areas of the body are being damaged by nutritional insufficiency resulting from inadequate cardiac output'. The essential physiological defect in shock is a marked reduction of cardiac output. Haemorrhage is but one of many causes of this syndrome, although an important and, in the early stages at any rate, a relatively easily treated one.

(It has been suggested that shock may, in fact, occur in the presence of a normal, or even increased, cardiac output (Udhoji and Weil, 1965). Most of the

ACP–8*

patients in whom this occurs appear to have marked arterio-venous shunting from such conditions as Paget's disease and hepatic cirrhosis; they therefore have inadequate tissue perfusion, even in the presence of an apparently normal cardiac output. Cohn et al. (1968) suggest that in some forms of septic shock large numbers of arterio-venous anastomoses open up in the peripheral systemic circulation, with the result that much of the heart's output by-passes the capillaries, and tissue perfusion in a functional sense is therefore inadequate even in the presence of a cardiac output which is considerably above normal.)

Clinical manifestations

The clinical manifestations of shock are due either to haemodynamic abnormalities or to the intense sympathetic and adrenal medullary overactivity which occurs as the body attempts to maintain adequate perfusion of vital organs such as the brain and heart.

Sympathetic activity is especially marked to the skin, kidneys, and splanchnic areas; the patient has a cold sweaty skin, pale mucosae, and marked oliguria. The pulse is rapid, but of small volume ('thready') due to severe reduction of stroke volume resulting from the tachycardia and reduced cardiac output.

Arterial blood pressure is low, therefore cerebral blood flow may be reduced, especially if the head is raised or the cerebral vessels are diseased so that their ability to autoregulate (*see* page 92) is impaired. Initially, there may be restlessness due to cerebral hypoxia; later, there is central nervous depression with apathy, stupor and insensitivity to pain.

The patient often complains of severe thirst due to the fact that cardiovascular receptors on the venous side of the circulation detect the hypovolaemia and cause stimulation of the hypothalamic 'thirst centres'.

Compensated versus deteriorating shock

Provided that the initial physiological insult is not too great, the body's compensatory mechanisms are able to maintain blood flow to vital organs, despite a fairly severe reduction of cardiac output. This is the condition of *compensated shock*. If the physiological stress is more severe, however, the compensatory mechanisms may be able to maintain the function of vital organs for a time, but sooner or later the patient's condition begins to deteriorate. He then enters the vicious circle in which shock generates more shock until, unless energetic treatment is initiated, death ensues. This is the condition of *deteriorating shock*.

Some of the compensating mechanisms which are responsible for keeping the patient alive during moderate or early shock may themselves be the cause of his death from severe or prolonged shock (*see* page 231).

The classification of shock into compensated and deteriorating is in no way limited to haemorrhagic shock, although most available quantitative information refers to this state. For example, Hinshaw et al. (1961) found that, in previously healthy young adults, the acute loss of 10 per cent of the total blood volume reduced arterial blood pressure by 7 per cent and cardiac output by 21 per cent;

the loss of 20 per cent of the blood volume reduced arterial pressure by 15 per cent and cardiac output by 41 per cent.

In compensated shock, arterial pressure may be relatively normal in the presence of a mild or moderate decrease of cardiac output. This situation, however, is dependent on the body's compensatory mechanisms which may be stretched almost to their limit. A slight additional physiological insult (for example, a small additional haemorrhage) may overcome the body's remaining compensating ability, and be accompanied by a marked clinical deterioration. The dividing line between a patient who is in the relatively stable condition of compensated shock and one who is in the unstable condition of deteriorating shock is narrow. Arterial blood pressure is a poor guide to the condition of the cardiovascular system; in particular, it gives little information about the extent to which the body's compensatory mechanisms are being called into play, that is, about how much reserve compensatory power is available.

Mechanisms involved in compensated shock

The negative-feedback mechanisms which tend to maintain cardiac output and arterial pressure in compensated shock have been considered in detail previously (*see* page 124). A fall of mean arterial pressure, or of arterial pulse pressure, causes compensatory responses throughout the cardiovascular system. These responses depend mainly on an increase of sympathetic tone to the veins, the heart and the arterioles, and to increased secretion of catecholamines from the adrenal medullae. Venoconstriction raises the mean systemic pressure; cardiac stimulation increases the heart rate and force of myocardial contraction; arteriolar constriction restores arterial pressure partially or completely to normal, and diverts the reduced cardiac output away from relatively unimportant regions, such as the skin, to the brain and heart. Even if mean arterial pressure is restored to normal, pulse pressure is usually still reduced. This diminution of pulse pressure is detected by the baroreceptors which are insensitive to changes of the pulsatile component of arterial pressure as well as to its mean value (*see* page 97).

Reversible versus irreversible shock

Shock may also be classified as reversible or irreversible. This is a bad classification because the term 'irreversible' implies that the condition is not amenable to any form of treatment. This is not necessarily the case because, although the treatment of irreversible shock may be difficult, and often unsuccessful, it is taking too nihilistic a view to assume that the condition must inevitably be fatal. For this reason some workers prefer the term 'refractory shock'.

The classification into reversible and irreversible really applies to haemorrhagic shock, and to whether this condition can be reversed simply by restoration of blood volume. If the blood volume of a patient with early haemorrhagic shock, particularly a young adult, is restored to normal, he is usually quickly restored to health. However, if the patient is allowed to remain in a severely shocked state for some time, quantitative replacement of the shed blood often results in a purely temporary restoration of cardiac output and, without further treatment, is followed by deterioration of the patient and ultimately by his death. This is irreversible shock.

The treatment which is required to prevent death in irreversible shock is considered later in this chapter (*see* page 227).

Normovolaemic versus hypovolaemic shock

Cardiac output may be reduced either because of a reduction of the efficiency of the cardiac pump (*see* page 124) or because the mean systemic pump pressure, m.s.p. (*see* page 119), is below normal. In the former case blood volume is usually normal, therefore this condition is classified as normovolaemic shock. The commonest cause of the second type of shock is haemorrhage; blood volume is below normal, therefore this condition is classified as hypovolaemic shock.

It is, of course, also possible to develop shock due to a low m.s.p. in the presence of a normal blood volume. If the capacitance vessels become dilated, m.s.p. is reduced despite a normal blood volume. This condition may occur, for example, as a result of wide-spread bacterial infection (bacteraemic or septic shock).

Deteriorating shock

The pathways involved in deteriorating shock are complex, and it is usually impossible to be dogmatic about the precise pathway or pathways which lead to a fatal outcome in any individual patient. This depends to a large extent on the aetiology of the shocked state, and on the patient's pre-existing physiological weaknesses.

The body possesses various compensatory mechanisms which, in compensated shock, help to maintain cardiac output, and to divert blood away from less vital organs to the heart and brain. Although in the short term these mechanisms may be beneficial to the body as a whole, they may ultimately damage the ischaemic tissues, with the result that toxic products are liberated into the general circulation to damage organs which are not themselves hypoxic.

IRREVERSIBLE SHOCK

Although irreversible shock is not necessarily irreversible in the strict sense of the word (*see* page 223), there is no doubt that this condition is difficult to treat, and even energetic therapy is all too often followed by death. The precise pathogenesis of this condition is uncertain and probably varies from patient to patient. At the present time, however, three mechanisms appear to be of particular importance, although there are almost certainly others.

Impairment of cardiac function

A prolonged period of non-cardiogenic shock is sooner or later followed by deterioration of cardiac function, and by aggravation of the patient's shocked state. This deterioration has been demonstrated by many workers (for example, Crowell and Guyton, 1962; Regan et al., 1965) since it was first postulated by Wiggers and Werle in 1942.

Most experimental work on this problem has inevitably been on animals; and this has the disadvantage that, although the condition may be better controlled than spontaneously-occurring human shock, the two conditions are not necessarily comparable. There does, however, appear to be evidence that, in man also, impaired cardiac function may complicate haemorrhagic shock; this is suggested by the beneficial effects which have been claimed for digitalization of patients with irreversible shock (Lillehei et al., 1964b). Also reversible ECG changes have been reported in human haemorrhagic shock by Master et al. (1947).

The cause of such myocardial deterioration is uncertain. Amongst other factors, it is probably due to myocardial ischaemia and hypoxia, and to the systemic acidosis which almost inevitably accompanies severe shock (*see* page 220). Although the body's compensatory mechanisms are designed to direct as much as possible of the reduced cardiac output to the vital organs, a very severe reduction of cardiac output must be accompanied by some decrease of myocardial blood flow. If arterial pressure falls to such an extent that autoregulatory vasodilatation of the coronary vessels can no longer keep pace with the arterial hypotension, myocardial ischaemia must result.

The myocardium is unfortunately particularly vulnerable to hypoxia because its ratio of oxygen consumption to oxygen supply is normally the highest in the body—the coronary arterio-venous oxygen content difference is approximately 12 ml 100 ml^{-1} (Wade and Bishop, 1962).

Bing (1961) showed that myocardial metabolism was abnormal during both the hypovolaemic and subsequent normovolaemic (after transfusion) phases of experimental irreversible shock. The picture was similar to that found in myocardial hypoxia from other causes, such as ventricular fibrillation or extreme ventricular tachycardia. There was a decrease of myocardial oxygen consumption accompanied by decreased extraction of glucose, pyruvate and lactate from the coronary blood. The precise relationship between these biochemical abnormalities and a demonstrable impairment of myocardial performance, however, remains to be clarified.

It is known also that myocardial function is impaired by the metabolic acidosis which accompanies shock, although again the precise manner in which acidosis interferes with myocardial function is not known. An increased hydrogen ion concentration is thought to decrease the myocardial response to sympathetic stimulation and to circulating sympathomimetic amines. Other circulating toxins, such as bacterial endotoxins or high concentrations of potassium, may also impair myocardial contractility.

Changes in the microcirculation

In the early stages of shock the small vessels in organs such as the gut are severely constricted. Later, however, these vessels may become dilated, although blood flow remains greatly reduced. Microscopic examination of such congested, hyperaemic tissues suggests that the precapillary sphincters are relaxed while the post-capillary venules are constricted (Lillehei, Longerbeam and Rosenberg, 1962), thus allowing the capillaries to become overfilled with blood. Lewis and Mellander (1962) suggest that, in conditions of reduced tissue perfusion, vasodilator metabolites accumulate locally and cause relaxation of afferent arterioles and precapillary sphincters; the post-capillary venules, however, are less sensitive to such substances, therefore they remain firmly constricted.

In severe shock, therefore, there may be a large increase in the amount of blood contained in the capillaries, perhaps up to 5 or 10 per cent of the total blood volume. In addition there may be an increase of capillary hydrostatic pressure which causes increased loss of plasma into the tissue spaces and thus depletes the circulating blood volume still further. The sequestered blood in the tissue capillaries and plasma in the interstitial spaces accounts for what Cannon (1923) referred to as 'the blood which is out of currency'.

The increase of blood viscosity which occurs as a result of haemoconcentration is accentuated by further increase due to the non-Newtonian behaviour of blood (*see* page 10). Blood viscosity is increased at low shear-rates, therefore a vicious circle is established, whereby slowing of blood flow through the microcirculation causes an increase of viscosity, which causes a further reduction of flow, and so on.

Intravascular 'sludging' and thrombosis

Ultimately the vessels of the microcirculation become filled with a 'sludge' of erythrocytes, which seriously impedes capillary blood flow. Such flow as persists in tissues such as the gut by-passes the true exchange vessels via arteriovenous anastomoses; functional blood flow in these tissues is therefore virtually zero. The rationale for using low molecular weight dextran (Gelin and Ingelman, 1961) for the treatment of irreversible shock was based on the hope that it might coat the erythrocytes and vessel walls with electronegatively charged molecules, and thus reduce intravascular sludging.

Hardaway (1962) suggests that blood flow may be so sluggish that there may actually be transient intravascular microcirculatory thrombosis. This would, of course, considerably intensify any pre-existing stagnant hypoxia. The cause of the hypercoagulability which Hardaway postulates is probably multiple: acidosis, circulating bacterial toxins and circulating catecholamines have all been suggested as possible factors. The results of treatment with heparin or fibrinolysins are, however, disappointing.

Circulating toxins

Acidosis

There is little doubt that one of the most important circulating toxins in shock is lactic acid, produced by anaerobic metabolism in ischaemic tissues (*see* page 220). It should be pointed out, however, that not all workers have been able to confirm the precise relationship between mortality and oxygen debt found by Crowell and Guyton (1962)—*see* page 221. Nevertheless, the correction of nonrespiratory acidosis by infusion of sodium bicarbonate solution plays an important part in the clinical management of most forms of shock, whether haemorrhagic or cardiogenic.

Bacterial toxins

Some workers suggest that intestinal bacteria play a major role in the pathogenesis of severe shock, whether primarily haemorrhagic or cardiogenic. They suggest that the visceral ischaemia which occurs as a result of intense sympathetic activity damages the integrity of the intestinal mucosa, thus allowing bacteria and bacterial toxins to enter the blood stream to damage remote organs. It is known that gnotobiotic (germ-free) animals survive haemorrhagic shock better than normal controls (Carter and Einheber, 1966), although the importance of such a postulated septic element in human shock is uncertain.

Other toxins

Potassium ions may leak out of damaged cells, and increase the plasma potassium concentration sufficiently to cause impairment of cardiac function. Cellular damage in ischaemic tissues may permit the release of intracellular proteolytic enzymes; among the most important of these are hydrolytic enzymes called lysosomes (Janoff, 1964). These intracellular enzymes are normally surrounded by a lipoprotein membrane, but when the cell is damaged they may be liberated into the cytoplasm to cause cellular autolysis. Leakage of autolytic products from dead or injured cells may then propagate the injury from cell to cell.

PHYSIOLOGICAL PRINCIPLES OF TREATMENT

The treatment of a fit young adult suffering from haemorrhagic shock of recent onset is straightforward. Replacement of the blood volume deficit (guided preferably by measurement of central venous pressure—*see* page 278), correction of acid-base balance, and surgery to prevent further blood loss will quickly restore the patient to health. In the case of an older patient, however, or when the shocked state has persisted for some hours, restoration of blood volume may result in a purely temporary improvement of cardiac output, followed by deterioration of the patient's physiological state, and, without treatment, by his eventual death. This is the condition of 'irreversible' shock (*see* page 223). The permanent restoration of cardiac output in such patients presents a complex therapeutic problem which present physiological knowledge is often insufficient to answer.

The first essential in the treatment of shock is the restoration of a satisfactory cardiac output. This is usually, but not necessarily, accompanied by a simultaneous increase of arterial blood pressure (*see* page 212). An increase of blood pressure without, at the same time, an increase of cardiac output, has little effect on the patient's chances of survival; indeed, a rise of arterial pressure induced by sympathomimetic amines may sometimes cause a paradoxical deterioration of the patient's condition (*see* page 230). Cannon (1923) wrote: 'Merely a higher arterial pressure is not the *desideratum* in the treatment of shock, but a higher pressure which provides an increased nutritive flow through the capillaries all over the body'.

Is arterial pressure important?

This is not to say, of course, that maintenance of arterial blood pressure above a certain minimum level is of no importance. This is clearly not the case: there is a limit to the extent to which even normal blood vessels can dilate and, if the fall of arterial pressure outstrips this vasodilatation, tissue perfusion must suffer. The extent to which vascular dilatation is affected by pathological processes such as arteriosclerosis is unknown, as, therefore, is the minimum permissible blood pressure under any given circumstances. It is possible that, in some patients, vessels in certain tissues may be so rigid that little vasodilatation can occur; under these circumstances a fall of blood pressure, even of moderate degree, must be accompanied by a marked reduction of perfusion in the affected tissue(s).

In the kidneys a sufficient head of pressure is necessary for glomerular filtration to take place against the oncotic pressure of the plasma proteins. In shock, blood is diverted from the kidney by vasoconstriction of glomerular arterioles; this tends to cause a severe reduction of glomerular capillary pressure even though pressure in the large arteries may be reasonably normal. It is fortunate that the kidney is not essential for the short-term economy of the body; the loss of renal function for a few hours is usually unaccompanied by serious physiological consequences, unless there is cortical necrosis due to prolonged renal ischaemia.

Sympathomimetic amines

The receptor theory of adrenergic transmission was considered briefly in Chapter 3. The clinically-used sympathomimetic amines may conveniently be classified as alphamimetic, betamimetic or alphabetamimetic, according to whether their action is predominantly on the α receptors, the β receptors or on both (*Figure 9.4*). (There is actually, of course, a continuous spectrum of activity from an almost pure alphamimetic drug such as phenylephrine to an almost pure betamimetic agent such as isoprenaline.)

Briefly, stimulation of α receptors causes contraction of vascular smooth muscle and vasoconstriction; stimulation of β receptors causes relaxation of smooth muscle and vasodilatation. In the veins there is some dispute about the type of receptor present (*see* page 88); most sympathomimetic amines, however, appear to cause venoconstriction. Stimulation of the β receptors of the heart increases its rate, excitability and force of contraction.

Although all tissues probably contain both types of receptor, one usually predominates in any given tissue (Vickers, 1966). The response of a tissue to an

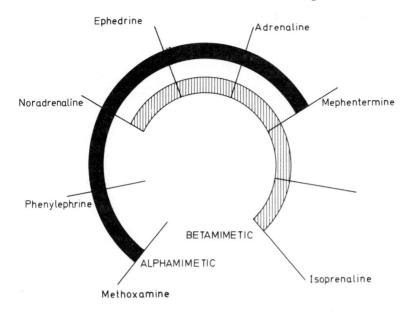

Ephedrine
Adrenaline
Noradrenaline
Mephentermine
Phenylephrine
BETAMIMETIC
ALPHAMIMETIC
Isoprenaline
Methoxamine

Figure 9.4. Alphamimetic and betamimetic synpathomimetic amines (relative potencies after Howitt, 1966)

amine which stimulates both α and β receptors is, therefore, that of stimulation of the predominant type of receptor. The receptors of resistance vessels in skin, kidney and gut are mainly α, therefore most sympathomimetic amines cause vasoconstriction in these regions. In contrast, the cardiac receptors are β, therefore the heart is stimulated to some extent by almost all sympathomimetic amines except those, such as phenylephrine, which have a purely alphamimetic action.

Alphamimetic drugs

The most important of the alphamimetic drugs are phenylephrine and methoxamine. Kukovetz et al. (1959) found that phenylephrine, in very large doses, stimulated the isolated rat heart, whereas methoxamine had no such action. These drugs cause intense arteriolar constriction in tissues which are well supplied with α receptors. They therefore raise arterial blood pressure by increasing total peripheral resistance and divert blood from the gut, kidney and skin to the heart and brain. They also cause venoconstriction and may, therefore, induce a slight increase of cardiac output, even though they have no clinically-significant effect on myocardial contractile force (*see* Chapter 4).

Angiotensin has a chemical structure different from that of the sympathomimetic amines. It has, however, a pharmacological action very similar to that of phenylephrine, and causes marked arteriolar constriction accompanied by a rise of arterial blood pressure, with little change of cardiac output. This action is not blocked by sympatholytic agents such as phenoxybenzamine.

Betamimetic drugs

An important betamimetic drug which is sometimes used in the treatment of shock is isoprenaline; this drug markedly increases the rate and force of cardiac contraction, and causes some venoconstriction. Its administration therefore usually causes a significant increase of cardiac output. In the case of the arterioles, isoprenaline causes dilatation rather than constriction, particularly in tissues well supplied with β receptors; it therefore causes a reduction of total peripheral resistance. Indeed, betamimetic drugs may often cause a decrease of arterial blood pressure even in the presence of an increased cardiac output.

Alphabetamimetic drugs

Many vasopressor drugs in common use, such as metaraminol, are alphabetamimetic in action. They therefore cause an increase of cardiac output, accompanied by some increase of arterial blood pressure. It is said that, in small amounts, their action is mainly betamimetic (Foster, 1966).

Use of sympathomimetic amines

One of the chief controversies in the treatment of severe shock centres around the use of sympathomimetic and sympatholytic drugs. On the one hand there is the school of thought which suggests that vasoconstrictor agents should be administered to supplement the body's own sympathetic activity; on the other hand some workers take the view that intense vasoconstriction from natural sympathetic activity may, in many cases, do more harm than good (*see* below), and correct treatment therefore requires administration of sympatholytic drugs to reverse spontaneous vasoconstriction. The situation is further complicated by the fact that many clinically-used sympathomimetic agents act on both α and β receptors (*see* above).

The vasoconstrictor school of thought

The protagonists of the vasoconstrictor school of thought point out that the body's normal response to severe blood loss is an increase of sympathetic activity and adrenal medullary catecholamine secretion. However, the body's physiological response to haemorrhage is geared more to restoration of arterial blood pressure than to restoration of cardiac output; and it has already been pointed out that such restoration of blood pressure may be detrimental to the perfusion of certain tissues, and is, therefore, not necessarily in the best interests of the body as a whole.

There is also some evidence that the inotropic effects of certain sympathomimetic amines may cause a decrease of myocardial efficiency, that is, an increase of myocardial oxygen consumption at the same work load (Waldhausen, Kilman and Abel, 1965). Therefore, even though such drugs may improve myocardial perfusion by increasing arterial blood pressure, they may increase cardiac oxygen requirements proportionately more; and as a result, the myocardium may become hypoxic. Anaerobic metabolism may then cause a local acidosis with a resultant decrease of myocardial contractile force, and a fall of cardiac output.

The vasodilator school of thought

The vasodilator school of thought is represented by workers such as Nickerson (1962) who point out that death from irreversible shock often occurs as a result of ischaemic changes in severely vasoconstricted tissues. They suggest that vasodilators should be given to reduce the intense vasoconstriction present in certain organs, in the hope that the deleterious effects of tissue ischaemia may thus be averted. It was demonstrated many years ago that spinal anaesthesia or sympathectomy could improve visceral blood flow, and reduce mortality in experimental shock (Eversole et al., 1944). More recently it has been shown that direct splanchnic denervation may also improve survival under similar circumstances (Palmerio et al., 1963).

Most workers at the present time prefer to induce vasodilatation by means of systemically-acting vasodilator drugs such as phenoxybenzamine (*see* page 72) rather than by the injection of local anaesthetics.

Of course, arteriolar vasodilatation with constant cardiac output must divert blood away from vital organs such as the brain and heart to the previously vasoconstricted tissues. It appears, however, that reduction of arterial blood pressure consequent on a decrease of total peripheral resistance may reduce the work of the heart (which may be damaged by acidosis, ischaemia, and so on) sufficiently to allow cardiac output to increase, thus preventing cerebral or myocardial ischaemia. The situation is thus rather analogous to the way in which peripheral vasodilatation may permit an increase of cardiac output during halothane anaesthesia (*see* page 117).

It is important to stress that vasodilator drugs dilate the capacitance (*see* page 88) as well as the resistance vessels. They therefore tend to cause a decrease of mean systemic pressure even though blood volume remains constant. Untreated this would cause a severe, and perhaps fatal, fall of cardiac output. The administration of vasodilator drugs must therefore be preceded and accompanied by adequate fluid replacement. The volume of blood or other fluid which needs to be transfused under these circumstances exceeds that which would be required in the absence of vasodilatation; and it is almost a *sine qua non* that fluid replacement in such patients is monitored by measurement of CVP in order that the hazards of relative hypovolaemia and reduction of mean systemic pressure may be minimized.

Much experimental work has been done on the value of vasodilator drugs in the treatment of shock. Most has been with sympatholytic agents such as phenoxybenzamine (*see* for example, Bloch, Pierce and Lillehei, 1966). This is chiefly an alpha-sympathetic blocking agent, although it may have other nonspecific actions which enhance its value in the treatment of shock. Chlorpromazine and massive doses of adrenal cortical steroids (Lillehei et al., 1964a) have also been used for this purpose.

Collins, Jaffe and Zahony (1964) showed that the administration of chlorpromazine could significantly reduce mortality from clinical irreversible shock. The precise mode of action of this drug is uncertain, but its beneficial effects appear to be due partly at least to vasodilatation. Some workers in fact use chlorpromazine to assess the adequacy of fluid replacement—the 'CPZ test' (Zahony et al., 1964). If chlorpromazine causes a fall of arterial pressure—presumably due to decrease of cardiac output, consequent on reduction of mean systemic pressure—this is assumed to indicate hypovolaemia which needs further transfusion.

The mode of action of adrenal cortical steroids in shock is again not precisely known, although it appears to be due partly to peripheral vasodilatation. It was at one time suggested that adrenal cortical secretion is depressed in shock, and that the therapeutic efficiency of adrenal steroids in this condition is due to correction of a hypothetical adrenal insufficiency. It is now known, however, that, except in Addison's disease and similar conditions, the plasma concentrations of adrenal glucocorticoids are high, and the adrenals respond normally to ACTH stimulation (Davies and Davies, 1968).

RECOMMENDED FURTHER READING

Anon. (1970). 'Septic Shock.' *Br. med. J.* **1**, 3
Anon. (1970). 'Loss of Blood.' *Br. med. J.* **2**, 251
Anon. (1974). 'Bacteraemic Shock.' *Lancet* i, 296
Barrett, A. M. and Einstein, R. (1975). 'Catecholamines and the Cardiovascular System.' In Oliver, M. F., *Modern Trends in Cardiology*, ch. 2. London; Butterworths
Bloch, J. H., Dietzman, R. H., Pierce, C. H. and Lillehei, R. C. (1966). 'Theories of the Production of Shock. A Review of their Relevance to Clinical Practice.' *Br. J. Anaesth.* **38**, 234
Bloch, J. H., Pierce, C. H. and Lillehei, R. C. (1966). 'Adrenergic Blocking Agents in the Treatment of Shock.' *Ann. Rev. Med.* **17**, 483
Chien, S. (1967). 'Role of the Sympathetic Nervous System in Haemorrhage.' *Physiol. Rev.* **47**, 214
Davies, J. and Davies, I. J. T. (1968). 'The Pathogenesis and Treatment of Shock.' *Hosp. Med.* **2**, 686
Dietzman, R. H. and Lillehei, R. C. (1968). 'The Nature and Treatment of Shock.' *Hosp. Med.* **2**, 300
Fine, J. (1965). 'Shock and Peripheral Circulatory Insufficiency. In *Handbook of Physiology, Circulation*, Vol. III, p. 2037. Washington; American Physiological Society
Fowle, A. S. E. (1968). 'The Physiology of Shock.' *Hosp. Med.* **2**, 307
Foster, R. W. (1966). 'The Pharmacology of Pressor Drugs.' *Br. J. Anaesth.* **38**, 690
Guyton, A. C., Jones, C. E. and Coleman, T. G. (1973). *Cardiac Output and its Regulation*, 2nd edn, ch. 21. Philadelphia; W. B. Saunders
Hershey, S. G., del Guercio, L. R. M. and McConn, R. (1971). *Septic Shock in Man*. Edinburgh; Churchill Livingstone
Hershey, S. G. and Altura, B. M. (1973). 'Vasopressors and Low-flow States.' In Zauder, H. L., *Clinical Anaesthesia: Pharmacology of Adjuvant Drugs*, p. 31. Philadelphia; F. A. Davis
Howitt, G. (1966). 'Therapy with Adrenergic Drugs and their Antagonists.' *Br. J. Anaesth.* **38**, 719
Kelman, G. R. (1969). 'Cardiac Output in Shock.' *Int. Anesth. Clin.* **7**, 4
Kelman, G. R. (1975). 'Shock and Peripheral Circulatory Failure.' In *Physiology—A Clinical Approach*, 2nd edn, ch. 2. Edinburgh; Churchill Livingstone
Moore, F. D. (1973). 'Systemic Indicators of the Low-flow State: Biochemistry and Metabolism during Tissue Hypoperfusion.' In Wells, R., *The Microcirculation in Clinical Medicine*, p. 195. London; Academic Press
Novelli, G. P. (1975). 'Physiology of the Shock-state.' In *Physiological Basis of Anaesthesiology*, p. 265. Padua; Piccin Medical Books

Shoemaker, W. C. (1971). 'Cardiorespiratory Patterns in Complicated and Uncomplicated Septic Shock.' *Ann. Surg.* **174**, 119

Shoemaker, W. C. (1975). 'Pathophysiology and Therapy of Shock.' In Walker, W. F. and Taylor, D. E. M., *Intensive Care.* Edinburgh; Churchill Livingstone

Smith, N. T. and Corbasio, A. N. (1970). 'The Use and Misuse of Pressor Agents.' *Anesthesiology* **33**, 58

Chapter 10 Chronic Heart Failure

Paul Wood defined heart failure as 'a state in which the heart fails to maintain an adequate circulation for the needs of the body despite a satisfactory venous filling pressure'. This definition excludes low cardiac outputs which occur as a result of reduced mean systemic pressure (*see* page 119), but applies equally to acute heart failure in cardiogenic shock (*see* page 126), and to chronic heart failure occurring as a result of, for example, valvular heart disease, hypertension or chronic myocardial ischaemia. Acute heart failure is considered in Chapter 9; chronic heart failure forms the subject of the present chapter.

In chronic heart failure there is, in addition to an inadequate cardiac output, a marked retention of water and electrolytes, chiefly sodium; this leads to expansion of the extracellular fluid space, and often to systemic and pulmonary oedema. The cause of this fluid and electrolyte retention is disputed (*see* page 239), but is probably due in the main to increased secretion of aldosterone from the adrenal cortex. Many of the manifestations of chronic heart failure are due more to abnormal fluid retention than to the inadequate cardiac output *per se.*

The anatomical distribution of the water and electrolyte excess is influenced by the nature of the causative lesion, by whether the failure affects primarily the left or right ventricle. In left ventricle failure the majority of fluid retention occurs in the pulmonary circulation; this causes decreased pulmonary compliance and dyspnoea, first during exercise and later at rest. In right ventricular failure the retention causes predominantly systemic oedema.

CARDIAC OUTPUT AND PERIPHERAL BLOOD FLOW

Cardiac output

In most cases of chronic heart failure cardiac output is slightly below normal; Stead, Warren and Brannon (1948), for example, found a mean resting value of $3.8\,l\,min^{-1}$ in patients with congestive cardiac failure. In mild cases, however, cardiac output may lie within the normal range at rest, although it does not increase adequately under the stress of exercise. In very severe failure, particularly that due to valvular stenosis, cardiac output may be markedly reduced at rest, and increases but slightly, or not at all, during exercise (*see* page 169).

High-output failure

In some conditions the body requires a cardiac output which is considerably above normal; this may occur, for example, as a result of anaemia, thyrotoxicosis, and arterio-venous fistulae. Under these circumstances heart failure may occur with a cardiac output which is above the normal range (high-output heart failure). (An analogous state of affairs occurs in some forms of shock. In the presence of arterio-venous anastomoses, the shock syndrome may occur in the presence of a normal or even raised cardiac output—*see* page 222.)

The disparity between cardiac output and the body's metabolic requirements is reflected in the composition of the mixed-venous blood. Epstein, S. E. et al. (1966) found that, in chronic heart failure, the amount of oxygen returning to the heart each minute (the product of cardiac output and mixed-venous oxygen content) was decreased from a normal resting value of 375 ml $min^{-1} m^{-2}$ body surface to 181 ml $min^{-1} m^{-2}$ in patients with failure. Despite the obvious physiological importance of a reduction of cardiac output, however, there is a rather poor correlation between the severity of a patient's subjective symptoms and the apparent inadequacy of his cardiac output. This suggests that additional (unknown) factors are concerned in producing the symptoms of cardiac failure.

Peripheral blood flow

Although the chronically failing heart is unable to provide a normal cardiac output, it is able to maintain an almost normal arterial blood pressure. This means, of course, that the total peripheral resistance must be increased by vasoconstriction in certain tissues. This vasoconstriction diverts blood to the remainder of the body in precisely the same way as it does in acute heart failure or in hypovolaemic shock (*see* page 217). Many of the clinical manifestations of heart failure, including probably the retention of water and electrolytes, is due to chronic ischaemia of various peripheral tissues.

This decrease of tissue blood flow is particularly marked in the kidney, gut and limbs. The kidney is particularly affected; Wade and Bishop (1962) quote a mean renal blood flow of 231 ml $min^{-1} m^{-2}$ body surface in patients with congestive failure, compared with 660 ml $min^{-1} m^{-2}$ in normal subjects. On a percentage basis this reduction is considerably greater than the concomitant reduction of cardiac output. Donald, Bishop and Wade (1955) found that arm blood flow at rest was markedly reduced in patients with rheumatic heart disease, and that there was a good correlation between the local decrease of blood flow and the reduction of cardiac output. And Ferrer et al. (1965) found that the splanchnic blood flow was reduced in chronic heart failure by roughly the same proportion as cardiac output.

The average distribution of cardiac output in chronic heart failure given by Wade and Bishop (1962) is shown in *Figure 10.1.*

This increase of vascular resistance is presumably due in part to increased sympathetic activity. It appears, however, that other factors may also be involved, because it has been found that reactive hyperaemia after vascular occlusion is reduced in patients with congestive failure (Mason, 1966). This finding suggests that there may be actual physical changes in the arteriolar walls

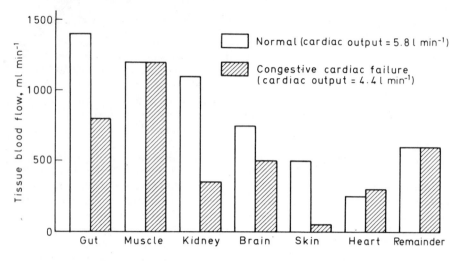

Figure 10.1. Distribution of total cardiac output (4.4 l min⁻¹) in a resting patient with congestive cardiac failure (figures from Wade and Bishop, 1962)

of such patients; the nature of these postulated changes is, however, unknown at present.

THE CARDIAC DEFECT IN CHRONIC HEART FAILURE

The syndrome of chronic heart failure is due primarily to inability of the heart to pump a sufficient quantity of blood for the body's metabolic needs. In some cases the reason for the impairment of cardiac function is clear enough; in other cases its cause is entirely speculative. Olson (1964) divided cardiac failure into two major groups: patients in whom myocardial energy production is inadequate, e.g. those with myocardial ischaemia; and those in whom energy production is normal, but its utilization is impaired. Most patients with chronic congestive failure fall into the second group.

In coronary heart disease part of the myocardium may be replaced by fibrous tissue, so that it is unable to contract with normal vigour; in myocarditis the heart is unable to contract normally because the myocardium is obviously diseased; in beri-beri cardiac metabolism is deranged because of a lack of vitamin B, which is essential for normal carbohydrate metabolism; in infiltrative disease, myocardial function is directly impaired by the infiltrative process. In most cases, however, the cause of the defective function is not at all obvious, and the myocardium appears macroscopically and microscopically normal.

Most forms of chronic heart failure are preceded by a period of increased cardiac work. This increased load may, for example, be hypertension, valvular stenosis or incompetence, or a chronic increase of the body's metabolic requirements as in thyrotoxicosis. It leads to myocardial hypertrophy as a result of which the heart is able, for a time, to deal satisfactorily with the increased load imposed upon it. Sooner or later, however, the myocardium becomes unable to maintain a sufficient cardiac output for the body's needs, and chronic heart failure develops. Myocardial contraction is then clearly abnormal, although the precise biochemical or biophysical defect has, as yet, not been precisely defined.

Cardiac contraction may be considered to consist of three stages (*see* page 41): energy liberation, energy storage and energy conversion (the conversion of chemical into mechanical energy). The defect in cardiac failure appears to be in the last stage.

Energy liberation

The myocardium derives its energy from the breakdown of a variety of substrates (*see* page 42). In congestive failure, myocardial uptake of glucose, pyruvate, fatty acids and ketones appears to be normal (Kako and Bing, 1958). Myocardial oxygen consumption is also normal at rest, and during moderate exercise, although some patients with cardiac failure from chronic myocardial ischaemia may develop myocardial hypoxia during heavy exercise. Under most conditions, therefore, cardiac failure does not appear to be due to defective energy production by the heart.

Energy storage

The evidence about the normality or otherwise of energy storage in cardiac failure is conflicting. The majority view, however, appears to be that the defect in chronic heart failure is in energy utilization rather than in energy storage. Some workers have demonstrated a decreased myocardial concentration of high energy phosphate compounds in experimental heart failure; the relevance of this finding to spontaneously-occurring failure in man is, however, uncertain.

Energy conversion

Although there is little direct microscopic evidence of physical abnormality of the contractile proteins in human heart failure, it has been found that the contractility of actomyosin bands taken from patients dying of congestive failure is impaired, and may be partially restored by the addition of digoxin and calcium ions (Kako and Bing, 1958). Abnormalities of the myocardial contractile proteins have also been found in animals subjected to experimental heart failure; and Bing, Wu and Gudbjarnason (1964) suggest that there may be a deficiency of the enzymes which are involved in protein synthesis, so leading in time to functional impairment of the myocardial contractile apparatus.

There is also depletion of the myocardial stores of noradrenaline, so that the heart is unable to respond normally to sympathetic stimulation. The action of exogenous catecholamines is, however, relatively unimpaired. Guanethidine causes severe depletion of myocardial catecholamines, and may precipitate heart failure in patients with hypertensive heart disease (Braunwald et al., 1963). Tyrosine hydroxylase catalyses a rate-limiting step in the synthesis of noradrenaline, and it has recently been shown that this enzyme is markedly reduced in experimental heart failure (Pool et al., 1967).

Leonard (1966) suggests that myocardial function in chronic heart failure is deficient because of impairment of the mechanisms which control the passage of calcium ions through the cell membrane. This hypothesis is supported by the fact that digitalis is thought to act partly by increasing the number of calcium ions which are liberated in the vicinity of the intracellular contractile proteins when the cell membrane is depolarized.

Objective evidence of impaired myocardial function is provided by the fact that, in heart failure, the maximum rate of rise of intraventricular pressure (*see* page 45) is considerably below normal (Miller, Kirklin and Swan, 1965).

VENTRICULAR FUNCTION IN CONGESTIVE CARDIAC FAILURE

The retention of water and electrolytes which occurs in chronic heart failure expands the extracellular fluid compartment, thus increasing the mean systemic pressure (*see* page 119) and right atrial pressure, and restoring cardiac output partially or completely to normal (*see* Chapter 4). Myocardial function is depressed, therefore the heart is able to produce a given cardiac output only at a higher right atrial pressure than normal. This increase of pressure is responsible for the neck-vein distension which is a characteristic clinical feature of chronic congestive cardiac failure. It should be noted, however, that acute hypervolaemia causes only a transient increase of venous pressure (Warren et al., 1948); therefore in heart failure there is probably also an increase of venous tone. Clinically it has been shown that venous distensibility increases when cardiac failure responds to treatment (Wood, Litter and Wilkins, 1956). (It should be noted that in some forms of heart failure, particularly when this is associated with marked ventricular hypertrophy, the compliance of the ventricular wall may be considerably decreased, with the result that atrial pressure may be increased even when the functional ability of the myocardium is relatively normal—Braunwald and Ross, 1963.)

If the defect of cardiac function is limited mainly to the left side of the heart, fluid retention occurs chiefly in the pulmonary circulation, thus raising the left atrial pressure to maintain the output of the left ventricle. Guyton's graphical analysis, which is discussed in Chapter 4, may be applied independently to both sides of the heart, but the procedure is then unfortunately too cumbersome to be of much value in helping the intuitive understanding of cardiac regulation.

Increase of atrial pressure causes an increase of ventricular output by the Frank-Starling mechanism (*see* page 49). It leads also to some degree of ventricular dilatation, as a result of which the heart is able to expel a given quantity of blood with a smaller muscular contraction than when ventricular volume is normal. This mechanical advantage is, however, partially offset by the fact that the tension which myocardial fibres must produce to cause a given intraventricular pressure is greater at larger ventricular volumes (Laplace's Law, *see* page 12).

If ventricular dilatation becomes excessive, ventricular function may be impaired rather than enhanced. This is often attributed to over-extension of the sarcomeres (*see* page 25), but Linzbach (1960) suggests that the muscle fibres of the dilated heart are not, in fact, overstretched; and that the sarcomere length is the same as in the normal heart, the dilatation being due to sliding of the muscle fibres relative to each other. When the heart becomes very large, functional incompetence of the atrioventricular valves may cause severe impairment of cardiac efficiency.

CAUSE OF FLUID AND ELECTROLYTE RETENTION IN CHRONIC HEART FAILURE

The increase of blood volume found in chronic heart failure is not due solely to water and electrolyte retention. There is also an increase of red cell mass, which returns to normal after successful treatment (Samet et al., 1957). The cause of this polycythaemia is unknown; it may, perhaps, be due to stimulation of the bone-marrow as a result of stagnant hypoxia.

In severe heart failure, plasma volume may be increased above normal by as much as 30 per cent. One of the most important factors in the causation of this fluid and electrolyte retention is defective renal function, but the precise physiological defect responsible is uncertain. It is known that both renal blood flow and glomerular filtration rate are reduced in chronic heart failure. Experimental reduction of glomerular filtration, however, usually causes a purely temporary retention of water and electrolytes. Moreover, in some forms of intrinsic renal disease glomerular filtration may be reduced to levels comparable to those found in chronic heart failure with but little fluid and electrolyte retention. Similarly, acute compression of the renal veins causes an increase of local venous pressure, comparable to that found in chronic heart failure, but again induces a purely temporary decrease of water and electrolyte excretion.

The primary renal defect is, in fact, probably diminished sodium re-absorption from the tubules rather than decreased filtration by the glomeruli. The evidence on this point is, however, conflicting. Aldosterone excretion is known to be increased in patients with congestive heart failure (Luetscher and Johnson, 1954) and, more recently, increased concentrations of this hormone have been found in the plasma of such patients. It is, however, well known that very high aldosterone concentrations may occur in cirrhotic patients without fluid retention; also oedema is not a prominent feature of primary hyperaldosteronism. Moreover, spironolactone, an aldosterone antagonist, may be ineffective in inducing diuresis in patients with chronic heart failure.

The renin–angiotensin theory of the control of aldosterone release was considered briefly in Chapter 4. Increased amounts of both renin and angiotensin II have been found in the renal venous blood in congestive heart failure; and in experimental heart failure there is increased granularity of the juxtaglomerular apparatus (Tobian, 1960). This region of the kidney is thought to be concerned with the regulation of renin secretion.

It is known that the administration of sympatholytic agents to patients with chronic failure may induce diuresis. This suggests that the fluid and electrolyte retention in these patients may be due to sympathetically-induced spasm of the renal afferent arterioles, with resultant stimulation of the juxtaglomerular apparatus. Sodium excretion is said to be increased in normal subjects by the administration of guanethidine which reduces sympathetically-induced vasoconstriction.

RECOMMENDED FURTHER READING

Ayres, S. M. (1971). 'Metabolic and Nutritional Heart Disease.' In Ayres, S. M. and Gregory, J. J., *Cardiology: A Clinicophysiologic Approach*, p. 613. London; Butterworths

Beller, B. M. (1973). 'Digitalis and Anesthesia: A Comprehensive Review of the Chemistry, Pharmacology, and Clinical Use of the Cardiac Glycosides in Anesthesia.' In Zauder, H. L., *Pharmacology of Adjuvant Drugs*. Philadelphia; F. A. Davis

Bing, R. J., Wu, C. and Gudbjarnason, S. (1964). 'Mechanism of Heart Failure.' *Circulation Res.* **15** (Suppl. 2), 64

Davis, J. O. (1965). 'The Physiology of Congestive Heart Failure.' In *Handbook of Physiology, Circulation*, Vol. III, p. 2071. Washington; American Physiological Society

Hajdu, S. and Leonard, E. (1959). 'The Cellular Basis of Cardiac Glycoside Action.' *Pharmacol. Rev.* **11**, 173

Henderson, A. H. (1975). 'Contractile Basis of Heart Failure.' In Oliver, M. F., *Modern Trends in Cardiology*, 3rd edn, ch. 7. London; Butterworths

Howitt, G. (1971). 'The Pharmacology of the Normal and Diseased Heart in Relation to Cardiac Surgery.' *Br. J. Anaesth.* **43**, 261

Guyton, A. C., Jones, C. E. and Coleman, T. G. (1973). *Cardiac Output and its Regulation*, 2nd edn, chps 26 and 27. Philadelphia; Saunders

Kelman, G. R. (1975). 'Heart Failure.' In *Physiology: A Clinical Approach*, 2nd edn. Edinburgh; Churchill Livingstone

Martinez-Mojares, M. A., Gudbjarnason, S. and Bing, R. J. (1969). 'Myocardial Metabolism.' In Morgan Jones, A., *Modern Trends in Cardiology*, 2nd edn. London; Butterworths

Oakley, C. M. (1976). 'Correlation between Structure and Function in Heart Disease.' *Proc. roy. Soc. Med.* **69**, 199

Olson, R. E. (1964). 'Abnormalities of Myocardial Metabolism.' *Circulation Res.* **15** (Suppl. 2), 109

Peters, T. J., Wells, G., Brooksby, I. A. B., Jenkins, B. S., Webb-Peploe, M. M. and Coltart, D. J. (1976). 'Enzymic Analysis of Cardiac Biopsy Material from Patients with Valvular Heart-disease.' *Lancet* i, 269

Rushmer, R. F. (1971). 'The Cardiac Reserve and Congestive Heart Failure.' In *Cardiovascular Dynamics*, 3rd edn, ch. 15. Philadelphia; Saunders

Scheuer, J. (1970). 'Metabolism of the Heart in Cardiac Failure.' *Prog. cardiovasc. Dis.* **13**, 24

Zelis, R. and Longhurst, J. (1975). 'The Circulation in Congestive Heart Failure.' In Zelis, R. M., *The Peripheral Circulations*. New York; Grune and Stratton

Chapter 11   Hypertension

In health, arterial blood pressure is maintained within fairly narrow limits by a variety of homeostatic mechanisms, of which the most important are the carotid and aortic baroreceptor reflexes (*see* page 97), and the mechanisms which control sodium balance (*see* later). It is true that some rise of arterial pressure may accompany the sympatho-adrenal overactivity of exercise and emotional stimulation; but this rise is relatively small, is readily reversed, and is entirely appropriate to the body's physiological requirements of the moment. Chronic hypertension represents a very different situation: there is then a breakdown of the body's homeostatic mechanisms, allowing the arterial pressure to become chronically elevated, a condition which may have serious, and often fatal, effects of several organs, particularly the heart, brain and kidney.

NORMAL BLOOD PRESSURE

It is not possible to make a definitive statement about what constitutes a 'normal' arterial blood pressure, since this varies considerably from minute to minute (*Figure 11.1*). The usual textbook normal resting value is 120/80 mm Hg (15.9/10.6 kPa). But this figure is probably too high for a young person, and is certainly too low for a middle-aged or elderly adult; blood pressure, as is well known, tends to increase with increasing age (*Table 11.1*). In medical students it is not uncommon to find arterial pressures as low as 110/65 mm Hg, or even lower when the subject is mentally and physically relaxed.

This increase of pressure with age does not, however, occur in isolated, non-Western communities, although it does if these communities adopt a Western way of life (Shaper et al., 1969).

In middle and old age the systolic pressure increases disproportionately compared with the diastolic pressure. The reason for this is the decrease of arterial elasticity which occurs with increasing age—'arteriosclerosis'. When the elasticity of the Windkessel vessels (*see* page 73) is decreased, the ejection of a given stroke volume from the left ventricle causes a larger than normal pulse pressure, and therefore a disproportionate increase of systolic pressure. The old adage that the systolic pressure is '100 + age' is thus a reasonable approximation to the truth.

In recent years small portable tape recorders have been developed which can be connected to indwelling arterial cannulae to provide a continuous 24-hour record of arterial blood pressure (Bevan, Honour and Stott, 1969). A typical record (*Figure 11.1*) shows the great variations of pressure which occur between the waking and sleeping states, and in response to emotional stimulation.

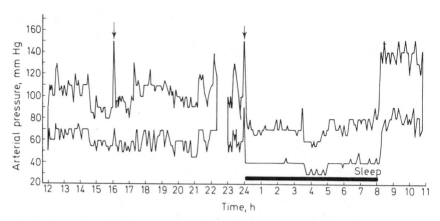

Figure 11.1. 24-Hour blood pressure recording of normal subject. Arrows indicate periods of emotional stress. (Reproduced with permission from Bevan, A. T., Honour, A. J. and Stott, F. M., 1969. Clin. Sci. **36**, *329)*

Table 11.1   AVERAGE ARTERIAL BLOOD PRESSURES (mm Hg) IN NORMAL ADULT MALES LIVING IN LONDON (FIGURES FROM PICKERING, 1974)

	Pressure	
Age	*Systolic*	*Diastolic*
20–24	123	74
30–34	123	74
40–44	127	77
50–54	134	82
60–64	154	88
70–74	161	87

Hypertension

As with many conditions, it is difficult to define precisely the border-line which separates a normal blood pressure from overt hypertension. Arterial blood pressure increases with age, even in normal people; and moreover there is, in any homogenous age group, a continuous gradation between the blood pressure of individuals who are clearly normal and of those who are unequivocally hypertensive. The frequency distribution curve of arterial blood pressure at any age is unimodal, therefore it is not possible to separate off a well-defined group of hypertensive patients, and to delimit these from their normal fellows (Pickering, 1968). The level of arterial blood pressure above which hypertension is considered to be present must be arbitrary.

THE FUNCTIONAL ABNORMALITY IN HYPERTENSION

As explained in an earlier section (*see* page 75) the mean arterial blood pressure is equal to the product of the cardiac output and the so-called peripheral resistance (systemic vascular resistance), i.e. the effective resistance of all the body's vascular beds connected in parallel between the arterial and venous sides of the circulation. The resistance of an individual vascular bed depends on the viscosity of the blood (*see* page 10), and the length and (particularly) the diameter of the individual vessels.

Theoretically therefore arterial hypertension could be due to increased cardiac output, increased blood viscosity, or decreased vascular calibre. In practice, however, most forms of systemic hypertension appear to be due to narrowing of the peripheral resistance vessels (Frolich, Tarazi and Dustan, 1969). (It is well recognized, of course, that polycythaemia may be accompanied by mild hypertension, presumably as a result of increased blood viscosity. Also, the mild hypertension of exercise (*see* page 174) is due to an increased cardiac output, the total peripheral resistance being considerably below its resting value. Increased pulmonary blood flow may cause *pulmonary* hypertension in certain forms of congenital heart disease.)

There is debate about whether the increased resistance to peripheral blood flow is due to structural or functional abnormality of the affected vessels. It is known, however, that in some tissues at any rate, the vascular resistance remains increased even under conditions of maximal vasodilatation (Sivertsson and Olander, 1968: Folkow, 1971), indicating some degree of structural abnormality. Also, it is, of course, well recognized that arteriolar hypertrophy is a common histological feature of most forms of hypertension.

It has been argued, particularly by Folkow (*see* Recommended Further Reading), that the response of such hypertrophied vessels to vasoconstrictor influences is increased because contraction of the outer layers of the hypertrophied walls forces the inner layers inwards, so encroaching on the vascular lumen. And it is thus possible to explain both the vessels' increased resistance under conditions of maximal vasodilatation, and also their increased responsiveness to neurogenic or chemical vasoconstrictor influences.

Renin, angiotensin and sodium metabolism

There is no doubt that hypertension and sodium metabolism are intimately related—*see* Recommended Further Reading, particularly Swales (1975). But there is, as yet, no clear consensus of opinion on this subject.

The body's sodium balance is largely under the control of the hormone aldosterone, the secretion of which is modulated both by the plasma sodium (and probably also potassium) concentration, and indirectly by the plasma renin level (*see* page 130).

Renin is an enzyme which acts on an α_2-globulin in the plasma to produce a decapeptide, angiotensin I, which is then converted in the blood to the octapeptide angiotension II. This is an extremely powerful pressor agent, molecule-for-molecule being 40 times as powerful as noradrenaline. Angiotensin also causes release of aldosterone from the glomerulosa cells of the adrenal medulla, and so induces sodium retention, a response which is probably involved in restoring the blood volume after haemorrhage.

The plasma renin concentration is usually elevated in renal hypertension (*see* below); in essential hypertension, however, the plasma renin concentration is usually normal, although it may be high or low (Löwenstein, 1972). High plasma renin levels are characteristic of malignant hypertension.

SECONDARY HYPERTENSION

In the majority of cases systemic hypertension is of unknown etiology. But in a minority—the size of which depends to some extent on how intensively the patient is investigated—it is secondary to some other condition; and in a few patients the primary causative condition is remediable by surgery. (It is, however, well recognized that in some patients the blood pressure remains elevated even when the primary cause of the hypertension has been removed. It is thought, also, that hypertension from any cause ultimately produces vascular changes which are themselves capable of perpetuating the hypertensive state. Possibly malignant hypertension is an accelerated form of the self-perpetuating process.)

Endocrine causes

The hypertension which occurs with a phaeochromocytoma is readily understood. Such tumours arise from chromaffin tissue either in the adrenal medulla or in adrenal rests elsewhere in the body. They secrete the catecholamines adrenaline and noradrenaline—usually intermittently—and so cause hypertension, often in the form of paroxysms in which the blood pressure rises precipitously, and there are accompanying signs and symptoms of adrenal oversecretion: pallor of the extremities, tremor, anxiety, tachycardia, and sweating. The diagnosis can be confirmed by measuring the 24-hour excretion of adrenaline and noradrenaline, or of their metabolic endproducts vanillomandelic acid (VMA) or met-noradrenaline.

Primary aldosteronism—Conn's syndrome (Conn, 1955)

Over-secretion of aldosterone by a tumour of the adrenal cortex produces mild or moderate hypertension, although the precise cause of the raised blood pressure is less certain than with a phaeochromocytoma. The hypertension is, however, probably related to sodium retention, which occurs as a result of the action of aldosterone on the distal part of the nephron (*see* below). For the same reason there is excessive loss of potassium and hydrogen ions in the urine, with a consequent hypokalaemic metabolic alkalosis.

Plasma renin levels in this condition are low unless the hypertension has entered a 'malignant' phase.

Cushing's syndrome

Cushing's syndrome is due to oversecretion of cortisol from the adrenal cortex, either as a result of hypertrophy or tumour formation, or of oversecretion of ACTH from the anterior pituitary. As with primary hyperaldosteronism the cause of the hypertension in Cushing's syndrome is debated, but again is probably due in part to sodium retention.

Renal hypertension

The relationship between hypertension and renal disease has been known since the original description of 'Bright's disease' early in the nineteenth century. It is now well recognized that not only may primary renal disease cause hypertension, but hypertension itself will sooner or later result in renal damage, so setting up a vicious circle in which the hypertension gradually becomes more severe.

The relationship between the kidney and hypertension is perhaps best seen in the classical experiments of Goldblatt et al. (1934) in which he showed that partial occlusion of one or both renal arteries resulted in an increased systemic blood pressure. The clinical counterpart of these experiments is unilateral renal artery stenosis, a condition which may sometimes be amenable to surgery. Such unilateral renal artery stenosis usually results in increased renin secretion from the ischaemic kidney, as may be determined by renal vein catheterization.

In the main there are three hypotheses about the pathogenesis of hypertension in renal disease:

1. that it is due to renin oversecretion,
2. that it is due to sodium and water retention,
3. that the normal kidney prevents the development of hypertension either by producing an (unknown) vasodilator chemical, or by breaking down some (unknown) vasoconstrictor chemical.

None of these hypotheses is, however, entirely satifactory, and probably— as so often happens in physiology and medicine—more than one mechanism acts simultaneously. Of the three, the one which is least favoured at the moment is the last because it has been shown that removal of both (diseased) kidneys in man does *not* result in hypertension *provided that sodium and water overload is prevented* (Merrill, Giorando and Heetderks, 1961). There is good evidence that partial obstruction of one renal artery may cause increased renin/angiotensin levels in the blood (Bianchi, Tenconi and Lucca, 1970); but the levels which are found in many forms of renal disease do not appear to be sufficient to explain the observed hypertension simply in terms of the known pharmacological actions of angiotensin. It is, however, known that sodium and water retention may enhance the blood vessels' sensitivity to vasoconstrictor influences; and it may, therefore, be that some forms of renal hypertension are due to mechanisms (1) and (3) acting synergistically.

It has been suggested on the basis of experimental work in anephric man that sodium and water retention at first causes hypertension by producing an increase of cardiac output by the Starling mechanism (*see* page 49), but that in time the output of the heart returns to normal, and the hypertension is then maintained by an increase of peripheral resistance (Coleman et al., 1970).

ESSENTIAL HYPERTENSION

If the pathogenesis of renal hypertension is unclear, still more so is that of so-called 'essential' hypertension (which is in any case unlikely to be a single disease entity). Many physiological abnormalities—for example, of baroreceptor sensitivity (Sleight, Gribbin and Pickering, 1971), of renal sodium handling

ACP—9

(Brown et al., 1974), and of renin/angiotension secretion (Laragh et al., 1972) have been found in patients with essential hypertension; but it is almost impossible to say with any degree of authority whether these changes are primary or secondary (*see* Recommended Further Reading—Hypertension: The Chicken and the Egg). As already mentioned, renin secretion in patients with essential hypertension may be high, normal, or low; although it appears that patients may respond differently to treatment according to whether they are renin hyper- or hyposecretors.

A plausible hypothesis

A plausible hypothesis has been put forward, albeit with some differences of detail, by several groups of workers. It goes somewhat along the following lines: in its early stages hypertension is intermittent, and is due mainly to an increase of cardiac output; however, sooner or later the body reacts to the effects of the intermittently raised blood pressure, and as a result the hypertension becomes permanent.

Ledingham, for example (Ledingham, 1971) has suggested that intermittent sympatho-adrenal overactivity causes renal vasoconstriction, and that this leads to sodium retention, expansion of the extracellular fluid volume, and increased cardiac output. This increase of cardiac output then tends to cause an increase of blood flow to various tissues resulting in an autoregulatory increase of peripheral resistance to maintain tissue blood flow within normal limits. The changes in the affected blood vessels then sooner or later become irreversible causing the hypertension to become permanent.

Folkow's interpretation (Folkow et al., 1973) is very similar except that—by analogy with what happens to the walls of veins which are exposed to increased intravascular pressures as a result of an arteriovenous fistula—he takes the view that the increased pressure *per se* causes medial hypertrophy of the resistance vessels, and that this hypertrophy leads both to an increased peripheral resistance and to increased vascular reactivity (*see* page 243).

The attractive feature of this hypothesis is that it explains the well-known observation that hypertension may be caused by psychological stress, although constitutional factors undoubtedly influence the degree to which the body reacts to a given amount of stress. Folkow, for example, considers that hypertension is relatively more common in mesomorphic individuals whose mesenchymal tissues appear to be particularly well able to hypertrophy in the face of increased functional demands.

ANAESTHESIA IN HYPERTENSIVE PATIENTS

Prys-Roberts et al. (*see* Recommended Further Reading) have made a series of valuable investigations into the effect of general anaesthesia on the cardio-vascular system of hypertensive patients. All practising anaesthetists should consult the original articles, which are summarized briefly here.

Both in treated and untreated hypertensive patients general anaesthesia with thiopentone, halothane and nitrous oxide, and spontaneous ventilation, caused a marked fall in arterial blood pressure which in some cases was sufficient to cause ECG changes suggestive of myocardial ischaemia (Prys-Roberts, Meloche and Foëx, 1971a). The fall in cardiac output (about 30 per cent) was not significantly different from that found in a control group of non-hypertensive patients of the same age; and the hypotension was thus attributed to a decrease of the (abnormally high) systemic vascular resistance.

In an investigation into the effects of different induction agents on blood pressure the same workers (1971b) found that hypertensive patients were particularly prone to develop (relative) hypertension during induction of anaesthesia. No method of induction was entirely satisfactory, but neuroleptanalgesia with a combination of phenoperidine and droperidol had less tendency to cause hypotension than the other agents investigated. Propanidid (200–300 mg) and diazepam (10–20 mg) caused severe hypotension in some patients.

Equally alarming were the *increases* of blood pressure which occurred during laryngoscopy and intubation, and which were sometimes accompanied by disturbing cardiac dysrhythmias. In untreated patients arterial blood pressure during intubation sometimes exceeded the pre-anaesthetic level, perhaps a reflection of the greater reactivity of the peripheral resistance vessels in such patients (*see* earlier). These upward swings of pressure were also commonly accompanied by ECG evidence of myocardial ischaemia.

Similar large falls of blood pressure were found in hypertensive patients anaesthetized with nitrous oxide, and artificially ventilated to a mean Pa_{CO_2} of 23 mm Hg (Prys-Roberts et al., 1971a). Addition of 1 per cent halothane caused a further fall of arterial pressure, with a decrease of cardiac output and a small increase of systemic vascular resistance. During the nitrous oxide/halothane/hyperventilation phase of the study all six of the untreated patients showed T wave abnormalities, and three showed ST segment changes. ECG abnormalities were also seen in some of the treated patients. The incidence of ECG abnormalities was much less during anaesthesia with nitrous oxide (and hyperventilation) alone.

As a result of these findings Prys-Roberts and colleagues recommend that: (1) low arterial P_{CO_2} should be avoided during anaesthesia of hypertensive patients, (2) halothane and hypocapnia seems to be a particularly undesirable combination, and (3) hypertensive patients should be adequately treated before elective surgery.

The same workers (1973) also investigated the effects of the beta-blocking drug practolol (now withdrawn from general use) on the cardiovascular system of hypertensive patients. They found that, provided bradycardia was avoided by administration of adequate doses of atropine (0.02 mg kg^{-1}), the use of such beta-blockers did not appear to have deleterious consequences on the cardiovascular system, cardiac output being higher and systemic vascular resistance lower than in companion studies on non-beta-blocked patients. At the same time the use of adequate doses of practolol seemed to protect the patient from the excessive swings of arterial pressure and the cardiac dysrhythmias which were commonly found during intubation of hypertensive patients (*see* above).

RECOMMENDED FURTHER READING

Anon. (1971). 'Renal Hypertension.' *Lancet* i, 483
Anon. (1975). 'When to Measure Renin.' *Lancet* i, 783

Anon. (1976). 'Hypertension—The Chicken and the Egg.' *Lancet* i, 345

Brown, J. J., Lever, A. F., Robertson, J. I. S. and Schalekamp, M. A. (1974). 'Renal Abnormality of Essential Hypertension.' *Lancet* ii, 320

Brown, J. J., Lever, A. F., Robertson, J. I. S. and Schalekamp, M. A. (1976). 'Pathogenesis of Essential Hypertension.' *Lancet* i, 1217

Conway, J. (1975). 'Beta Adrenergic Blockade and Hypertension.' In Oliver, M. F., *Modern Trends in Cardiology,* 3rd edn, ch. 13. London; Butterworths

Davis, J. O. (1971). 'Review: What Signals the Kidney to Release Renin.' *Circulation Res.* **28**, 301

Dustan, H. P., Tarazi, R. C. and Bravo, E. L. (1972). 'Physiologic Characteristics of Hypertension.' *Am. J. Med.* **52**, 610

Foëx, P. and Prys-Roberts, C. (1974). 'Anaesthesia and the Hypertensive Patient.' *Br. J. Anaesth.* **46**, 579

Folkow, B. and Neil, E. (1971). *Circulation,* ch. 31. Oxford University Press

Frolich, E. D. (1975). 'Cardiovascular Pathophysiology of Essential Hypertension.' In Zelis, R., *The Peripheral Circulations.* New York; Grune and Stratton

Havard, C. W. H. (1973). 'Aldosterone and Hyperaldosteronism.' In *Frontiers of Medicine.* London; Heinemann

Hickler, R. B. (1973). 'The Microcirculation in Hypertension.' In Wells, R., *The Microcirculation in Clinical Medicine.* London; Academic Press

Hickler, R. B. and Vandam, L. D. (1970). 'Hypertension.' *Anesthesiology* **33**, 214

Kelman, G. R. (1975). 'Hypertension.' In *Physiology: A Clinical Approach,* 2nd edn, ch. 3. Edinburgh; Churchill Livingstone

Ledingham, J. M. (1971). 'The Etiology of Hypertension.' *Practitioner* **207**, 5

Mulrow, P. J. (1971). 'Hypertension XIX, Salts, Hormones and Hypertension.' *Circulation Res.* **28** (Suppl. 2)

Pickering, G. (1974). *Hypertension, Causes, Consequences and Management,* 2nd edn. London; Churchill Livingstone

Prys-Roberts, C., Foëx, P., Green, L. T. and Waterhouse, T. D. (1972). 'Studies of Anaesthesia in Relation to Hypertension.IV. The Effect of Artificial Ventilation on the Circulation and Pulmonary Gas Exchanges.' *Br. J. Anaesth.* **44**, 335

Prys-Roberts, C., Foëx, P., Biro, G. P. and Roberts, J. G. (1973). 'Studies of Anaesthesia in Relation to Hypertension.V. Adrenergic Beta-receptor Blockade.' *Br. J. Anaesth.* **45**, 671

Prys-Roberts, C., Green, L. T., Meloche, R. and Foëx, P. (1971b). 'Studies of Anaesthesia in Relation to Hypertension: Haemodynamic Consequences of Induction and Endotracheal Intubation.' *Br. J. Anaesth.* **43**, 531

Prys-Roberts, C. Meloche, R. and Foëx, P. (1971). 'Studies of Anaesthesia in Relation to Hypertension. I. Cardiovascular Responses of Treated and Untreated Patients.' *Br. J. Anaesth.* **43**, 122

Ross, E. J., Pritchard, B. N. C., Kaufman, L., Robertson, A. I. G. and Harries, B. J. (1967). 'Pre-operative and Operative Management of Patients with Phaeochromocytoma.' *Br. Med. J.* **1**, 191

Swales, J. D. (1975). *Sodium Metabolism in Disease.* London; Lloyd-Luke

Swales, J. D. (1976). 'The Hunt for Renal Hypertension.' *Lancet* i, 1976

Tobian, L. (1960). 'Interrelationship of Electrolytes, Juxtaglomerular Cells and Hypertension.' *Physiol. Rev.* **40**, 280

Chapter 12   Cardiovascular Measurements

This chapter describes the techniques available for the measurement of cardiac output, blood volume, and arterial and central venous blood pressures in man. The methods commonly used for measurement of blood flow in peripheral tissues are described in Chapter 5.

Many of these techniques are inconvenient or difficult, therefore circulatory monitoring during anaesthesia is usually limited to feeling the pulse, to intermittent measurement of arterial blood pressure by sphygmomanometry, to the estimation (or guesstimation) of the amount of blood lost at operation, and to clinical assessment of the adequacy or otherwise of the cutaneous circulation. When rapid blood loss is anticipated these measurements may be supplemented by measurement of the venous pressure by a central venous catheter, and occasionally, in major procedures, by continuous monitoring of arterial blood pressure via an indwelling arterial cannula. The measurement of cardiac output, total blood volume, and tissue blood flow are still research procedures which play little part in routine clinical management.

ELECTRICAL HAZARDS

Most modern techniques of measurement involve the use of electronic black boxes which are connected to the patient by electrically-conducting leads. Many investigators fail to realize that incorrect use of such apparatus may risk electrocution of the patient. Bousvaros, Don and Hopps (1962) describe the accidental induction of ventricular fibrillation from this cause in a patient undergoing right heart catheterization and other incidents have almost certainly occurred in which the cause of the cardiac arrest has not been realized. Users of complex electronic equipment should be familiar with the potential hazards, and with the ways in which these may be minimized.

The electrical induction of ventricular fibrillation can occur only if a current of sufficient magnitude passes through the myocardium. The current required varies according to the phase of the cardiac cycle and, in the case of alternating current, to the frequency. The heart is most vulnerable to fibrillation at the beginning of the ECG T wave; it is, unfortunately, particularly sensitive to alternating currents of mains frequency (50 Hz in Great Britain, 60 Hz in North America). A current as low as 20 μA at this frequency may induce ventricular fibrillation in the dog, and 150 μA induces fibrillation in man during open-heart surgery. The minimum current which gives rise to cutaneous sensation is approximately 1 mA, that is 8 times that required to cause fibrillation.

For a current to flow there must be a source of electrical potential difference (voltage) and a pathway for the current to follow. In any circuit, current is equal to the quotient of voltage divided by total electrical resistance (or, in the case of alternating currents, impedance) of the circuit. A large current can flow either with a high voltage source or with a low resistance pathway.

Normally the body's tissues present a relatively high electrical resistance; therefore voltages applied to its surface must be fairly large before they can cause ventricular fibrillation. Further, even if the total current passing through the body is large, the current density through the myocardium is much less because only a small part of the total current takes this path. But when part of the body's resistance is by-passed by an electrically-conducting catheter introduced directly into the heart, relatively large currents can flow with quite moderate external voltages. This may happen with a saline-filled catheter or, still more, if an electrical conductor is introduced into the right heart to record the intracardiac electrocardiogram. Perhaps more important is the fact that, under these circumstances, current is concentrated in the region of the myocardium where high local current densities may easily induce ventricular fibrillation.

Prevention

To prevent any possibility of electrocution, it is necessary to ensure that there is a limit to the current which can pass through the body, and particularly through the myocardium.

Because of explosion hazards from static electricity anaesthetized patients are usually placed on electrically-conducting surfaces, so that any accumulated electrical charge may leak away to earth. There is then a conducting pathway through the body to earth should any high voltage source come in contact with its surface. To minimize such current, specifications have been laid down by the Ministry of Health for the minimum resistance of electrically-conducting rubber mattresses and of the electrical resistance of operating room floors (*see,* for example, Hill, 1972). For the same reason the lead to the indifferent diathermy electrode is connected, not directly to ground, but via a 0.01 μF capacitor; this provides negligible electrical resistance for currents of diathermy frequency (which are too high to induce ventricular fibrillation) but provides a barrier to direct currents and to currents of mains frequency.

In Great Britain all metalwork on electronic apparatus is connected to earth via a separate low-resistance conductor which runs with the mains lead to the third ('earth') pin of the wall socket. Electrical leakage from components inside the apparatus cannot appreciably raise the potential of such earthed metalwork because the resistance between it and ground is so low. But if the earth lead should become disconnected, or develop a high electrical resistance due to corrosion, then the electrical potential of the case may rise sufficiently to produce an electrocution danger. This is particularly so if an additional earth lead, for example that of an electrocardiogram, is connected to the patient, for then the leakage current passes to earth through the patient's body, with possible fatal consequences. For this reason it is now recommended (Hospital Technical Memorandum No. 8, revised 1969) that monitoring apparatus for use in hospitals should include isolating circuits designed to prevent appreciable leakage currents from passing through the patient. In view of the very small current which can induce fibrillation when introduced directly into the heart (*see* above) the design of such equipment presents a considerable technical challenge, and is inevitably expensive.

In some countries, equipment is connected to the mains by two leads only, and the metalwork is connected to one of these leads. Since one side of the mains is earthed this system is safe, provided the mains plug is correctly inserted into its socket, that is, with the chassis of the apparatus connected to the earthy side of the mains. If the connections are reversed, however, the full mains voltage appears on the metal parts of the equipment, causing a potentially dangerous situation. For this reason two-pin mains outlets should be avoided whenever possible, especially for medical use.

The precautions to be taken in the design of medical electronic equipment have been laid down by the Ministry of Health (Hospital Technical Memorandum, No. 8, revised 1969). It is also desirable that equipment should be checked by a competent engineer at regular intervals, and that no attempt should be made to use equipment which is in a faulty condition. Unexplained electrical interference may indicate failure of electrical insulation in some part of the apparatus.

MEASUREMENT OF CARDIAC OUTPUT

Until recently, the most accurate method of determining cardiac output in man was the direct Fick technique using oxygen. This method was made possible by Forssmann's (1929) heroic demonstration of the safety and feasibility of percutaneous right heart catheterization. In recent years, the Fick technique has been challenged by the indicator dilution method; this has the advantage that it does not require sampling of mixed-venous blood, nor measurement of the body's oxygen consumption, a difficult measurement to make during general anaesthesia (*see* below).

Both the Fick and indicator dilution techniques are based on the principle of Conservation of Matter. The assumption is made that, over any appreciable period of time, the amount of some substance—usually oxygen or carbon dioxide with the Fick technique, a dye with the indicator dilution technique— which enters a given region of the body is equal to the amount which leaves during the same period (plus any which accumulates or is metabolized).

Indicator dilution technique

With the indicator dilution technique a bolus of indicator, commonly a dye, is rapidly injected into the venous side of the circulation, and the resulting indicator concentration-time profile is measured down-stream on the arterial side of the circulation. Cardiac output is calculated from the mass of indicator injected and the area under the curve of indicator concentration against time.

Derivation of indicator dilution formula

Consider the diagrammatic representation of the heart and pulmonary circulation shown in *Figure 12.1*. The rapid injection of indicator at point *A* causes a sudden, transient high concentration of indicator in the venous blood. By the time the indicator has reached the arterial side of the circulation, however, this concentration profile has become flattened and prolonged, because different particles of blood take different pathways through the pulmonary circulation and therefore have different pulmonary transit times. (It is, in fact, possible to determine the distribution of transit times through the pulmonary circulation by analysis of the concentration-time profiles as the indicator enters and leaves the pulmonary vascular bed. The mean pulmonary transit time may also be calculated; and, from knowledge of this parameter and of cardiac output, it is possible to estimate the pulmonary blood volume—*see* Zierler, 1962.)

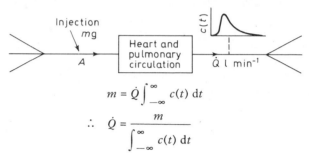

$$m = \dot{Q} \int_{-\infty}^{\infty} c(t)\, dt$$

$$\therefore \quad \dot{Q} = \frac{m}{\int_{-\infty}^{\infty} c(t)\, dt}$$

Figure 12.1. Derivation of indicator dilution formula

If it is assumed that blood flow through the system is constant ($\dot{Q}$ l min^{-1}), the amount of indicator leaving the system during a small time interval Δt is $\dot{Q}c\Delta t$, where c is the indicator concentration at time t. Then, using standard calculus techniques, it is possible to derive the formula:

$$m = \dot{Q} \int_{-\infty}^{\infty} c(t)\, dt$$

where m is the mass of dye injected and $c(t)$ is the concentration-time profile at the sampling site.

Since no indicator can leave before any has been injected, the lower limit may be replaced by $t = 0$, that is:

$$m = \dot{Q} \int_{0}^{\infty} c(t)\, dt$$

Rearrangement gives the relationship:

$$\dot{Q} = \frac{m}{\int_{0}^{\infty} c(t)\, dt}$$

$\int_{0}^{\infty} c(t)\, dt$ is, of course, the area under the curve of indicator concentration against time.

An intuitive understanding of the indicator dilution technique may be obtained by considering a system in which no mixing occurs, that is, one in which all particles have identical transit times. Suppose in *Figure 12.2* that m g of indicator are injected at point A over a period of t minutes. During injection, the concentration of indicator leaving the injection site is $m/\dot{Q}t$ g l^{-1}; this concentration is subsequently measured down-stream at point B (*see Figure 12.2*), where the area under the concentration-time curve is $m/\dot{Q}$. Flow ($\dot{Q}$) therefore equals m/area.

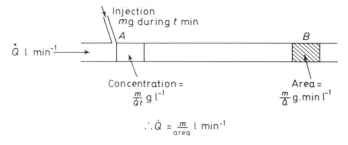

Figure 12.2. Derivation of indicator dilution formula for flow down a long straight tube (uniform transit time)

Effects of peripheral sampling and injection

Figure 12.1 fails to represent the actual circulation in two important respects. Firstly, it has but a single inlet and outlet, secondly no recirculation can occur. In practice, the injection is sometimes made not into the right atrium (which corresponds to the single inlet of *Figure 12.1*), but into a peripheral vein. Also, it is usual to measure indicator concentration peripherally, rather than at the aortic root.

The first objection is not important. In *Figure 12.3*, if indicator is injected at A' rather than at A, the mass balance condition on which the technique depends is still obeyed, provided the injectate all passes the sampling point B. Also, if the indicator concentration is measured not at the aortic root (B) but in a peripheral artery (B'), then, provided there is no change of concentration-time profile other than a simple time delay between B and B', the calculated cardiac output will again be correct (not, however, the mean circulation time).

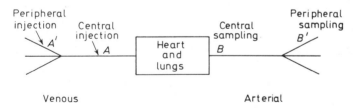

Figure 12.3. Possible causes of inaccuracy with the indicator dilution technique (see text)

Effects of recirculation

Recirculation presents a more serious problem. A typical indicator dilution curve (*Figure 12.4*) has two or even three peaks, because the injected bolus passes the sampling point more than once. The effects of recirculation may, however, be minimized by extrapolating the curve from before the point at which recirculation starts. This extrapolation is facilitated by the fact that, before the onset of recirculation, the dye concentration falls exponentially, so that, if the curve is replotted on semi-logarithmic graph paper (logarithm of dye concentration against time), this exponential segment becomes linear (Kinsman, Moore and Hamilton, 1929)—*see Figure 12.5.*

ACP–9*

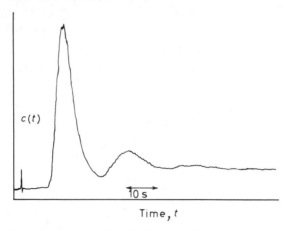

Figure 12.4. Typical dye dilution curve (indocyanine green)

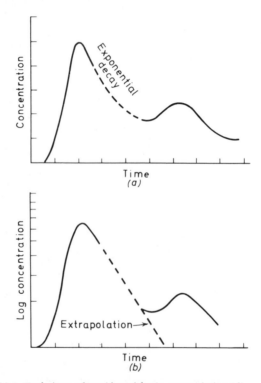

Figure 12.5. Technique of semi-logarithmic extrapolation (diagrammatic)

Early recirculation in low output states   It has been shown that, when cardiac output is considerably reduced, as in shock (*see* page 212), blood flow through certain regions of the circulation may be relatively normal, so that some recirculation may occur relatively early, and be unrecognized (Oriol, Sekelj and McGregor, 1967). The curve then still decays exponentially but its apparent decay constant is incorrect and the calculated cardiac output is correspondingly reduced. It is possible that this phemonenon may account in part for some of the very low outputs which have been reported during general anaesthesia in man.

What does the indicator dilution technique measure?

It is important to discuss precisely what is being measured by the indicator dilution technique. This is especially so in the presence of intrapulmonary and intracardiac shunts, when the outputs of the two ventricles may not be identical. Provided the aortic valve is competent, and all the injected indicator passes through it, then it follows from the way in which the dilution formula is derived (*see* page 252) that the technique must measure flow through the aortic valve, that is, left ventricular output. The only circumstance under which this would not be the case would be if indicator were able to pass from the venous to the arterial side of the circulation without passing the sampling point; this does not, however, occur because the pressures are in the wrong direction.

Choice of indicator

The most frequently used indicator is a dye, the plasma concentration of which may be measured photoelectrically. The technique is, however, by no means limited to dyes: it is possible to use a bolus of cold saline ('coolth'), and to estimate its blood concentration by a thermistor or thermocouple (Branthwaite and Bradley, 1968), or to use ^{131}I-tagged serum albumin (RISA), or red cells labelled with radioactive chromium. There are, however, theoretical objections to the use of heat as indicator (*see* page 256), while radioactive measurements unfortunately require sophisticated and expensive equipment, plus the services of a competent medical physicist or specialist in clinical measurement.

Indocyanine green   Probably the best indicator for general use is the green dye indocyanine green (Cardiogreen). This dye has its peak absorption in the infra-red region of the spectrum at 805 nm, which is an isobestic wavelength * for oxyhaemoglobin and reduced haemoglobin. It is therefore possible to

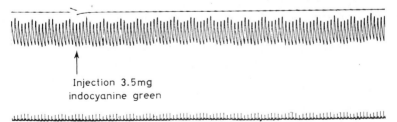

Injection 3.5mg
indocyanine green

Figure 12.6. Heart rate and blood pressure before and after injection of 3.5 mg indocyanine green—no change

* At an isobestic wavelength the optical densities of oxyhaemoglobin and reduced haemoglobin are identical.

estimate the dye without interference from changes of oxyhaemoglobin saturation. This is particularly important when measuring cardiac output in hypoxic patients, whose arterial saturation may vary markedly during the respiratory cycle.

Indocyanine green is non-toxic even in large doses (Merriman et al., 1958), and in the dose used for output determinations, has no demonstrable effect on the cardiovascular system (*Figure 12.6*). It becomes firmly bound to plasma protein, and therefore remains in the circulation during its passage through the pulmonary capillaries; and it is then rapidly excreted by the liver. This prevents the build-up of high concentrations during multiple output determinations. (The rate of clearance of indocyanine green from the plasma may also be used as a test of hepatic function, or for the estimation of hepatic blood flow—*see* page 150).

Cold saline ('coolth')   Cold saline is a useful indicator; it is cheap, non-toxic and avoids problems from recirculation because the 'coolth' becomes distributed throughout the body tissues during a single circulation. For the same reason, multiple, rapidly-repeated determinations of cardiac output are possible. In addition, estimation is easy and requires only simple apparatus.

However, the accuracy of the technique depends on the assumption that no loss of 'coolth' occurs between the injection and measuring points, and there is an inevitable loss of indicator through the walls of the injection catheter. Most workers use an empirical correction factor to compensate for this loss. Douglas et al. (1975) have recently compared the thermal dilution technique and the standard technique with indocyanine green.

Radioactive indicators   Cardiac output may be estimated with a radioactive indicator, the intracardiac concentration of which is estimated by an external counter sited over the praecordium (Veall, 1968). Lorimer et al. (1968) used RISA (radioactive iodinated serum albumin) or 99 m technetium with a suitably collimated scintillation counter. Although the reproducibility of this technique was good, it systematically over-estimated cardiac output, especially at low values; and therefore this technique should, at present, probably be regarded as qualitative rather than quantitative.

The Fick technique

The other standard method for the measurement of cardiac output is the direct Fick technique with oxygen. This technique, however, requires catheterization of the right heart in order to obtain samples of mixed-venous blood, a disadvantage which has led to attempts to determine the mixed-venous oxygen or carbon dioxide content by 'indirect' means, such as by rebreathing or breath-holding. These techniques are discussed later.

Derivation of the Fick formula

Consider the diagrammatic representation of the pulmonary circulation shown in *Figure 12.7*. If the blood flow through the system is $\dot{Q}$ l min^{-1}, the amount of oxygen entering the system each minute in the venous blood is $\dot{Q} \times C\bar{v}o_2$, and the amount leaving in the same time in the arterial blood is $\dot{Q} \times Cao_2$, where Cao_2 and $C\bar{v}o_2$ are, respectively, the concentrations of oxygen in the arterial and mixed-venous blood. The rate of oxygen removal from the lungs by the blood is therefore $\dot{Q}(Cao_2 - C\bar{v}o_2)$, and when the body is in a steady state this equals the oxygen consumption measured at the mouth ($\dot{V}o_2$). Cardiac output therefore equals $\dot{V}o_2/(Cao_2 - C\bar{v}o_2)$.

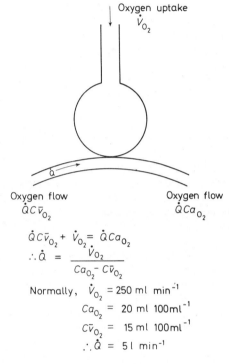

Figure 12.7. Derivation of Fick equation

$$\dot{Q}C\bar{v}_{o_2} + \dot{V}_{o_2} = \dot{Q}Ca_{o_2}$$

$$\therefore \dot{Q} = \frac{\dot{V}_{o_2}}{Ca_{o_2} - C\bar{v}_{o_2}}$$

$$\text{Normally, } \dot{V}_{o_2} = 250 \text{ ml min}^{-1}$$

$$Ca_{o_2} = 20 \text{ ml } 100\text{ml}^{-1}$$

$$C\bar{v}_{o_2} = 15 \text{ ml } 100\text{ml}^{-1}$$

$$\therefore \dot{Q} = 5 \text{ l min}^{-1}$$

The insertion of typical values into this equation—$\dot{V}o_2 = 250$ ml min^{-1}, $Cao_2 = 20$ ml 100 ml^{-1}, $C\bar{v}o_2 = 15$ ml 100 ml^{-1}—gives a calculated cardiac output of 5 l min^{-1}.

Validity of the equation

The Fick equation assumes that pulmonary oxygen consumption is neglible compared with the oxygen consumption of the body as a whole. This assumption has been disputed in the past, but is now generally accepted by most workers. The other assumption is that the rate of oxygen removal from the lungs by the blood equals the rate of oxygen uptake at the mouth. This condition does *not* apply at the start of exercise, nor immediately after a change of respiratory minute volume or inspired gas composition. If the pulmonary oxygen stores are not constant throughout the measurement period, the calculated cardiac output must be inaccurate.

(Inaccuracy may also arise if the composition of the arterial or mixed-venous blood varies during the respiratory or cardiac cycle. Under these circumstances a representative blood sample can be obtained only by withdrawing blood at a rate proportional to the instantaneous rate of blood flow. This is virtually impossible. Phasic variations in the composition of mixed-venous blood are fortunately not great, but the composition of arterial blood varies with respiration sufficiently to cause errors in the calculated output of up to 4 per cent at rest, and considerably more during exercise (Wood et al., 1955). This difficulty of determining the mean composition of a moving fluid, the composition of which varies from instant to instant, will be familiar to respiratory physiologists, who often need to calculate the mean composition of inspired or expired gas. If the rate at which gas flows past the sampling point is not constant, its mean composition cannot be obtained simply by averaging the instantaneous composition over a complete respiratory cycle; it is necessary first to weight the instantaneous composition by the instantaneous flow rate.)

Measurement of oxygen consumption

Oxygen consumption is measured at the mouth as the difference between the amount of oxygen inspired and the amount expired over a given period of time (at least 1 minute). Oxygen consumption ($\dot{V}_{O_2}$) is calculated from the formula:

$$Fi_{O_2} \dot{V}i - Fe_{O_2} \dot{V}e, \text{ where}$$

Fi_{O_2} is the inspired fractional concentration of oxygen,
Fe_{O_2} is the mixed-expired fractional concentration of oxygen,
$\dot{V}i$ is the inspired minute volume, and
$\dot{V}e$ is the expired minute volume.

It is often unnecessary to measure both inspired and expired minute volumes because, if the body is in nitrogen equilibrium, these are related by the equation:

$$Fi_{N_2} \dot{V}i = Fe_{N_2} \dot{V}e,$$

where Fi_{N_2} and Fe_{N_2} are, respectively, the inspired and mixed-expired fractional nitrogen concentrations. Fi_{N_2} is, of course, equal to 1 minus the sum of the fractional concentrations of the other gases present in the inspired gas mixture; a similar relationship applies to Fe_{N_2}. The inspired or expired minute volume may then be conveniently measured either with a calibrated Wright respirometer or with a dry gas meter.

When the body is not in nitrogen equilibrium, it is necessary to measure both inspired and expired minute volumes independently, or to measure accurately the difference between them with a bag-in-box spirometer, such as that described by Nunn and Pouliot (1962). This additional complexity is unfortunately required during the uptake or elimination of gaseous anaesthetic agents. With Nunn's technique the subject inspires an appropriate gas mixture from a rigid airtight box, and then expires into a bag contained within the box. The change of volume of the total box-bag system gives a measure of the difference between inspired and expired minute volume, while the volume change of the system during a single breath gives the inspired or expired tidal volume. The chief difficulty with this apparatus is its sensitivity to temperature fluctuations which may be wrongly interpreted as changes of gas volume.

Measurement of arterial and mixed-venous oxygen content

Arterial blood may be obtained by percutaneous puncture of the radial or brachial artery. Mixed-venous blood, however, can be obtained only by catheterization of the right heart, and true mixed-venous blood is found only in the right ventricle or pulmonary artery, because mixing of separate streams from the SVC, IVC, and coronary sinus is not complete in the right atrium. (The oxygen content of coronary sinus blood may be as low as 9 ml 100 ml^{-1} (Rowe, 1959), compared with the normal mixed-venous oxygen content of 14–16 ml 100 ml^{-1}.)

The van Slyke apparatus   The classical method for determination of oxygen content (oxygen concentration) uses the manometric van Slyke apparatus. With this technique oxygen is liberated from combination with haemoglobin by a solution of saponin and potassium ferricyanide, which haemolyses the blood and converts its haemoglobin into methaemoglobin. The volume of gas liberated is estimated by measurement of the pressure increase which it causes at constant volume. This technique is the yardstick against which all others must be checked and calibrated. Unfortunately, however, it requires considerable skill and experience; and it is usual for routine use to employ other, less accurate but more convenient techniques such as the polarographic method described by several groups of workers, for example, Linden, Ledsome and Normal (1965).

Calculation from the oxygen tension   If great accuracy is not required, oxygen content (C_{O_2}) may be calculated from oxygen tension (P_{O_2}) and haemoglobin concentration by the expression:

$$C_{O_2} = \alpha P_{O_2} + 0.0139\, S_{O_2}\, \text{Hb, where}$$

α is the solubility of oxygen in whole blood, that is, approximately 0.003 ml 100 ml^{-1} mm Hg^{-1} at body temperature,
S_{O_2} is the percentage oxyhaemoglobin saturation, and
Hb is the haemoglobin concentration in g 100 ml^{-1}.
The proportionality factor 0.0139 arises from the fact that 1 g of haemoglobin combines with 1.39 ml of oxygen (STPD) when fully saturated.

This conversion has recently been simplified by tables which relate oxygen tension and content over a wide range of haemoglobin concentrations, temperatures and acid-base states (Kelman and Nunn, 1968–*Figure 12.8*).

Indirect Fick techniques

The direct Fick technique requires sampling of mixed-venous blood, a difficult and possibly dangerous procedure. There is, therefore, a considerable interest in various 'bloodless' modifications of this technique, which attempt to estimate mixed-venous oxygen or, more usually, carbon dioxide tension indirectly. O_2 or CO_2 tension can then be converted into concentration by tables or nomograms, and cardiac output calculated either from the oxygen Fick equation (*see* page 257) or from the analogous equation for carbon dioxide:

$$\dot{Q} = \frac{\dot{V}_{CO_2}}{C\bar{v}_{CO_2} - Ca_{CO_2}}$$

Temp = 37°C, PCO_2 = 40 mm Hg, pH = 7.40

Hb g 100 ml⁻¹ PO_2	6	7	8	9	10	11	12	13	14	15	16	17	18	19	20
2	0.09	0.10	0.11	0.13	0.14	0.15	0.17	0.18	0.19	0.21	0.22	0.24	0.25	0.26	0.28
5	0.29	0.34	0.38	0.43	0.47	0.52	0.57	0.61	0.66	0.70	0.75	0.80	0.84	0.89	0.93
10	0.82	0.96	1.09	1.22	1.35	1.49	1.62	1.75	1.88	2.02	2.15	2.28	2.41	2.55	2.68
15	1.79	2.08	2.37	2.66	2.96	3.25	3.54	3.83	4.12	4.41	4.70	4.99	5.28	5.57	5.87
20	2.88	3.35	3.82	4.29	4.76	5.23	5.70	6.17	6.64	7.11	7.58	8.05	8.52	8.99	9.47
25	3.90	4.54	5.18	5.81	6.45	7.09	7.73	8.37	9.00	9.64	10.28	10.92	11.55	12.19	12.83
30	4.82	5.61	6.40	7.18	7.97	8.76	9.55	10.34	11.13	11.91	12.70	13.49	14.28	15.07	15.85
35	5.62	6.54	7.46	8.38	9.30	10.22	11.14	12.06	12.98	13.90	14.82	15.74	16.66	17.58	18.50
40	6.30	7.33	8.36	9.39	10.42	11.45	12.48	13.51	14.54	15.57	16.60	17.63	18.66	19.69	20.72
45	6.84	7.96	9.08	10.19	11.31	12.43	13.55	14.67	15.78	16.90	18.02	19.14	20.25	21.37	22.49
50	7.25	8.43	9.62	10.80	11.99	13.17	14.35	15.54	16.72	17.90	19.09	20.27	21.45	22.64	23.82
55	7.55	8.78	10.02	11.25	12.48	13.71	14.94	16.17	17.40	18.64	19.87	21.10	22.33	23.56	24.79
60	7.77	9.04	10.31	11.57	12.84	14.10	15.37	16.63	17.90	19.17	20.43	21.70	22.96	24.23	25.49
65	7.94	9.23	10.52	11.81	13.10	14.39	15.68	16.97	18.26	19.55	20.84	22.13	23.42	24.71	26.00
70	8.06	9.37	10.68	11.98	13.29	14.60	15.91	17.22	18.53	19.83	21.14	22.45	23.76	25.07	26.38
75	8.15	9.48	10.80	12.12	13.44	14.76	16.08	17.41	18.73	20.05	21.37	22.69	24.01	25.34	26.66
80	8.23	9.56	10.89	12.23	13.56	14.89	16.22	17.55	18.88	20.22	21.55	22.88	24.21	25.54	26.87
85	8.29	9.63	10.97	12.31	13.65	14.99	16.33	17.67	19.01	20.35	21.69	23.03	24.37	25.71	27.05
90	8.35	9.69	11.04	12.38	13.73	15.07	16.42	17.77	19.11	20.46	21.80	23.15	24.50	25.84	27.19
95	8.39	9.74	11.09	12.44	13.79	15.15	16.50	17.85	19.20	20.55	21.90	23.25	24.60	25.95	27.30
100	8.43	9.79	11.14	12.50	13.85	15.21	16.56	17.92	19.27	20.63	21.98	23.34	24.69	26.05	27.40
110	8.50	9.86	11.22	12.58	13.95	15.31	16.67	18.03	19.39	20.75	22.11	23.48	24.84	26.20	27.56
120	8.56	9.92	11.29	12.66	14.02	15.39	16.76	18.12	19.49	20.85	22.22	23.59	24.95	26.32	27.69
130	8.61	9.98	11.35	12.72	14.09	15.46	16.83	18.20	19.57	20.94	22.31	23.68	25.05	26.42	27.79
140	8.66	10.03	11.40	12.77	14.15	15.52	16.89	18.26	19.64	21.01	22.38	23.75	25.13	26.50	27.87
150	8.70	10.07	11.45	12.82	14.20	15.57	16.95	18.32	19.70	21.07	22.45	23.82	25.20	26.57	27.95
160	8.74	10.12	11.49	12.87	14.25	15.62	17.00	18.38	19.75	21.13	22.51	23.88	25.26	26.64	28.01
170	8.78	10.16	11.54	12.91	14.29	15.67	17.05	18.43	19.80	21.18	22.56	23.94	25.32	26.70	28.07
180	8.82	10.20	11.58	12.95	14.33	15.71	17.09	18.47	19.85	21.23	22.61	23.99	25.37	26.75	28.13
190	8.85	10.23	11.61	12.99	14.38	15.76	17.14	18.52	19.90	21.28	22.66	24.04	25.42	26.80	28.18

Oxygen tension (mm Hg)

Oxygen tension (mm Hg)

O₂ tension															
200	8.89	10.27	11.65	13.03	14.41	15.80	17.18	18.56	19.94	21.32	22.70	24.08	25.47	26.85	28.23
220	8.96	10.34	11.72	13.11	14.49	15.87	17.25	18.64	20.02	21.40	22.79	24.17	25.55	26.93	28.32
240	9.02	10.41	11.79	13.18	14.56	15.94	17.33	18.71	20.10	21.48	22.86	24.25	25.63	27.02	28.40
260	9.09	10.47	11.86	13.24	14.63	16.01	17.40	18.78	20.17	21.55	22.94	24.32	25.71	27.09	28.48
280	9.15	10.54	11.92	13.31	14.70	16.08	17.47	18.85	20.24	21.62	23.01	24.39	25.78	27.17	28.55
300	9.22	10.60	11.99	13.38	14.76	16.15	17.53	18.92	20.31	21.69	23.08	24.46	25.85	27.24	28.62
350	9.37	10.76	12.15	13.53	14.92	16.31	17.70	19.08	20.47	21.86	23.24	24.63	26.02	27.41	28.79
400	9.53	10.91	12.30	13.69	15.08	16.47	17.85	19.24	20.63	22.02	23.41	24.79	26.18	27.57	28.96
450	9.68	11.07	12.46	13.84	15.23	16.62	18.01	19.40	20.79	22.17	23.56	24.95	26.34	27.73	29.12
500	9.83	11.22	12.61	14.00	15.39	16.77	18.16	19.55	20.94	22.33	23.72	25.11	26.50	27.88	29.27
550	9.98	11.37	12.76	14.15	15.54	16.93	18.32	19.71	21.09	22.48	23.87	25.26	26.65	28.04	29.43
600	10.13	11.52	12.91	14.30	15.69	17.08	18.47	19.86	21.25	22.64	24.02	25.41	26.00	28.19	29.58
650	10.29	11.67	13.06	14.45	15.84	17.23	18.62	20.01	21.40	22.79	24.18	25.57	26.96	28.34	29.73
700	10.44	11.83	13.21	14.60	15.99	17.38	18.77	20.16	21.55	22.94	24.33	25.72	27.11	28.50	29.89
750	10.59	11.98	13.37	14.75	16.14	17.53	18.92	20.31	21.70	23.09	24.48	25.87	27.26	28.65	30.04
800	10.74	12.13	13.52	14.91	16.29	17.68	19.07	20.46	21.85	23.24	24.63	26.02	27.41	28.80	30.19
900	11.04	12.43	13.82	15.21	16.60	17.99	19.38	20.76	22.15	23.54	24.93	26.32	27.71	29.10	30.49
1000	11.34	12.73	14.12	15.51	16.90	18.29	19.68	21.07	22.46	23.85	25.23	26.62	28.01	29.40	30.79
1100	11.64	13.03	14.42	15.81	17.20	18.59	19.98	21.37	22.76	24.15	25.54	26.93	28.32	29.70	31.09
1200	11.94	13.33	14.72	16.11	17.50	18.89	20.28	21.67	23.06	24.45	25.84	27.23	28.62	30.01	31.40
1300	12.24	13.63	15.02	16.41	17.80	19.19	20.58	21.97	23.36	24.75	26.14	27.53	28.92	30.31	31.70
1400	12.54	13.93	15.32	16.71	18.10	19.49	20.88	22.27	23.66	25.05	26.44	27.83	29.22	30.61	32.00
1500	12.84	14.23	15.62	17.01	18.40	19.79	21.18	22.57	23.96	25.35	26.74	28.13	29.52	30.91	32.30
1600	13.14	14.53	15.92	17.31	18.70	20.09	21.48	22.87	24.26	25.65	27.04	28.43	29.82	31.21	32.60
1700	13.44	14.83	16.22	17.61	19.00	20.39	21.78	23.17	24.56	25.95	27.34	28.73	30.12	31.51	32.90
1800	13.74	15.13	16.52	17.91	19.30	20.69	22.08	23.47	24.86	26.25	27.64	29.03	30.42	31.81	33.20
1900	14.04	15.43	16.82	18.21	19.60	20.99	22.38	23.77	25.16	26.55	27.94	29.33	30.72	32.11	33.50
2000	14.34	15.73	17.12	18.51	19.90	21.29	22.68	24.07	25.46	26.85	28.24	29.63	31.02	32.41	33.80
2100	14.64	16.03	17.42	18.81	20.20	21.59	22.98	24.37	25.76	27.15	28.54	29.93	31.32	32.71	34.10
2200	14.94	16.33	17.72	19.11	20.50	21.89	23.28	24.67	26.06	27.45	28.84	30.23	31.62	33.01	34.40

Oxygen content

Figure 12.8. Table relating oxygen tension (mm Hg) and content (ml 100 ml⁻¹) at different haemoglobin concentrations

where $\dot{V}co_2$ is the rate of carbon dioxide production by the body, and $C\bar{v}co_2$ and $Caco_2$ are, respectively, the carbon dioxide contents of mixed-venous and arterial blood.

Three such techniques will be considered: the CO_2-rebreathing technique, the O_2-rebreathing technique, and a breath-holding technique.

CO_2-rebreathing technique   The subject rebreathes from a bag containing a mixture of carbon dioxide and oxygen until gas exchange in his lungs ceases. At this point the Pco_2 of the gas in the bag is assumed to be the same as the CO_2 tension of the mixed-venous blood. However, it has been shown by Denison et al. (1969), and by other workers, that during the alveolar plateau the arterial Pco_2 is *not* the same as the alveolar Pco_2; and this experimental finding has cast doubt on the validity of the CO_2 rebreathing technique. The cause of this 'downstream effect' is disputed; it cannot, however, be explained in terms of inhomogeneity of pulmonary ventilation (Kelman, unpublished).

The rebreathing bag initially contains a mixture of carbon dioxide in oxygen with a Pco_2 a few mm Hg higher than the expected $P\bar{v}co_2$. During the initial mixing period the carbon dioxide in the bag is diluted by gas of lower Pco_2 from the subject's pulmonary alveoli and dead space, therefore the Pco_2 of the bag-lung system rapidly approximates to that of mixed-venous blood. Carbon dioxide transfer then occurs between the mixed-venous blood and the bag-lung system until a constant carbon dioxide tension is reached; this plateau lasts for several seconds until the onset of recirculation, when the Pco_2 starts to rise. The approach to the plateau is monitored at the mouth by a fast-response CO_2 analyser (*Figure 12.9*).

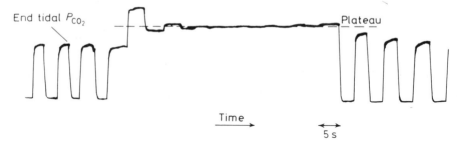

Figure 12.9. Estimation of mixed-venous Pco_2 by rebreathing technique

Before cardiac output can be calculated, mixed-venous Pco_2 must be converted into CO_2 content. This is conveniently done by the Singer-Hastings nomogram (Singer and Hastings, 1948). It should be noted, however, that the measured CO_2 tension is that of blood which has been equilibrated with almost 100 per cent oxygen; and allowance must be made for this fact when performing the conversion. It is also possible to use tables relating Pco_2 and Cco_2 similar to those available for the interconversion of Po_2 and Co_2 shown in *Figure 12.8*. An example is shown in *Figure 12.10*.

Arterial carbon dioxide tension may be estimated by monitoring the instantaneous expired carbon dioxide tension, and assuming that arterial Pco_2 equals alveolar Pco_2, derived from the end-tidal plateau. Provided the lungs are sufficiently healthy for a plateau to be reached, this assumption is reasonably valid. However, the presence of an increased physiological dead space due to ventilated but not perfused alveoli lowers the P_{CO_2} of mixed-alveolar gas, thus causing an appreciable $(A-a)\ P_{CO_2}$ difference.

O_2-rebreathing technique (Cerretelli et al., 1966)   This method is based on principles similar to the CO_2-rebreathing technique. The subject rebreathes from a bag containing a mixture of 7 or 8 per cent carbon dioxide in *nitrogen*. If the volume of the bag is chosen appropriately, that is, approximately equal to the subject's functional residual capacity, a plateau is rapidly reached where the gas composition (both oxygen and carbon dioxide) in the bag-lung system is equal to that of mixed-venous blood.

Spence and Ellis (1970) have recently cast doubt on the validity of the O_2-rebreathing technique by demonstrating that an apparent plateau can often be obtained, but that its level depends on the size of the rebreathing bag, a finding which suggests that the plateau is due to mixing in the lung-bag system and not to true equilibration between it and the mixed-venous blood. The analytical resolution required to distinguish this type of spurious plateau from a true plateau is beyond the accuracy of many measuring instruments (*see also* Kelman, 1972).

The method of Kim, Rahn and Farhi (1966)   During breath-holding, gas exchange in the alveoli continues: the P_{CO_2} of the alveolar gas rises as carbon dioxide leaves the mixed-venous blood, and its P_{O_2} falls as oxygen passes into the arterial blood. During this process, as a result of the flatness of the oxygen dissociation curve, the oxygen saturation (and therefore content) of the arterial blood is almost unchanged, whereas its carbon dioxide content rises continuously. As a result the instantaneous respiratory exchange ratio falls:

$$\dot{V}_{CO_2}/\dot{V}_{O_2} = (C\bar{v}_{CO_2} - Ca_{CO_2})/(Ca_{O_2} - C\bar{v}_{O_2})$$

Gas exchange during breath-holding is shown diagrammatically in *Figure 12.11*. The normal arterial and mixed-venous points are represented by *a* and $\bar{v}$ respectively. During breath-holding (before the onset of recirculation) the venous point remains unchanged but the arterial point moves to the right along the dissociation curve for oxygenated blood. The exchange ratio falls progressively as the CO_2 content difference between the mixed-venous and arterial blood falls. When the arterial point is vertically below the mixed-venous point (at point a'), the ratio has the value 0.32; at this point the change of blood P_{CO_2} due to equilibration of mixed-venous blood with alveolar gas is just balanced by the opposing change due to increased oxygen saturation, and therefore decreased affinity of haemoglobin for CO_2—the Haldane effect (Christiansen, Douglas and Haldane, 1914).

The P_{CO_2} at point a' is, of course, equal to the P_{CO_2} of the normal mixed-venous blood. At point a'' the carbon dioxide content of the arterial and mixed-venous bloods are identical, that is, the exchange ratio is zero. The carbon dioxide tension at this point is that of oxygenated mixed-venous blood (the tension estimated by the standard CO_2-rebreathing technique).

The breath-holding technique is used in practice by asking the subject to make a prolonged expiration (which is physiologically equivalent to breath-holding except that the volume of the lungs is not constant), and measuring the oxygen and carbon dioxide tensions of successive samples of exhaled alveolar

Hcrit = 40%, Temp. = $37°C$

Base excess mmol l^{-1}	−15	−10	−5
PCO_2			
12	15.74(0.05)15.19	20.15(0.08)19.37	25.43(0.11)24.36
14	17.06(0.06)16.49	21.68(0.08)20.87	27.17(0.11)26.06
16	18.30(0.06)17.70	23.10(0.08)22.26	28.77(0.11)27.63
18	19.47(0.06)18.85	24.43(0.09)23.57	30.26(0.12)29.10
20	20.58(0.06)19.94	25.69(0.09)24.80	31.67(0.12)30.48
22	21.64(0.07)20.98	26.88(0.09)25.98	32.99(0.12)31.78
24	22.66(0.07)21.98	28.03(0.09)27.10	34.26(0.02)33.02
26	23.64(0.07)22.95	29.12(0.09)28.18	35.46(0.13)34.21
28	24.59(0.07)23.88	30.18(0.10)29.22	36.62(0.13)35.35
30	25.51(0.07)24.79	31.20(0.10)30.22	37.73(0.13)36.44
32	26.40(0.07)25.67	32.18(0.10)31.19	38.81(0.13)37.50
34	27.26(0.07)26.52	33.14(0.10)32.14	30.84(0.13)38.53
36	28.11(0.08)27.35	34.07(0.10)33.05	40.85(0.13)39.52
38	28.93(0.08)28.17	34.97(0.10)33.94	41.82(0.13)40.48
40	29.74(0.08)28.96	35.85(0.10)34.81	42.77(0.14)41.42
42	30.53(0.08)29.74	36.71(0.11)35.66	43.70(0.14)42.33
44	31.30(0.08)30.51	37.55(0.11)36.49	44.60(0.14)43.22
46	32.06(0.08)31.26	38.38(0.11)37.31	45.48(0.14)44.09
48	32.80(0.08)31.99	39.18(0.11)38.10	46.34(0.14)44.94
50	33.54(0.08)32.71	39.97(0.11)38.88	47.18(0.14)45.77
52	34.25(0.08)33.42	40.75(0.11)39.65	48.00(0.14)46.59
54	34.96(0.08)34.12	41.51(0.11)40.40	48.81(0.14)47.39
56	35.66(0.08)34.81	42.26(0.11)41.14	49.60(0.14)48.17
58	36.34(0.09)35.49	42.99(0.11)41.87	50.38(0.14)48.94
60	37.02(0.09)36.16	43.71(0.11)42.59	51.14(0.14)49.70
62	37.68(0.09)36.82	44.43(0.11)43.29	51.89(0.15)50.44
64	38.34(0.09)37.47	45.13(0.11)43.99	52.63(0.15)51.18
66	38.99(0.09)38.11	45.82(0.11)44.67	53.36(0.15)51.90
68	39.63(0.09)38.75	46.50(0.12)45.35	54.08(0.15)52.61
70	40.26(0.09)39.37	47.17(0.12)46.02	54.78(0.15)53.31
72	40.89(0.09)39.99	47.84(0.12)46.67	55.48(0.15)54.00
74	41.51(0.09)40.61	48.49(0.12)47.32	56.16(0.15)54.68
76	42.12(0.09)41.21	49.14(0.12)47.97	56.84(0.15)55.35
78	42.72(0.09)41.81	49.78(0.12)48.60	57.51(0.15)56.01
80	43.32(0.09)42.41	50.41(0.12)49.23	58.17(0.15)56.67
82	43.91(0.09)43.00	51.04(0.12)49.58	58.82(0.15)57.31
84	44.50(0.09)43.58	51.66(0.12)50.46	59.46(0.15)57.95
86	45.08(0.09)44.15	52.27(0.12)51.07	60.10(0.15)58.59
88	45.66(0.09)44.73	52.87(0.12)51.67	60.72(0.15)59.21
90	46.23(0.09)45.29	53.47(0.12)52.27	61.35(0.15)59.83
92	46.79(0.09)45.85	54.07(0.12)52.86	61.96(0.15)60.44
94	47.35(0.09)46.41	54.65(0.12)53.44	62.57(0.15)61.04
96	47.91(0.09)46.96	55.24(0.12)54.02	63.17(0.15)61.64
98	48.46(0.10)47.51	55.81(0.12)54.59	63.77(0.15)62.23
100	49.01(0.10)48.05	56.38(0.12)55.16	64.36(0.15)62.82

(left margin, rotated) CO_2 Tension (mm Hg)

CO_2 content (ml 100 ml^{-1})

Figure 12.10. Table relating carbon dioxide tension (mm Hg) and content (ml 100 ml^{-1}) for different values of base excess (mmol l^{-1}). Left-hand figure applies to fully reduced blood;

+0	+5	+10
31.63(0.14)30.20	38.75(0.19)36.87	46.74(0.24)44.35
33.57(0.15)32.09	40.87(0.19)38.95	49.01(0.24)46.57
35.34(0.15)33.83	42.80(0.20)40.85	51.07(0.25)48.60
36.99(0.15)35.45	44.58(0.20)42.60	52.96(0.25)50.47
38.53(0.16)36.96	46.23(0.20)44.23	54.71(0.25)52.19
39.97(0.16)38.39	47.78(0.20)45.76	56.34(0.25)53.81
41.34(0.16)39.74	49.25(0.20)47.20	57.87(0.25)55.32
42.65(0.16)41.02	50.63(0.21)48.57	59.32(0.26)56.76
43.90(0.16)42.25	51.95(0.21)49.87	60.69(0.26)58.12
45.09(0.17)43.43	53.21(0.21)51.12	62.00(0.26)59.41
46.24(0.17)44.56	54.42(0.21)52.32	63.25(0.26)60.65
47.35(0.17)45.66	55.59(0.21)53.47	64.45(0.26)61.85
48.42(0.17)46.72	56.71(0.21)54.58	65.60(0.26)62.99
49.45(0.17)47.74	57.79(0.21)55.65	66.71(0.26)64.09
50.46(0.17)48.73	58.84(0.21)56.69	67.78(0.26)65.16
51.44(0.17)49.70	59.85(0.22)57.70	68.82(0.26)66.19
52.39(0.17)50.64	60.84(0.22)58.67	69.82(0.26)67.19
53.31(0.18)51.56	61.80(0.22)59.63	70.80(0.26)68.17
54.22(0.18)52.45	62.73(0.22)60.55	71.75(0.26)69.11
55.10(0.18)53.33	63.64(0.22)61.46	72.67(0.26)70.03
55.96(0.18)54.18	64.53(0.22)62.34	73.57(0.26)70.93
56.81(0.18)55.02	65.40(0.22)63.20	74.45(0.26)71.80
57.63(0.18)55.84	66.25(0.22)64.05	75.31(0.26)72.66
58.44(0.18)56.64	67.08(0.22)64.87	76.14(0.26)73.49
59.24(0.18)57.43	67.89(0.22)65.68	76.96(0.27)74.31
60.02(0.18)58.21	68.69(0.22)66.48	77.76(0.27)75.11
60.78(0.18)58.97	69.47(0.22)67.25	78.55(0.27)75.90
61.54(0.18)59.72	70.24(0.22)68.02	79.32(0.27)76.67
62.28(0.18)60.45	70.99(0.22)68.77	80.08(0.27)77.42
63.01(0.18)61.18	71.74(0.22)69.51	80.82(0.27)78.16
63.73(0.18)61.89	72.47(0.22)70.24	81.55(0.27)78.89
64.43(0.18)62.59	73.18(0.22)70.95	82.26(0.27)79.61
65.13(0.18)63.29	73.89(0.22)71.65	82.97(0.27)80.31
65.82(0.18)63.97	74.58(0.22)72.35	83.66(0.27)81.01
66.49(0.19)64.64	75.27(0.22)73.03	84.34(0.27)81.69
67.16(0.19)65.31	75.95(0.22)73.71	85.02(0.27)82.36
67.32(0.19)65.96	76.61(0.22)74.37	85.68(0.27)83.02
68.47(0.19)66.61	77.27(0.22)75.03	86.33(0.27)83.68
69.11(0.19)67.25	77.92(0.22)75.67	86.97(0.27)84.32
69.75(0.19)67.88	78.56(0.22)76.31	87.61(0.27)84.96
70.38(0.19)68.51	79.19(0.22)76.94	88.23(0.26)85.58
71.00(0.19)69.13	79.81(0.22)77.56	88.85(0.26)86.20
71.61(0.19)69.74	80.43(0.22)78.18	89.46(0.26)86.81
72.22(0.19)70.34	81.04(0.22)78.79	90.06(0.26)87.42
72.82(0.19)70.94	81.64(0.22)79.39	90.66(0.26)88.01

CO_2 content (ml 100 ml^{-1})

right-hand figure applies to fully oxygenated blood; figure in brackets is 0.1 times difference, and is used to facilitate interpolation at intermediate saturations gas. The points obtained are plotted on an O_2–CO_2 diagram and the corresponding values of respiratory exchange ratio calculated from the slope of the curve linking these points. The value of P_{CO_2} corresponding to an R value of 0.32—the true mixed-venous carbon dioxide tension—may then be determined by interpolation. If required, the P_{CO_2} of oxygenated mixed-venous blood may be estimated by extrapolating the relationship between R and P_{CO_2} to an exchange ratio of zero.

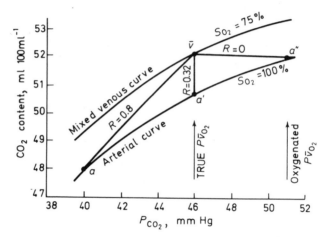

Figure 12.11. Estimation of true mixed-venous P_{CO_2} and oxygenated mixed-venous P_{CO_2} by breath-holding technique (see text for explanation)

If the value of R for the whole body before the start of breath-holding is known (R' say) it is possible to estimate Pa_{CO_2} by similarly extrapolating the curve relating P_{CO_2} and R to R'.

The technique just described is based on the assumption that the changes of alveolar gas tension observed during prolonged expiration are due solely to the fact that successive samples of expired air have been in contact with mixed-venous blood for a longer period. It is specifically assumed that the observed variations of gas composition are not due to sequential emptying of alveoli with different O_2 and CO_2 tensions caused by differences of ventilation/ perfusion ratio. This assumption is probably valid for normal lungs; its applicability in patients is, however, dubious (*see also* Hlastala, Wranne and Lenfant, 1972).

Other techniques for measuring cardiac output

Inert gas uptake

If the concentration of an inert gas in the mixed-venous blood is zero, its rate of uptake from the lungs is equal to the product of pulmonary capillary blood flow and the gas concentration in the pulmonary capillary blood. This concentration is equal to the product of alveolar tension and the blood-solubility of the gas. Pulmonary capillary blood flow ($\dot{Q}c$) may then be calculated from the equation:

$$\dot{Q}c = \dot{V}/\lambda P_A, \text{ where}$$

$\dot{V}$ is the rate of uptake of inert gas,

P_A is its alveolar tension, and

λ is its solubility in pulmonary capillary blood.

Of course, after the start of recirculation, the mixed-venous gas concentration is no longer zero; and this simple equation then no longer holds.

The ideal gas for this purpose would be one which does not recirculate. It should also have a high solubility in blood, so that its uptake is reasonably rapid; its solubility in the lung tissues should, however, not be so great that local solution produces an artificially high apparent rate of uptake. In addition, the gas should be non-toxic in the concentration used, and have no pharmacological action on the heart or circulation.

Two gases which have been used in the past are acetylene and nitrous oxide. It has also been suggested recently that the refrigerent gas Freon 22 (mono-chlorodifluoromethane) is so lipid-soluble that its concentration in the mixed-venous blood is low enough to be neglected. Klausen (1965) has shown that, with care, a good correlation can be obtained between cardiac output determined by the CO_2-rebreathing and the acetylene uptake techniques. Values so obtained agree well with those found by standard methods such as the Fick technique.

Pulse contour technique

There is clearly a relationship between left ventricular stroke volume and the variation of aortic blood pressure during the cardiac cycle. An increase of stroke volume would be expected to be accompanied by an increase of pulse pressure (systolic minus diastolic pressure); and by continuously recording the pressure in the aorta throughout the cardiac cycle. It should, therefore, theoretically be possible to obtain a continuous estimate of left ventricular stroke volume, and so of cardiac output. The attraction of this method is that it gives a beat-by-beat estimate of cardiac output; other methods, such as the Fick or indicator dilution techniques, give a mean value averaged over at least several seconds.

Unfortunately, most attempts to define the precise mathematical relationship between stroke volume and pulse pressure have proved unsatisfactory. This is chiefly because of the difficulty of measuring such parameters as the compliance of the aortic reservoir and of defining the way in which they vary with changes of mean arterial pressure.

The formulae which have been developed by different workers vary greatly in complexity. Basically, however, they all make the assumption that the rate of aortic 'run off', that is, the rate at which blood leaves the aortic reservoir, depends at each instant on the aortic pressure, and that there is a well-defined relationship between aortic pressure and the volume of the aortic reservoir. The situation is, of course, complicated by the fact that the pulse wave takes a finite time to travel from the aortic root to the periphery of the arterial tree (*see* page 77), therefore the instantaneous pressure available for driving blood through the tissues is not identical to that measured at the aortic root.

The compliance of the arterial tree may be estimated by measuring the pulse-wave velocity, or determined by simultaneously measuring the aortic pressure contour and the cardiac output, and then calculating the compliance using the pulse formula in reverse. If it is then assumed that aortic compliance remains constant, the aortic pressure pulse may be used to give a second-by-second record of cardiac output under different physiological circumstances. Warner et al. (1953) obtained encouraging results with this method and have compared it with the Fick technique under a variety of conditions. They found that the variability between the two methods was less than 10 per cent (standard deviation). More recently, Graves et al. (1968) have described the clinical use of a similar technique in which the pulse pressure method is calibrated against a single indicator dilution estimation, and subsequent variations of cardiac output are calculated from changes of the aortic pressure pulse contour.

Catheter flowmeters

During the past few years several different types of catheter flowmeter have been developed. These can be introduced percutaneously into a large vessel, such as the aorta or pulmonary artery, where blood flow is closely related to total cardiac output. Although the use of such flow-probes is, at present, restricted mainly to research, they will probably become of more general use in the next few years, therefore they are mentioned here briefly.

Electromagnetic flowmeter　The normal type of electromagnetic flowmeter consists of a cuff which is placed round an exposed artery in an experimental animal or human at operation. However, Mills (1968) rather brilliantly turned such a flowmeter inside out (*Figure 12.12*), so that the blood flowed over the surface of the electromagnet instead of through it, as is the case with the conventional type of flowmeter. The flow of blood (which is, of course, a conductor of electricity) relative to the magnetic field causes an induced

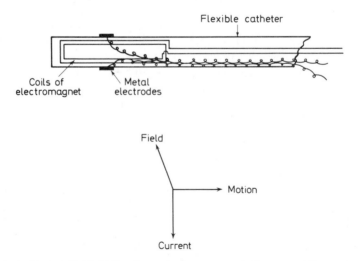

Figure 12.12. Mills' (1968) catheter-tip electromagnetic flowmeter (diagrammatic)

potential difference at the electrodes which is proportional to the flow velocity over the surface of the probe.

Of course, if blood flow velocity varies across the diameter of the vessel (as is the case with fully developed laminar flow, *see* page 6), the technique is valueless for the calculation of cardiac output, because it is necessary to know the position of the probe relative to the centre of the blood vessel. However, it appears that, with the type of flow-profile which occurs in large arteries such as the aorta and pulmonary artery, the velocity is relatively constant across the vessel, and in this case the radial position of the probe is clearly of little importance.

Thin-film flowmeters   It is also possible to measure blood flow velocity in a large artery by a thin-film probe. This consists of a thin metal film deposited on the end of a flexible catheter which can be introduced percutaneously into the aorta or pulmonary artery. An electric current passed through the film raises its temperature above that of its surroundings, while the flow of blood over its surface tends to remove heat by convection, and therefore to lower its temperature. The temperature of the film (and therefore its electrical resistance) thus gives a measure of blood flow velocity in the immediate vicinity of the probe.

A probe suitable for clinical use has recently been developed by Bellhouse et al. (1968).

Doppler flowmeter   If a beam of ultrasound is directed along the length of a flowing column of blood, the frequency of the reflected echo depends on the velocity of the blood flow relative to the probe (Doppler effect). Flow velocity may therefore be determined by comparison of the frequencies of the incident and reflected ultrasonic beams. This method has been used to assess peripheral blood flow; and it has recently been adapted by Light (1969) to estimate blood flow velocity in the aortic arch of intact man, and thus to obtain a continuous, albeit probably only semi-quantitative, record of cardiac output.

Ballistocardiography

As the ventricular contents are discharged into the arterial tree during systole, the remainder of the body experiences a force in the opposite direction, analogous to the 'kick' of a firearm. This force occurs as a result of Newton's third law of motion—action and reaction are equal and opposite. To look at the same process in another way, the headward ejection of blood attempts to shift the body's centre of gravity, but, because of inertia, this shift cannot occur instantaneously, therefore the remainder of the body moves in the opposite direction to maintain its centre of gravity in a constant position.

The forces arising from the heart's action may be recorded by placing the body on a horizontally suspended platform equipped with means of measuring either its movement or the applied force. The record obtained with such a system is known as a ballistocardiogram (BCG)—*Figure 12.13.*

Many workers have attempted to derive stroke volume from the magnitude of the BCG deflections because, theoretically, the force applied to the ballisto-cardiograph platform should be related to the amount of blood ejected during

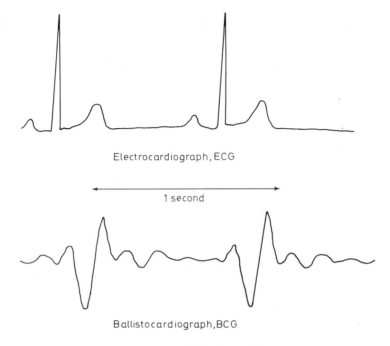

Electrocardiograph, ECG

1 second

Ballistocardiograph, BCG

Figure 12.13. A typical ballistocardiogram

ventricular systole. Most have, however, concluded that the relationship between stroke volume and magnitude of BCG deflection is qualitative rather than quantitative. Ballistocardiography can, however, undoubtedly give valuable information about the force of cardiac contraction.

The BCG is thus fundamentally different from the ECG. The latter gives virtually no information about the pumping ability of the heart. It is well recognized that cardiac output may fall to zero, seconds or even minutes before any ECG abnormality occurs.

Clinical experience has shown that the force of systolic ejection may be considerably reduced before there is any reduction of cardiac output. The BCG may, therefore, be useful in the diagnosis of insipient heart disease, at a time when the patient is still fairly normal clinically. Similarly, it may be used to assess the efficiency of therapeutic measures in chronic heart disease. For example, it has been demonstrated by this technique that digitalization results in a considerable improvement of performance of the failing heart, even when it is in sinus rhythm, and that the dose of digitalis required to achieve maximum improvement is often considerably less than that usually recommended (Starr, 1967).

MEASUREMENT OF BLOOD VOLUME

The direct measurement of blood volume by exsanguination is of limited application in clinical practice, although the technique is said to have been used on executed criminals. The most practical method for routine use is the dilution technique in which a small quantity of tracer is injected into the circulation, and its final concentration determined after it has become completely distributed throughout the circulating blood volume. Blood volume (V) is calculated from the formula:

$$V = m/c, \text{ where}$$

m is the mass of tracer injected, and
c is its final concentration in the blood.

Because of uncertainty about the value of the whole-body haematocrit ratio, the most accurate determination of blood volume involves separate measurements of the plasma and red cell volumes by two different tracers. In routine practice, however, it is usual to determine either the red cell or plasma volume, and then to calculate the total blood volume using the peripheral haematocrit ratio which is assumed to be an accurate measure of the whole body ratio (*see also* below).

Criteria for a tracer for blood volume estimation

The criteria for a satisfactory tracer are similar to those for a suitable indicator to measure cardiac output by the dilution technique (*see* page 255). They are:

1. it should be possible to measure its blood concentration accurately and easily;
2. it should be possible to administer the tracer as a concentrated solution, so that blood volume is not artificially increased by the volume of the injectate;
3. the tracer should be non-toxic and without pharmacological action in the concentration used; nor should it react chemically with any component of the blood;
4. it should remain in the intravascular space for the duration of the measurement, and then be rapidly excreted or broken down so that repeated, serial determinations of blood volume can be performed. This ideal is approximated most closely by radioactive tracers.

Plasma volume

The tracers most commonly used for the estimation of plasma volume are Evans blue and radioactive iodinated (^{131}I) serum albumin (RISA). Evans blue dye is a small molecule, but after intravenous injection it is rapidly bound to plasma albumin so that it remains in the intravascular compartment for an adequate length of time.

The use of these tracers is complicated by the fact that labelled albumin has been shown experimentally to cross the capillary membrane into the interstitial fluid; RISA, for example, may be detected in the lymph a few minutes after its injection into the blood stream (Hollander, Reilly and Birrows, 1956). It is, however, possible to correct for such leakage by measuring the indicator concentration at various times after injection, and then extrapolating back to find what its concentration would have been before any loss had occurred. There are, however, doubts about the validity of this procedure and, although Evans blue and RISA give similar estimates of plasma volume, the value obtained is lower than that found by the use of a larger molecule such as high-molecular weight dextran (Craig and Waterhouse, 1957).

Red cell volume

Red cell volume may be determined by means of labelled erythrocytes. Several isotopes have been used for this purpose; the most suitable being ^{32}P and ^{51}Cr, because with these the erythrocytes may be labelled *in vitro*, so that it is possible to use the subject's own cells, and thus avoid problems of blood group incompatibility. ^{51}Cr is preferred because it is more easily estimated.

Total blood volume

The technique of measuring either red cell volume or plasma volume alone, and then calculating total blood volume from the haematocrit ratio is prone to error because the venous haematocrit is not identical to the whole-body ratio. Determinations of the latter, based on separate measurements of red cell and plasma volume, indicate that it is lower than the haematocrit of blood from a large artery or vein.

It is usual to correct for this discrepancy by multiplying the measured large vessel haematocrit by the (experimentally-determined) factor 0.91. (It is also necessary to correct for plasma trapped amongst the packed erythrocytes. The extent of this correction depends on the duration of centrifugation and on the acceleration (*g*) used. An average correction is about 4 per cent.)

It is not usually practicable to determine the ratio of the whole body haematocrit to large vessel haematocrit in an individual patient, therefore it is necessary to consider the conditions under which the factor 0.91 is likely to be applicable. This problem has been reviewed by Gregersen and Chien (1968) who suggest that the factor is unchanged after acute haemorrhage, but that it is reduced in patients with congestive heart failure, and is increased in pregnancy and in patients with splenomegaly.

Recently, semi-automatic instruments such as the Volumetron blood-volume computer have become available for clinical estimation of blood volume. With this instrument a bolus of radioactive albumin is injected into the patient, and the amount of injected radioactivity compared with that of a blood sample taken from a remote site 5 minutes later. Blood volume is then calculated automatically.

MEASUREMENT OF INTRAVASCULAR PRESSURES

Arterial pressure

The continuous assessment of arterial blood pressure plays an important role in the clinical management of seriously ill patients. There have been several attempts to develop a machine which will record arterial pressure at frequent intervals with an automatically-controlled sphygmomanometer. Such apparatus, however, unfortunately tends to be inconvenient, expensive and unreliable, so that it is probably better to use an electrical manometer, connected to an indwelling arterial cannula. Such a system causes little disturbance to the patient and is reasonably trouble-free in use. (It must not be forgotten, however, that blood *flow* is usually of more importance than blood pressure, and that oversedulous treatment of hypotension may at times have serious consequencies—*see* page 212).

Electromanometers

A typical electromanometer (*Figure 12.14*) consists of a small chamber which is connected to an arterial cannula by a saline-filled catheter. One wall of the chamber is formed by a flexible metal diaphragm and the arterial pressure, transmitted down the catheter, impinges on this diaphragm and deforms it. The deformation is then converted into an electrical signal; the greater the pressure, the greater is the electrical output of the manometer.

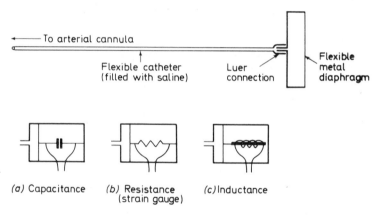

Figure 12.14. Blood pressure transducers (diagrammatic)

There are several ways in which diaphragmatic distortion may be detected and converted into an electrical signal; the diaphragm may form one plate of a capacitor, the capacitance of which varies with the imposed pressure; it may be connected to a resistance strain-gauge, the resistance of which varies; or it may be coupled to a small iron core inside an inductor, the inductance of which varies according to the applied pressure. The details are of no great importance in the present context; it is sufficient to note that the system produces an electrical signal which varies in a predictable manner with the pressure on the diaphragm—the sytem functions as a pressure/voltage transducer.*

A satisfactory electromanometer should have sufficient sensitivity and a linear response. A small change of pressure on the diaphragm should produce a sufficient change of output voltage for this to be easily measured, and the

* A transducer is a system which converts one form of energy into another.

voltage should vary in direct proportion to the applied pressure. In addition, the system should have a satisfactory dynamic response; it should be capable of following rapid changes of pressure without serious distortion of the pressure waveform. (This is mathematically the same as saying that the system should respond equally to the various frequency components of the pressure waveform, *see* below.)

Fundamental and harmonics

For most purposes arterial pressure may be considered as a periodic waveform which is repeated unchanged at regular intervals of time. It is a well-known physical principle that such periodic waveforms may be regarded as the sum of a constant term plus a series of sine waves (harmonics) of frequencies which are integral multiples of the frequency of the parent waveform (the fundamental frequency).

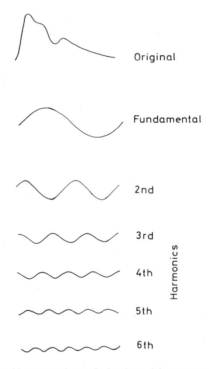

Figure 12.15. Fourier analysis of arterial pressure pulse

Fourier analysis

The analysis of a complicated periodic waveform into such a series of harmonics is known as Fourier analysis (*Figure 12.15*). This may be expressed in mathematical shorthand as:

$$F(t) = a_0 + a_1 \sin (ft + \phi_1) + a_2 \sin (2ft + \phi_2) + \ldots ,$$

where

F(t) is the periodic waveform under consideration,

f is the fundamental frequency,

a_0 is a constant (D.C.) term, and

a_n and ϕ_n are, respectively, the amplitude and phase angle of the nth harmonic (n = 1, 2, . . .).

In the case of arterial pressure, the mean pressure is represented by the D.C. component, a_0, and the presence of the higher harmonics represents the fact that the waveform is not a pure sinusoid. The fundamental frequency lies in the approximate range 1–3 Hz.

Deficiencies in manometer performance

A manometer may respond unequally to diffferent frequencies for two (interconnected) reasons: the system may be unable to follow rapidly fluctuating pressures because of viscous resistance in the connecting catheter; alternatively, the system may resonate around a certain frequency. If the manometer and its associated catheter are connected to a constant-amplitude sinusoidal pressure generator, the electrical output of the manometer varies with frequency in one of the ways shown in *Figure 12.16.* In the first case

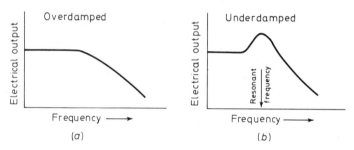

Figure 12.16. Frequency response of (a) overdamped, and (b) underdamped catheter-manometer system (diagrammatic)

(*Figure 12.16a*), the output decreases when the applied frequency is increased beyond a certain point because viscosity prevents sufficiently rapid movement of fluid in the catheter. In the second case (*Figure 12.16b*), the response is modified by the fact that the manometer diaphragm tends to vibrate at its own natural frequency, so that the frequency response curve has a peak around this resonant frequency.

Minimization of deficiencies

The effects of viscosity may be minimized, but not completely avoided, by choosing suitable dimensions for the coupling catheter. Resonance may be prevented by suitably damping the system, although it may in fact be necessary to choose a degree of damping which still gives a small resonance peak. It may be shown theoretically that an ideal catheter-manometer system has a damping coefficient of 0.7 of critical; this gives a flat frequency response up to 35 per cent of the system's natural frequency of oscillation (Harris and Heath, 1962).

Because of the effects of viscosity and damping, the natural frequency of the system should be as high as possible. It may be shown mathematically that this frequency is proportional to the square root of the pressure-volume modulus of the system, proportional to the cross-sectional area of the catheter, and inversely proportional to the square root of the catheter's length. Ideally, therefore, the manometer should have rigid walls with a stiff diaphragm, while the catheter should have uncompliant walls, a large cross-sectional area and short length. Unfortunately, these requirements are often incompatible with other demands on a system which is designed for recording intravascular pressures when the catheter may have to be long, flexible and of relatively narrow bore.

Some of the practical problems involved in determining the frequency response of catheter-electromanometer systems are considered by Addyman (1964) who also describes the frequency response of several commonly-used catheter-electromanometer combinations. A more detailed examination of two systems is given by MacMillan and Stott (1968), and some of the problems which arise at the patient-manometer interface are considered by Shirer (1962). Hughes and Prys-Roberts (1971) suggest the rule-of-thumb that the manometer and the patient should be interconnected by a stiff-walled tube not more than 60 cm in length, and that bubbles must be rigorously excluded.

Probably the ultimate form of manometer, which avoids many of the problems of catheter distortion, will be an electromanometer small enough to be introduced directly into the interior of the cardiovascular system. Intravascular manometers are currently available, but are, of course, very expensive. Gould, Trenholme and Kennedy (1973) have recently examined the performance of such a catheter-tip manometer.

Sphygmomanometry

Of course, in clinical practice most measurements of arterial blood pressure are made by a simple (Riva Rocci) sphygmomanometer. This has the advantage of cheapness and reliability, but needs a human operator. There have been a number of attempts to develop automatic techniques for recording arterial blood pressure by sphygmomanometry, using an automatically-operated cuff in conjunction with a means of electronically detecting either the Korotkow sounds or the arterial pressure pulse. These systems, however, tend to be expensive, and artefacts are a constant source of trouble. It can probably be argued that a patient who is sufficiently ill to need constant blood pressure measurements is also ill enough to require intra-arterial pressure measurements which have the additional advantage that samples of arterial blood are available for blood gas analysis.

Riva Rocci's method for determining arterial blood pressure is too well known to require detailed description. The method usually depends on the Korotkow sounds for the determination of systolic and diastolic pressures. There is some controversy about the best criterion for the diastolic pressure: the general view, however, is that this relates best to the pressure at which the Korotkow sounds disappear, rather than to the pressure at which they become muffled (Bordley et al., 1951); and that the point of muffling overestimates the pressure by 5–10 mm Hg.

One of the main difficulties with this technique is that pressures in the sphygmomanometer cuff are not identical to those at the arterial wall because, as a result of soft-tissue rigidity, cuff pressure exceeds arterial pressure by a variable amount. Inaccurate results are particularly liable to occur when the cuff is too narrow in relation to the thickness of the limb. A rough guide is that the cuff width should be one-third the limb's circumference. In many hospitals this is obviously a counsel for perfection because only a single size is available. The recommended technique for measuring arterial pressure by sphygmomanometry has recently been redefined by the American Heart Association (1967).

The oscillometer

Since physical access to the arm may be difficult during some operations, some workers prefer to use an oscillometer (of von Recklinghausen) instead of a simple sphygmomanometer. The oscillometer cuff consists of two cuffs arranged as in *Figure 12.17.* An aneroid manometer measures, via a two-way tap, either the pressure in the two cuffs connected together or the pressure difference between them. Initially, the cuffs are interconnected and pumped up above systolic pressure. The pressure is then allowed to fall slowly and, at intervals of 5 mm Hg or so, the manometer is switched to the differential mode to detect pressure differences between the cuffs.

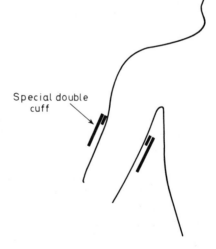

Figure 12.17. Oscillometer cuff (diagrammatic)

Special double cuff

At cuff pressures above systolic, no oscillations are transmitted below the small cuff, therefore there is no differential pressure, except for slight pulsation transmitted via the soft tissues. When the pressure lies between diastolic and systolic, a relatively large expansion occurs in the distal artery with each heart beat; this pulsation is detected by the differential manometer. When the pressure falls below diastolic, pressure swings no longer occur because the artery remains dilated throughout the cardiac cycle. The accuracy of the oscillometer for measuring arterial pressures has recently been examined by Corall and Strunin (1975).

ACP–10

CENTRAL VENOUS PRESSURE (CVP)

It has been increasingly realized that measurement of arterial blood pressure is of relatively little value in the functional assessment of the cardiovascular system. Not only may arterial pressure be relatively normal after a haemorrhage sufficient to cause a marked reduction of cardiac output, but a low arterial pressure may occur in the presence of adequate tissue perfusion (*see* Chapter 9). At the same time there has been a realization that central venous pressure—CVP (which for practical purposes is identical to the right atrial pressure so familiar to the physiologist, *see* page 109)—can give valuable information about the physiological state of the cardiovascular system (Sykes, 1963). Knowledge of the magnitude of CVP, plus clinical assessment of cardiac output gives information about the functional ability of the cardiac pump, and also about the degree to which the peripheral circulation is under- or over-filled with blood (Kelman, 1971). Measurement of CVP is of great importance in the assessment of the adequacy or otherwise of blood volume replacement during and after haemorrhage.

CVP is measured via a catheter with its tip in the SVC or intrathoracic IVC. This catheter may be inserted by several routes, but it is satisfactory for most purposes to introduce it percutaneously via an antecubital or jugular vein. The catheter is advanced until its tip lies in the thorax as indicated by the presence of marked respiratory pressure swings superimposed on the mean pressure. CVP is then measured either by a suitable pressure transducer or, more economically, by a saline manometer.

Because of the small absolute value of venous pressures, it is necessary when measuring CVP to consider differences of vertical height between the right atrium and the manometer. The measured pressure must be referred to a standard level such as the level of the right atrium. Unfortunately, there is no universal agreement about the best reference point; it is necessary, therefore, for the individual clinician to adopt his own reference level and to become familiar with the range of venous pressures which he encounters under different circumstances.

The interpretation of CVP measurements is considered in Chapter 4. The normal range is approximately 6–12 cm saline. A decrease below this level, in the presence of a low cardiac output, indicates inadequate filling of the peripheral circulation—a low mean systemic pressure (*see* page 119). A high CVP in the presence of a low cardiac output indicates decreased cardiac efficiency but does not, of course, rule out a concomitant deficiency of blood volume. The point is that a high CVP in the presence of a low blood volume means that the heart is unable to cope with the existing blood volume; further transfusion would probably result in deterioration of the patient's condition due to additional strain on an already failing heart.

A valuable review on the measurement and interpretation of CVP has recently appeared (Russell, 1974, *see* Recommended Further Reading). Also Gilbertson (1974) has reviewed the circumstances under which it may be inappropriate to measure CVP, that is, when it is better to measure the pulmonary artery wedge-pressure by means of a Swan-Ganz catheter.

RECOMMENDED FURTHER READING

Anon. (1974). 'Ultrasounding the Heart.' *Br. med. J.* **1**, 83

Anon. (1976). 'Ballistocardiography.' *Lancet* **i**, 347

Butler, J. (1965). 'Measurement of Cardiac Output using Soluble Gases.' In *Handbook of Physiology, Respiration,* Vol. II, p. 1489. Washington; American Physiological Society

Cliffe, P. (1974). 'Transducers for the Measurement of Pressure.' In Scurr, C. and Feldman, S., *Scientific Foundations of Anaesthesia.* London; Heinemann

Coltart, D. J. and Lewis, G. R. J. (1975). 'Non-invasive Methods of Evaluating the Cardiac Effect of Drugs.' *Br. J. clin. Pharmacol.* **2**, 193

Flynn, C. J. (1972). 'Non-invasive Monitoring. *Anesthesiology* **37**, 265

Gilbertson, A. A. (1974). 'Pulmonary Artery Catheterization and Wedge Pressure Measurement in the General Intensive Therapy Unit.' *Br. J. Anaesth.* **46**, 97

Hill, D. W. (1973). *Electronic Techniques in Anaesthesia and Surgery,* 2nd edn, chps 1, 2 and 4. London; Butterworths

Hopps, J. A. (1969). 'Shock Hazards in Operating Rooms and Patient-care Areas.' *Anesthesiology* **31**, 142

Guyton, A. C., Jones, C. E. and Coleman, T. G. (1973). *Cardiac Output and its Regulation,* 2nd edn. Philadelphia; W. B. Saunders

Leeming, N. M. (1973). 'Protection of the "Electrically Susceptible Patient".' *Anesthesiology* **38**, 370

Lowe, R. D. (1968). 'Problems in the Measurement of Blood Flow by Thermal Dilution.' In Bain, W. H. and Harper, A. M., *Blood Flow through Organs and Tissues.* Edinburgh; Livingstone

Monks, P. S. (1971). 'Safe Use of Electromedical Equipment.' *Anaesthesia* **26**, 264

Prampero, de P. E. (1975). 'Bloodless Methods for Measuring Cardiac Output.' In Mushin, W. W., Severinghaus, J. W., Tiengs, M. and Gorini, S., *Physiological Basis of Anaesthesiology.* Piccin Medical Books

Prys-Roberts, C. (1974). 'Arterial Manometry under Pressure. *Anesthesiology* **40**, 1

Pocock, S. N. (1972a). 'Earth-free Patient Monitoring.' *Bio-med. Eng.* **7**, 21

Pocock, S. N. (1972b). 'Faults found in Electromedical Instruments.' *Bio-med. Eng.* **7**, 533

Roberts, C. (1972). *Blood Flow Measurements.* London; Sector

Russell, W. J. (1974). *Central Venous Pressure.* London; Butterworths

Wayne, H. W. (1974). *Non-invasive Techniques in Cardiology.* London; Lloyd-Luke

Appendix I

Derivation of parabolic velocity profile under conditions of laminar flow

In *Figure A.1* the pressure difference between the ends of the tube of length l is ΔP. Consider the shaded cylinder of liquid of radius r. The force on this cylinder due to ΔP is $\pi r^2 \Delta P$ (pressure = force ÷ area—*see* page 1). This force acts to the left. The force due to viscosity (η) acts in the opposite direction and is equal to the surface area of the cylinder times the velocity gradient (dV/dr) at its surface. This force—$2\pi\, rl\, \eta\, dV/dr$—acts to the right.

At equilibrium, these two forces are equal and opposite,

that is
$$2\pi\, rl\eta\; dV/dr = -\pi r^2 \Delta P$$

whence
$$dV/dr = \frac{-r\Delta P}{2l\eta}$$

Integrating both sides with respect to r gives

$$V = \frac{-r^2 \Delta P}{4l\eta} + \text{constant.}$$

Now when $r = R$, $V = 0$, therefore constant $= \dfrac{R^2 \Delta P}{4l\eta}$, that is,

$$V = \frac{(R^2 - r^2)\,\Delta P}{4l\eta}$$

which is the formula used on page 6.

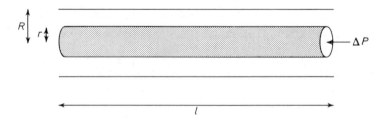

Figure A.1. Parabolic velocity profile under conditions of streamline flow

Appendix II

Critical closure

Consider a blood vessel, the wall of which is composed of a mixture of smooth muscle and elastic tissue. The total tension in the vascular wall must still be related to the transmural pressure by the Laplace relationship, but this total tension can be separated into a part due to contraction of the vascular smooth muscle and a part due to passive extension of elastic tissue (*Figure A.2*). The equilibrium position is represented by point X. If the active tension is increased by smooth muscle contraction, the vessel diameter decreases and the system comes to a new equilibrium with decreased vascular diameter and decreased wall tension (point X'). However, if the vessel diameter is decreased to such an extent that the two curves relating wall tension and vascular diameter become parallel (point Y), any further decrease of vessel diameter means that the transmural pressure can be resisted by a *smaller* total wall tension and by a *smaller* active tension, and this is an unstable situation which differs fundamentally from the stable situation represented by point X' where a small spontaneous decrease of vascular diameter causes a decrease of total wall tension, but requires a larger active tension for its maintenance. When the vessel is at point Y the excess active tension liberated, should the vessel decrease in diameter for any reason, is available to cause a further decrease of diameter so that the vessel collapses completely. This is the phenomenon of *critical closure*.

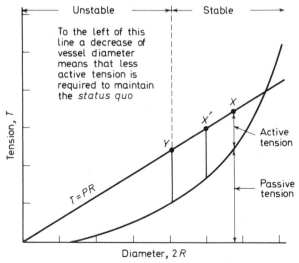

Figure A.2. Possible explanation for the phenomenon of critical closure. At X, the situation is stable; at Y, it is unstable, because a small, spontaneous decrease of vessel diameter allows the status quo to be maintained with a reduced amount of active wall tension. The tension which is no longer required is then available to cause a further decrease of vascular diameter, and so on, until the vessel closes completely

Appendix III

On page 45 it was argued that the inherent contractile ability of the myocardium is reflected in changes in the maximum velocity of shortening of its contractile element (dl/dt_{max}). In the Hill model of muscle contraction (*Figure 2.12*) it is possible to express the rate at which the muscle develops external tension (dT/dt) as the product of dT/dl and dl/dt, that is:

$$dT/dt = dT/dl \times dl/dt$$

where dT/dl is the stress–strain relationship of the series elastic element, and dl/dt is the velocity of shortening of the contractile element.

Experimentally, Parmley and Sonnenblick (1967) showed that the stress–strain relationship of the series elastic element was such that $dT/dl = kT + $ const. It follows therefore that $dl/dt = dT/dt \div (kT + $ const.$)$; so that, ignoring the constant, it is possible to say that the velocity of shortening of the contractile element (dl/dt) equals the time rate of change of external tension divided by the instantaneous developed tension. This expression is analogous to the index of myocardial contractility ($dP/dt_{max})/P$ used by Gersh et al. (*see* page 47).

References

Abbott, B. C. and Mommaerts, W. F. H. M. (1959). 'A Study of Inotropic Mechanisms in the Papillary Muscle Preparation.' *J. gen. Physiol.* **42**, 533

Adams, A. P., Economides, A. P., Finlay, W. E. I. and Sykes, M. K. (1970). 'The Effects of Variations of Inspiratory Flow Waveform on Cardiorespiratory Function during Controlled Ventilation in Normo-, Hypo- and Hypervolaemic Dogs.'*Br. J. Anaesth.* **42**, 818

Addyman, R. (1964). 'Frequency Response Curves; a Comparison of the Responses of Several Combinations of Catheter-electromanometer Blood Pressure Recording Systems.' *J. Soc. cardiol. Tech.* **6**, 119

Ahlquist, R. P. (1948). 'A Study of the Adrenotropic Receptors.' *Am. J. Physiol.* **153**, 586

Ahmad, G. and Nicoll, P. A. (1963). 'Chronotropic Response to Intravenous Infusion in the Anaesthetized Dog.' *Am. J. Physiol.* **204**, 423

Akers, R. P. and Lee, R. E. (1953). 'Peripheral Arteriolar Reactivity Gradient in the Hamster and Rat.' *Fedn Proc.* **12**, 3

Akester, J. M. and Brody, M. J. (1969). 'Mechanism of Vascular Resistance Changes produced in Skin and Muscle by Halothane.' *J. Pharmac. exp. Ther.* **170**, 287

Alexander, S. C., Cohen, P. J., Wollman, H., Smith, T. C., Reivich, M. and Molen, R. A. van der (1965). 'Cerebral Carbohydrate Metabolism during Hypocarbia in Man. Studies during Nitrous Oxide Anaesthesia.' *Anesthesiology* **26**, 624

American Heart Association (1967). 'Recommendations for Human Blood Pressure Determination by Sphygomanometers.' *Circulation* **36**, 980

Amory, D. W., Steffenson, J. L., Forsyth, R. P. (1971). 'Systemic and Regional Blood Flow Changes during Halothane Anesthesia in the Rhesus Monkey.' *Anesthesiology* **35**, 81

Anderson, F. L. and Brown, A. M. (1967). 'Pulmonary Vasoconstriction Elicited by Stimulation of the Hypothalamic Integrative Area for the Defense Reaction.' *Circulation Res.* **21**, 747

Arias-Stella, J. and Saldaña, M. (1963). 'Terminal Portion of the Pulmonary Arterial Tree in People Native to High Altitudes.' *Circulation* **28**, 915

Asmussen, E. and Nielson, M. (1951). 'The Arterial Blood Pressure on Transition from Rest to Work.' *Acta Physiol. scand.* (Suppl. 89), 5

Asmussen, E. and Nielson, M. (1952). 'The Cardiac Output in Rest and Work determined simultaneously by the Acetylene and the Dye Injection Methods.' *Acta Physiol. scand.* **27**, 217

Åstrand, P.-O., Cuddy, T. E., Saltin, B. and Stenberg, J. (1964). 'Cardiac Output during Submaximal and Maximal Work.' *J. appl. Physiol.* **19**, 268

Åstrand, P.-O., Ekblom, B., Messin, R., Saltin, B. and Stenberg, J. (1965). 'Intra-arterial Blood Pressure during Exercise with Different Muscle Groups.' *J. appl. Physiol.* **20**, 253

Åstrand, P.-O. and Saltin, B. (1961). 'Maximal Oxygen Uptake and Heart Rate in Various Types of Muscular Activity.' *J. appl. Physiol.* **16**, 977

Baez, S., Zauder, H. L. and Orkin, L. R. (1962). 'Effects of Various Anesthetic Agents on the Reaction of the Microcirculation.' *Fedn Proc.* **21**, 120

Bain, W. H., Lancaster, J. R. and Adams, W. E. (1965). 'Pulmonary Vascular Changes with Increased Oxygen Tensions.' In Ledingham, I. McA. *Hyperbaric Oxygenation: Proceeding of the Second International Congress,* p. 113. Edinburgh; Livingstone

Bainbridge, F. A. (1915). 'The Influence of Venous Filling upon the Rate of the Heart.' *J. Physiol.* **50**, 65

Banchero, N., Sime, F., Peñaloza, D., Cruz, J., Gamboa, R. and Marticorena, E. (1966). 'Pulmonary Pressure, Cardiac Output, and Arterial Oxygenation Saturation during Exercise at High Altitude and at Sea Level.' *Circulation* **33**, 249

Barron, J. N. and Veall, N. (1968). 'Some Applications of Blood Flow Measurements in Tube Pedicles and Flaps in Plastic Surgery.' I. Bain, W. H. and Harper, A. M., *Blood Flow Through Organs and Tissues,* p. 357. Edinburgh; Livingstone.

Bayliss, W. M. (1902). 'On the Local Reactions of the Arterial Wall to Changes of Internal Pressure.' *J. Physiol.* **28**, 220

Beck, L. and Brody, M. J. (1961). 'The Physiology of Vasodilatation.' *Angiology* **12**, 202

Bellhouse, B. J., Schultz, D. L., Karatzas, N. B. and Lee, G. de L. (1968). 'A Catheter Tip Method for the Measurement of the Pulsatile Blood Flow Velocity in Arteries.' In Bain, W. H. and Harper, A. M., *Blood Flow Through Organs and Tissues,* p. 43. Edinburgh; Livingstone

Bellhouse, B. J. and Talbot, L. (1969). 'The Fluid Mechanisms of the Aortic Valve.' *J. Fluid Mech.* **35**, 721

Bergel, D. H. and Milnor, W. R. (1965). 'Pulmonary Vascular Impedance in the Dog.' *Circulation Res.* **16**, 401

Berger, E. Y., Gladstone, M. and Horwitz, S. A. (1949). 'The Effect of Anoxic Anoxia in the Human Kidney.' *J. clin. Invest.* **28**, 648

Bergofsky, E. H., Bass, B. G., Ferretti, R. and Fishman, A. P. (1963). 'Pulmonary Vasoconstriction in Response to Precapillary Hypoxemia.' *J. clin. Invest.* **42**, 1201

Bergofsky, E. H., Lehr, D. E. and Fishman, A. P. (1962). 'The Effects of Changes in Hydrogen Ion Concentration on the Pulmonary Circulation.' *J. clin. Invest.* **41**, 1492

Bergström, J., Bucht, H., Ek, J., Josephson, B., Sundell, H. and Werkö, L. (1959). 'The Renal Extraction of Para-aminohippurate in Normal Persons and in Patients with Diseased Kidneys.' *Scand. J. clin. Lab. Invest.* **11**, 361

Berne, R. M. and Levy, M. N. (1967). *Cardiovascular Physiology,* 1st edn, p. 68. St Louis; C. V. Mosby.

Bernstein, R. L. and Orkin, L. R. (1965). 'Modified Valsalva Maneuver as a Test of Circulatory Integrity under Anaesthesia.' *Anesthesiology* **26**, 239

Beuren, A., Sparkes, C. and Bing, R. J. (1958). 'Metabolic Studies on the Arrested and Fibrillating Perfused Heart.' *Am. J. Cardiol.* **1**, 103

Bevan, A. T., Honour, A. J. and Stott, F. H. (1969). 'Direct Arterial Pressure Recording in Unrestricted Man.' *Clin. Sci.* **36**, 329

Bevegård, S. B. and Shephard, J. H. (1967). 'Regulation of the Circulation during Exercise in Man.' *Physiol. Rev.* **47**, 178

Bevegård, S. B. and Shepherd, J. T. (1966). 'Circulatory Effects of Stimulating the Carotid Arterial Stretch Receptors in Man at Rest and during Exercise.' *J. clin. Invest.* **45**, 132

Bianchi, G., Tenconi, L. T. and Lucca, R. (1970). 'Effect in the Conscious Dog of Constriction of the Renal Artery to a Sole Remaining Kidney on Haemodynamics, Sodium Balance, Body Fluid Volumes, Plasma Renin Concentration and Pressor Responsiveness to Angiotensin.' *Clin. Sci.* **38**, 741

Bing, R. J. (1961). 'Discussion.' In Proceedings of a Conference on Recent Progress and Present Problems in the Field of Shock. *Fedn Proc.* **20**(Suppl. 9), 72

Bing, R. J., Wu, C. and Gudbjarnason, S. (1964). 'Mechanism of Heart Failure.' *Circulation Res.* **15** (Suppl. 2), 64

Bird, A. D. and Telfer, A. B. M. (1965). 'The Effect of Increased Oxygen Tension on Peripheral Blood Flow.' In Ledingham, I. McA., *Hyperbaric Oxygenation: Proceedings of the Second International Congress.* p. 424. Edinburgh; Livingstone

Biscoe, T. J. and Millar, R. A. (1964). 'The Effect of Halothane on Carotid Sinus Baroreceptor Activity.' *J. Physiol.* **173**, 24

Biscoe, T. J. and Millar, R. A. (1966a). 'The Effects of Cyclopropane, Halothane and Ether on Central Baroreceptor Pathways.' *J. Physiol.* **184**, 535

Biscoe, T. J. and Millar, R. A. (1966b). 'The Effect of Cyclopropane, Halothane and Ether on Sympathetic Ganglionic Transmission.' *Br. J. Anaesth.* **38**, 3

Black, G. W., Linde, H. W., Dripps, R. D. and Price, H. L. (1959). 'Circulatory Changes accompanying Respiratory Acidosis during Halothane (Fluothane) Aaesthesia in Man.' *Br. J. Anaesth.* **31**, 238

Black, G. W. and McArdle, L. (1962). 'The Effects of Halothane on the Peripheral Circulation in Man.' *Br. J. Anaesth.* **34**, 2

Blackburn, J. P., Conway, C. M., Davies, R. M., Enderly, G. E. H., Edridge, A. W., Leigh, J. M., Lindop, M. J., Phillips, G. D. and Strickland, D. A. P. (1973). 'Valsalva Responses and Systolic Time Intervals during Anaesthesia and Induced Hypotension.' *Br. J. Anaesth.* **45**, 704

Blackburn, J. P., Conway, C. M., Leigh, J. M., Lindop, M. J. and Reitan, J. A. (1972). 'Pa_{CO_2} and the Pre-ejection Period: the Pa_{CO_2} Inotropy Response Curve.' *Anesthesiology* **37**, 268

Blackmon, J. R., Rowell, L. B., Kennedy, L. J., Twiss, R. D. and Conn, R. D. (1967). 'Physiological Significance of Maximal Oxygen Intake in "Pure" Mitral Stenosis.' *Circulation* **36**, 497

Blenkarn, G. D., Briggs, G., Bell, J. and Sugioka, K. (1972). 'Cognitive Function after Hypocapnic Hyperventilation.' *Anesthesiology* **37**, 381

Bloch, J. H., Pierce, C. H. and Lillehei, R. C. (1966). 'Adrenergic Blocking Agents in the Treatment of Shock.' *A. Rev. Med.* **17**, 483

Bloom, W. L. (1955). 'Demonstration of Diastolic Filling of Beating Excised Heart (Motion Picture).' *Am. J. Physiol.* **183**, 597

Bond, A. G. (1960). 'Variability of Haemoglobin Concentration during Anaesthesia.' *Br. J. Anaesth.* **41**, 947

Bonica, J. J., Berges, P. U. and Morikawa, K. (1970). 'Circulatory Effects of Peridural Block. I. Effects of Level of Analgesia and Dose of Lidocaine.' *Anesthesiology* **33**, 619

Boniface, K. J., Brodie, O. J. and Walton, R. F. (1953). 'Resistance Strain Gauge Arches for Direct Measurement of Heart Contractile Force in Animals.' *Proc. Soc. exp. Biol. Med.* **84**, 263

Boniface, K. J., Brown J. M. and Kronen, P. S. (1955). 'The Influence of some Inhalational Anaesthetic Agents on the Contractile Force of the Heart.' *J. Pharmac. exp. Ther.* **113**, 64

Bordley, J., Connor, C. A. R., Hamilton, W. F., Kerr, W. J. and Wiggers, C. J. (1951). 'Recommendations for Human Blood Pressure Determinations by Sphygomanometers.' *Circulation* **4**, 503

Bouckaert, J. J. and Leusen, I. (1951). 'Au Sujet des Influences Réflexe et Controle Directe du CO_2 sur le Système Vasomoteur.' *Archs. int. Pharmacodyn.* **87**, 393

Bousvaros, G. A., Don, C. and Hopps, J. A. (1962). 'An Electrical Hazard of Selective Angiocardiography.' *Can. med. Ass. J.* **87**, 286

Bradley, R. D. (1964). 'Diagnostic Right Heart Catheterisation with Miniature Catheters in Severely Ill Patients.' *Lancet* **ii**, 941

Brady, A. J. and Woodbury, J. W. (1960). 'The Sodium-Potassium Hypothesis as the Basis of Electrical Activity in Frog Ventricle.' *J. Physiol.* **154**, 385

Branthwaite, M. A. and Bradley, R. D. (1968). 'Measurement of Cardiac Output by Thermal Dilution in Man.' *J. appl. Physiol.* **24**, 434

Braunwald, E. and Chapman, C. B. (1963). 'Cardiovascular Dynamics: Basic and Applied Aspects.' In Grollman, A., *The Functional Pathology of Disease*, pp. 267. New York; McGraw-Hill

Braunwald, E., Chidsey, C. A., Harrison, D. C., Gaffney, T. E. and Kahler, R. L. (1963). 'Studies on the Function of the Adrenergic Nerve Endings in the Heart.' *Circulation* **28**, 958

Braunwald, E., Fishman, A. P. and Cournand, A. (1956). 'Time Relationship of Dynamic Events in the Cardiac Chambers, Pulmonary Artery and Aorta in Man.' *Circulation Res.* **4**, 100

Braunwald, E. and Ross, J. Jr. (1963). 'The Ventricular End-diastolic Pressure. Appraisal of its Value in the Recognition of Ventricular Failure in Man.' *Am. J. Med.* **34**, 147

Braunwald, E. and Ross, J. Jr. (1964). 'Applicability of Starling's Law of the Heart to Man.' *Circulation Res.* **15** (Suppl. 2), 169

Braunwald, E., Ross, J. Jr. and Sonnenblick, E. H. (1967). 'Mechanisms of Contraction of the Normal and Failing Heart.' *New Engl. J. Med.* **277**, 794

Brecher, G. A. (1956). 'Experimental Evidence of Ventricular Diastolic Suction.' *Circulation Res.* **4**, 513

Brecher, G. A. (1958). 'Critical Review of Recent Work on Ventricular Diastolic Suction.' *Circulation Res.* **6**, 554

Brenk, H. A. S. van den, Cass, N. M. and Chambers, R. D. (1956). 'Effects of Anaesthetic Agents and Relaxants on Vascular Tone Studies in Sandison-Clark Chambers.' *Br. J. Anaesth.* **28**, 98

Bristow, J. D., Prys-Roberts, C. and Fisher, A. (1969). 'Quantification of Baroreceptor Reflexes during Anaesthesia in Man.' *Br. J. Anaesth.* **41**, 556

Brock, R. C. (1952). 'The Surgical and Pathological Anatomy of the Mitral Valve. *Br. Heart J.* **14**, 489

Brown, B. R. and Crout, J. R. (1971). 'A Comparative Study of the Effects of Five General Anesthetics on Myocardial Contractility. I. Isometric Conditions.' *Anesthesiology* **34**, 236

Brown, J. J., Lever, A. F., Robertson, J. I. S., Schalekamp, M. A. (1974). 'Renal Abnormality of Essential Hypertension.' *Lancet* ii, 320

Bruns, D. L. (1959). 'The General Theory of the Causes of Murmurs in the Cardiovascular System.' *Amer. J. Med.* 27, 360

Burn, J. H. (1959). 'Pharmacological Testing of Anaesthetics.' *Proc. R. Soc. Med.* 52, 95

Burton, A. C. (1972). *Physiology and biophysics of the Circulation,* 2nd edn. Year Book Medical Publishers

Cannon, W. B. (1923). *Traumatic Shock.* New York; Appleton Century Crofts

Carlsten, A., Folkow, B., Grimby, G., Hamberger, C. A. and Thulesius, O. (1958). 'Cardiovascular Effects of Direct Stimulation of the Carotid Sinus Nerve in Man.' *Acta physiol. scand.* 44, 138

Carlsten, A., Folkow, B. and Hamberger, C. A. (1957). 'Cardiovascular Effects of Direct Vagal Stimulation in Man.' *Acta physiol. scand.* 41, 68

Carter, D. and Einheber, D. (1966). 'Intestinal Ischemic Shock in Germ Free Animals.' *Surgery Gynec. Obstet.* 122, 66

Cerretelli, P., Cruz, J. C., Farhi, L. E. and Rahn, H. (1966). 'Determination of Mixed Venous O_2 and CO_2 Tensions and Cardiac Output by a Rebreathing Method.' *Respir. Physiol.* 1, 258

Christensen, E. H. and Nielsen, M. (1942). 'Investigation of the Circulation in the Skin at Beginning of Muscular Work.' *Acta Physiol. scand.* 4, 162

Christensen, M. S., Høedt-Rasmussen, K. and Lassen, N. A. (1967). 'Cerebral Vasodilation by Halothane Anaesthesia in Man and its Potentiation by Hypotension and Hypercapnia.' *Br. J. Anaesth.* 39, 927

Christiansen, J., Douglas, C. G. and Haldane, J. S. (1914). 'The Absorption and Dissociation of Carbon Dioxide by Human Blood.' *J. Physiol.* 48, 244

Clarke, R. S. J. (1952). 'The Effect of Voluntary Overbreathing on the Blood Flow through the Human Forearm.' *J. Physiol.* 118, 537

Cohen, P. J., Alexander, S. C., Smith, T. C., Reivich, M. and Wollman, H. (1968). 'Cerebral Carbohydrate Metabolism of Man during Respiratory and Metabolic Alkalosis.' *J. appl. Physiol.* 24, 66

Cohn, J. D., Greenspan, M., Goldstein, C. R., Gudwin, A. L., Siegal, J. H. and Del Guercio, L. R. M. (1968). 'Arteriovenous Shunting in High Cardiac Output Shock Syndromes.' *Surgery Gynec. Obstet.* 127, 282

Coleman, T. G., Bower, J. D., Langford, H. G. and Guyton, A. C. (1970). 'Regulation of Arterial Pressure in the Anephric State.' *Circulation* 17, 509

Coleridge, H. M., Coleridge, J. C. G. and Kidd, C. (1964). 'Cardiac Receptors in the Dog, with Particular Reference to Two Types of Afferent Endings in the Ventricular Wall.' *J. Physiol.* 174, 323

Coleridge, J. C. G. and Kidd, C. (1963). 'Reflex Effects of Stimulating Baroreceptors in the Pulmonary Artery.' *J. Physiol.* 166, 197

Collins, V. J., Jaffe, R. J. and Zahony, I. (1964). 'Newer Attitudes in Management of Hemorrhagic Shock: The Use of Chlorpromazine as an Adjunct.' *Surg. Clins N. Am.* 44, 173

Conn, J. W. (1955). 'Primary Aldosteronism, a New Clinical Syndrome.' *J. Lab. clin. Med.* 45, 3

Cooper, K. E., Edholm, O. G. and Mottram, R. F. (1955). 'The Blood Flow in Skin and Muscle of the Human Forearm.' *J. Physiol.* 128, 258

Cooperman, L. H., Warden, J. C. and Price, H. L. (1968). 'Splanchnic Circulation during Nitrous Oxide Anesthesia and Hypocarbia in Normal Man.' *Anesthesiology* **29**, 254

Corall, M. and Strinin, L. (1975). 'Assessment of the von Recklinghausen Oscillotonometer.' *Anaesthesia* **30**, 59

Craig, A. B. and Waterhouse, C. (1957). 'The Volume of Distribution of High Molecular Weight Dextran and Its Relation to Plasma Volume in Man.' *J. Lab. clin. Med.* **49**, 165

Craythorne, N. W. B. and Darby, T. D. (1965). 'The Cardiovascular Effects of Nitrous Oxide in the Dog.' *Br. J. Anaesth.* **37**, 560

Cromwell, T. H., Stevens, W. C., Eger, E. I. II., Shakespeare, T. F., Halsey, M. J., Bahlman, S. H. and Fourcade, H. E. (1971). 'The Cardiovascular Effect of Compound 469 (Forane) during Spontaneous Ventilation and CO_2 Challenge in Man.' *Anesthesiology* **35**, 17

Crout, J. R. (1961). 'Effect of Inhibiting both Catechol-o-methyl Transferase and Monoamine Oxidase on Cardiovascular Responses to Norepinephrine.' *Proc. Soc. exp. Biol. Med.* **108**, 482

Crowell, J. W., Ford, R. G. and Lewis, V. M. (1959). 'Oxygen Transport in Hemorrhagic Shock as a Function of the Hematocrit Ratio.' *Am. J. Physiol.* **196**, 1033

Crowell, J. W. and Guyton, A. C. (1962). 'Further Evidence Favouring a Cardiac Mechanism in Irreversible Hemorrhagic Shock.' *Am. J. Physiol.* **203**, 248

Crowell, J. W. and Smith, E. E. (1964). 'Oxygen Deficit and Irreversible Hemorrhagic Shock.' *Am. J. Physiol.* **216**, 313

Cullen, B. F., Eger, E. I. II, Smith, N. T., Sawyer, D. C. and Gregory, G. A. (1971). 'The Circulatory Response to Hypercapnia during Fluroxene Anesthesia in Man.' *Anesthesiology* **34**, 415

Cullen, B. F., Eger, E. I. II, Smith, N. T., Sawyer, D. C., Gregory, G. A. and Joas, T. A. (1970). 'Cardiovascular Effects of Fluroxene in Man.' *Anesthesiology* **32**, 218

Cullen, D. J. and Eger, E. I., II (1974). 'Cardiovascular Effects of Carbon Dioxide in Man.' *Anesthesiology* **41**, 345

Cullen, D. J., Eger, E. I. II and Gregory, G. A. (1969a). 'The Cardiovascular Effects of Cyclopropane in Man.' *Anesthesiology* **31**, 398

Cullen, D. J., Eger, E. I. II and Gregory, G. A. (1969b). 'The Cardiovascular Effects of Carbon Dioxide in Man, Conscious and during Cyclopropane Anesthesia.' *Anesthesiology* **31**, 407

Daly, M. de B. and Scott, M. J. (1962). 'An Analysis of the Primary Cardiovascular Reflex Effects of Stimulation of the Carotid Body Chemoreceptors in the Dog.' *J. Physiol.* **162**, 555

Daniel, P. M., Peabody, C. N. and Prichard, M. M. L. (1951). 'Observations on the Circulation through the Cortex and the Medulla of the Kidney.' *Q. J. exp. Physiol.* **36**, 202

Davies, D. F. and Shock, N. W. (1950). 'Age Changes in Glomerular Filtration Rate, Effective Renal Plasma Flow, and Tubular Excretory Capacity in Adult Males.' *J. clin. Invest.* **29**, 496

Davies, J. and Davies, I. J. T. (1968). 'The Pathogenesis and Treatment of Shock.' *Hosp. Med. (London)* **2**, 686

Del Guercio, L. R. M., Coomaraswamy, R. P. and State, D. (1963). 'Cardiac Output and Other Hemodynamic Variables during External Cardiac Massage in Man.' *New Engl. J. Med.* **269**, 1398

Denison, D., Edwards, R. T. H., Jones, G. and Pope, H. (1969). 'Direct and Rebreathing Estimates of the O_2 and CO_2 Pressures in Mixed Venous Blood.' *Resp. Physiol.* 7, 326

Deutsch, S., Goldberg, M., Stephen, G. W. and Wu, W. H. (1966). 'The Effects of Halothane Anesthesia on Renal Function in Normal Man.' *Anesthesiology* 27, 793

Deutsch, S., Linde, H. W., Dripps, R. D. and Price, H. L. (1962). 'Circulatory and Respiratory Actions of Halothane in Normal Man.' *Anesthesiology* 23, 631

Deutsch, S., Pierce, E. C. Jr. and Vandam, L. D. (1967). 'Cyclopropane Effects on Renal Function in Normal Man.' *Anesthesiology* 28, 547

Dintenfass, L. (1963). 'Blood Rheology in Cardiovascular Diseases.' *Nature* 199, 813

Dintenfass, L. (1964). 'A Trolley Viscometer for Estimating Viscosity and Clotting of Blood in Hospital Wards.' *Lancet* ii, 567

Dintenfass, L., Julian, D. G. and Miller, G. (1966). 'Viscosity of Blood in Healthy Young Women, Effect of Menstrual Cycle.' *Lancet* i, 234

Djojosugito, A. M., Folkow, B., Öberg, B. and White, S. (1970). 'A Comparison of Blood Viscosity Measured *in vitro* and in a Vascular Bed.' *Acta Physiol. scand.*, 78, 70

Donald, D. E. and Shepherd, J. T. (1963). 'Response to Exercise of Dogs with Cardiac Denervation.' *Am. J. Physiol.* 205, 393

Donald, K. W., Bishop, J. M. and Wade, O. L. (1955). 'Changes in the Oxygen Content of Axillary Venous Blood during Leg Exercise in Patients with Rheumatic Heart Disease.' *Clin. Sci.* 14, 531

Douglas, I. H. S., MacDonald, J. A. E., Milligan, G. F., Mellon, A. and Ledingham, I. McA. (1975). 'A Comparison of Methods for the Measurement of Cardiac Output and Blood Oxygen Content.' *Br. J. Anaesth.* 47, 443

Drapanas, T., Kluge, D. N. and Schenk, W. G. Jr. (1960). 'Measurement of Hepatic Blood Flow by Bromsulphalein and by the Electromagnetic Flowmeter.' *Surgery* 48, 1017

Duke, H. N. (1957). 'Observations on the Effects of Hypoxia on the Pulmonary Vascular Bed.' *J. Physiol.* 135, 45

Dundee, J. W. and Moore, J. (1961). 'Zhiopentone and Methohexitol. A Comparison as Main Anaesthetic Agents for a Standard Operation.' *Anaesthesia* 16, 50

Eckenhoff, J. E., Hafkenschiel, J. H. and Landmesser, C. M. (1947). 'The Coronary Circulation in the Dog.' *Am. J. Physiol.* 148, 582

Edholm, O. G., Fox, R. H. and MacPherson, R. K. (1956). 'The Effect of Body Heating on the Circulation in Skin and Muscle.' *J. Physiol.* 134, 612

Eger, E. I. (1963). 'Application of a Mathematical Model of Gas Uptake.' In Papper, E. M. and Kitz, R. J., *Uptake and Distribution of Anesthetic Agents*, p. 88. New York; McGraw-Hill

Eger, E. I. (1964). 'Respiratory and Circulatory Factors in Uptake and Distribution of Volatile Anaesthetic Agents.' *Br. J. Anaesth.* 36, 155

Eger, E. I. II, Smith, N. T. and Cullen, D. J. (1971). 'A Comparison of the Cardiovascular Effects of Halothane, Fluoroxene, Ether and Cyclopropane in Man: A Resumé. *Anesthesiology* 34, 25

Eger, E. I. II, Smith, N. T., Stoelting, R. K., Cullen, D. J., Kadis, L. B. and Whitcher, C. E. (1970). Cardiovascular Effects of Halothane· in Man.' *Anesthesiology* **32**, 396

Egli, F. R. (1965). 'Betrachtungen zur Alveolär-arteriellen Sauerstoffdruck-differenz der Einfluss von CO_2 beim Narkotisierten Hund.' *Helv. physiol. pharmac. acta* **23** (Suppl. 15), 1

Ekblom, B. and Hermansen, L. (1968). 'Cardiac Output in Athletes.' *J. appl. Physiol.* **25**, 619

Ekelund, L. G. and Holmgren, A. (1964). 'Circulatory and Respiratory Adaptation during Long-term, Non-steady State Exercise, in the Sitting Position.' *Acta Physiol. scand.* **62**, 240

Elliott, T. R. (1912). 'The Control of the Suprarenal Glands by the Splanchnic Nerves.' *J. Physiol.* **44**, 374

Elmes, P. C. and Jefferson, A. A. (1942). 'The Effect of Anaesthesia on the Adrenaline Content of the Suprarenal Glands.' *J. Physiol.* **101**,355

Enderby, G. E. H. (1960). 'Halothane and Hypotension.' *Anaesthesia* **15**, 25

Epstein, R. M. (1964). 'Renal and Hepatic Blood Flow Methods.' In Price, H. L. and Cohen, P. J., *Effects of Anesthetics on the Circulation*, p. 225. Springfield; Charles C. Thomas

Epstein, R. M., Deutsch, S., Cooperman, L. H., Clement, A. J. and Price, H. L. (1966). 'Splanchnic Circulation during Halothane Anesthesia and Hyper-capnia in Normal Man.' *Anesthesiology* **27**, 654

Epstein, R. M., Wheeler, H. D., Frumin, M. J., Habif, D. V., Papper, E. M. and Bradley, S. E. (1961). 'The Effect of Hypercapnia on Estimated Hepatic Blood Flow, Circulating Splanchnic Blood Volume, and Hepatic Sulfobro-mophthaline Clearance during General Anesthesia in Man.' *J. clin. Invest.* **40**, 592

Epstein, S. E., Beiser, G. D., Stampfer, M., Robinson, B. F. and Braunwald, E. (1966). 'Two New and Sensitive Indices of Cardiac Performance: the Cardiac Output at a Mixed Venous O_2 Saturation of 30% and the Quantity of Unextracted O_2 Returned to the Lungs.' *Circulation* **34** (Suppl. 3), 97

Ernsting, J. and Parry, D. J. (1957). 'Some Observations on the Effect of Stimulating the Stretch Receptors in the Carotid Artery of Man.' *J. Physiol.* **137**, 45P

Etsten, B. E. and Li, T. H. (1962). 'Current Concepts of Myocardial Function during Anaesthesia.' *Br. J. Anaesth.* **34**, 884

Etsten, B. E., Rheinlander, H. F., Reynolds, R. N. and Li, T. H. (1953). 'Effect of Cyclopropane Anesthesia on Pulmonary Artery Pressure in Humans.' *Surg. Forum* **4**, 649

Etsten, B. E. and Shimosato, S. (1964). ' "Myocardial Contractility": Per-formance of the Heart during Anesthesia.' In Fabian, L. W., *Anesthesia and the Circulation*, p. 56. Philadelphia; F. A. Davis

Etsten, B. E. and Shimosato, S. (1965). 'Halothane Anesthesia and Cate-cholamine Levels in a Patient with Pheochromocytoma.' *Anesthesiology* **26**, 688

Euler, U. S. von (1954). 'Adrenaline and noradrenaline: Distribution and Action.' *Pharmac. Rev.* **6**, 15

Euler, U. S. von and Liljestrand, G. (1946). 'Observations on the Pulmonary Arterial Blood Pressure in the Cat.' *Acta physiol. scand.* **12**, 301

Euler, U. S. von, Liljestrand, G. and Zotterman, Y. (1939). 'The Excitation

Mechanism of the Chemoreceptors of the Carotid Body.' *Skand. Arch Physiol.* **83**, 132

Eversole, W. J., Kleinberg, W., Overman, R. R., Remington, J. W. and Swingle, W. W. (1944). 'Nervous Factor in Shock Induced by Muscle Trauma in Normal Dogs.' *Am. J. Physiol.* **140**, 490

Fahraeus, R. and Lindqvist, T. (1931). 'The Viscosity of the Blood in Narrow Capillary Tubes.' *Am. J. Physiol.* **96**, 562

Falck, B., Nielson, K. C. and Owman, C. (1968). 'Adrenergic Innervation of the Pial Circulation. *Scand. J. clin. Lab. Invest.* **22** (Suppl. 102) VI B

Farhi, L. E., Chinet, A., Haab, P. (1966). 'Pression Partielle d'Oxygène du Sang Veineux Mêlé chex d'Homme, en Plaine et Haute Altitude.' *J. Physiol. (Paris)* **58**, 516

Fawez, G. (1951). 'The Mechanism by which N-N-dibenzylchlorethylamine Protects Animals against Cardiac Arrhythmias induced by Sympathico-mimetic Amines in Presence of Cyclopropane and Chloroform.' *Br. J. Pharmac.* **6**, 492

Fazekas, J. F., Alman, R. W. and Bessman, A. N. (1952). 'Cerebral Physiology of the Aged.' *Am. J. med. Sci.* **223**, 245

Feigl, E. O. (1967). 'Sympathetic Control of Coronary Circulation.' *Circulation Res.* **20**, 262

Felder, D. A., Linton, R. R., Todd, D. P. and Banks, C. (1951). 'Changes in the Sympathectomized Extremity with Anaesthesia.' *Surgery* **29**, 803

Fencl, V., Vale, J. R. and Brock, J. R. (1968). 'Cerebral Blood Flow and Pulmonary Ventilation in Metabolic Acidosis and Alkalosis. *Scand. J. clin. Lab. Invest.* **22** (Suppl. 102), VIII B

Fermoso, J., Richardson, T. Q. and Guyton, A. C. (1964). 'Mechanism of Decrease in Cardiac Output Caused by Opening the Chest.' *Am. J. Physiol.* **207**, 1112

Ferrer, M. I., Bradley, S. E., Wheeler, H. O., Enson, Y., Preisig, R. and Harvey, R. M. (1965). 'The Effect of Digoxin on the Splanchnic Circulation in Ventricular Failure.' *Circulation* **32**, 524

Finnerty, F. A. Jr., Witkin, L. and Fazekas, J. F. (1954). 'Cerebral Hemo-dynamics during Cerebral Ischemia induced by Acute Hypotension.' *J. clin. Invest.* **33**, 1227

Fishman, A. P., Fritts, H. W. Jr. and Cournand, A. (1960). 'Effect of Acute Hypoxia and Exercise on the Pulmonary Circulation.' *Circulation* **22**, 204

Flacke, W. and Alper, M. H. (1962). 'Actions of Halothane and Norepinephrine in the Isolated Mammalian Heart.' *Anesthesiology* **23**, 793

Fleming, J. S. (1969). 'Evidence for a Mitral Valve Origin of the Left Ventricular Third Heart Sound. *Br. Heart J.* **31**, 192

Flickinger, H., Fraimow, W., Cathcart, R. T. and Nealon, T. F. (1961). 'The Effect of Thiopental Induction on Cardiac Output in Man.' *Anesth. Analg. curr. Res.* **40**, 693

Foëx, P. and Prys-Roberts, C. (1975). 'Effect of CO_2 on Myocardial Contractility and Aortic Input Impedance During Anaesthesia.' *Br. J. Anaesth.* **47**, 669

Folkow, B. (1960a). 'Range of Control of the Cardiovascular System by the Central Nervous System.' *Physiol. Rev.* **40**, Part II, 93

Folkow, B. (1960b). 'Role of the Nervous System in the Control of Vascular Tone.' *Circulation* **21**, 760

Folkow, B. (1971). 'The Haemodynamic Consequences of Adaptive Structural Changes of the Resistance Vessels in Hypertension.' *Clin. Sci.* **41**, 1

Folkow, B., Gelin, L. E., Lindell, S. E., Stenberg, K. and Thore, O. (1962). 'Cardiovascular Reactions during Abdominal Surgery.' *Ann. Surg.* **156**, 905

Folkow, B. and Halicka, H. D. (1968). 'A Comparison between 'Red' and 'White' Muscle with respect to Blood Supply, Capillary Surface Area and Oxygen Uptake during Rest and Exercise.' *Microvasc. Res.* **1**, 1

Folkow, B., Hallback, M., Lundgren, Y., Sivertsson, R. and Weiss, L. (1973). 'Importance of Adaptive Changes in Vascular Design for Establishment of Primary Hypertension, studied in Man and in Spontaneously Hypertensive Rats.' *Circulation Res.* **32** (Suppl. 1), 2

Folkow, B. and Neil, E. (1971). *Circulation.* Oxford University Press

Forrest, A. L., Laurson, J. I. M. and Otton, P. E. (1974). 'A Non-invasive Technique of Comparing Myocardial Performance following Epidural Blockade and Casopressor Therapy.' *Br. J. Anaesth.* **46**, 662

Forssmann, W. (1929). 'Die Sondierung des Rechten Hertzens.' *Klin. Wschr.* **8**, 2085

Foster, R. W. (1966). 'The Pharmacology of Pressor Drugs.' *Br. J. Anaesth.* **38**, 690

Fowler, N. O. (1969). 'The Normal Pulmonary Arterial Pressure-flow Relationship during Exercise.' *Am. J. Med.* **47**, 1

Fox, R. H. and Hilton, S. M. (1958). 'Bradykinin Formation in Human Skin as a Factor in Heat Vasodilation.' *J. Physiol.* **141**, 219

Frank, O. (1895). 'Zur Dynamik des Herzmuskels.' *Z. Biol.* **32**, 370

Freeman, J. (1966). 'Oxygen Measurements in Shock.' In Payne, J. P. and Hill, D. W., *Oxygen Measurements in Blood and Tissues*, p. 221. London; Churchill

Freeman, J. and Nunn, J. F. (1963). 'Ventilation-perfusion Relationships after Haemorrhage.' *Clin. Sci.* **24**, 135

Fritts, H. W. Jr., Odell, J. E., Harris, P., Braunwald, E. W. and Fishman, A. P. (1960). 'Effects of Acute Hypoxia on the Volume of Blood in the Thorax.' *Circulation* **22**, 216

Frohlich, E. D., Tarazi, R. C. and Dustan, H. P. (1969). 'Re-examination of the Hemodynamics of Hypertension.' *Am. J. med. Sci.* **257**, 9

Fry, D. L. (1962). 'Implications of Muscle Mechanics in the Heart. Discussion.' *Fedn Proc.* **21**, 991

Furnival, C. M., Linden, R. J. and Snow, H. M. (1967). 'An Assessment of the Sympathetic Nerves to the Heart.' *J. Physiol.* **191**, 60P

Galindo, A. (1965). 'Hepatic Circulation and Hepatic Function during Anaesthesia and Surgery. II. The Effects of Various Anaesthetic Agents.' *Can. Anaesth. Soc. J.* **12**, 337

Gall, F. (1965). 'Incompetence of the Atrioventricular Valves during Cardiac Massage.' *J. cardiovasc. Surg.* **6**, 356

Ganong, F. W. (1973). *Review of Medical Physiology.* 6th edn, p. 286. Los Altos; Lange

Gelin, L. E. and Ingelman, B. (1961). 'Rheomacrodex—a New Dextran Solution for Rheological Treatment of Impaired Capillary Flow.' *Acta. chir. scand.* **122**, 294

Gersh, B. J. (1970). 'Ventricular Function and Haemodynamics in the Dog during Anaesthesia.' Ph.D. Thesis; University of Oxford

Gersh, B. J., Prys-Roberts, C., Reuben, S. R. and Schultz, D. L. (1972). 'The Effects of Halothane on the Interactions between Myocardial Contractility, Aortic Impedance and Left Ventricular Performance. II. Aortic Input Impedance and the Distribution of Energy during Ventricular Ejection.' *Br. J. Anaesth.* **44**, 767

Giebisch, G. and Lozano, R. (1959). 'The Effects of Adrenal Steroids and Potassium Depletion on the Elaboration of the Osmotically Concentrated Urine.' *J. clin. Invest.* **38**, 843

Gilbertson, A. A. (1974). 'Pulmonary Artery Catheterization and Wedge Pressure Measurement in the General Intensive Therapy Unit.' *Br. J. Anaesth.* **46**, 97

Goldblatt, H., Lynch, J., Hanzal, R. F. and Summerville, W. W. (1934). 'Studies on Experimental Hypertension. I. The Production of Persistent Elevation of Systolic Blood Pressure by means of Renal Ischemia.' *J. exp. Med.* **59**, 347

Goodwin, G. M., McCloskey, D. I. and Mitchell, J. H. (1972). 'Cardiovascular and Respiratory Responses to Changes in Central Command during Isometric Exercise at Constant Muscle Tension.' *J. Physiol.* **226**, 173

Gould, K. L., Trenholme. S. and Kennedy, J. W. (1973). '*In vivo* Comparison of Catheter Manometer Systems with the Catheter-tip Micromanometer.' *J. appl. Physiol.* **34**, 263

Graf, K., Ström, G. and Wåhlin, Å. (1963). 'Circulatory Effects of Succinylcholine in Man.' *Acta anaesth. scand.* **7** (Suppl. 14), 1

Granata, L., Olsson, R. A., Huvos, A. and Gregg, D. E. (1965). 'Coronary Inflow and Oxygen Usage following Cardiac Sympathetic Nerve Stimulation in Unanesthetized Dogs.' *Circulation Res.* **16**, 114

Graves, C. L., Stauffer, W. M., Klein, R. L. and Underwood, P. S. (1968). 'Aortic Pulse Contour Calculation of Cardiac Output.' *Anesthesiology* **29**, 580

Green, H. D. and Kepchar, J. H. (1959). 'Control of Peripheral Resistance in Major Systemic Vascular Beds.' *Physiol. Rev.* **39**, 617

Greenbaum, R. (1969). 'The Blood and Transfusion Fluids in Shock.' In Freeman, J. (Ed.), *Physiological and Practical Aspects of Shock. International Anaesthesiology Clinics* **7**, 775

Greene, N. M. (1958). *Physiology of Spinal Anesthesia.* Baltimore; Williams and Wilkins

Greene, N. M. (1962). 'Physiology of Sympathetic Denervation.' *Ann. Rev. Med.* **13**, 87

Greenfield, A. D. M. (1960). 'Venous Occlusion Plethysmography.' *Meth. med. Res.* **8**, 293

Gregersen, M. I. and Chien, S. (1968). 'Blood Volume.' In Mountcastle, V. B., *Medical Physiology,* p. 244. St. Louis; C. V. Mosby

Gregg, D. E. (1963). 'Physiology of the Coronary Circulation.' *Circulation* **27**, 1128

Gregory, G. A., Eger, E. I. II, Smith, N. T., Cullen, B. F. and Cullen, D. J. (1971). 'The Cardiovascular Effects of Diethyl Ether in Man.' *Anesthesiology* **34**, 19

Grimby, G. (1965). 'Renal Clearances during Prolonged Supine Exercise at Different Loads.' *J. appl. Physiol.* **20**, 1294

Grindlay, J. H., Herrick, J. F. and Mann, F. C. (1941). 'Measurement of the Blood Flow of the Liver.' *Am. J. Physiol.* **132**, 489

Guyton, A. C. (1955). 'Determination of Cardiac Output by equating Venous Return Curves with Cardiac Response Curves.' *Physiol. Rev.* **35**, 123

Guyton, A. C. (1963). 'A Concept of Negative Interstitial Pressure Based on Pressure in Implanted Perforated Capsules.' *Circulation Res.* **12**, 399

Guyton, A. C. (1968). 'Regulation of Cardiac Output.' *Anesthesiology* **29**, 314

Guyton, A. C., Armstrong, G. G. Jr. and Chipley, P. L. (1956). 'Pressure-volume Curves of the Entire Arterial and Venous Systems in the Living Animal.' *Am. J. Physiol.* **184**, 253

Guyton, A. C., Jones, C. E. and Coleman, T. G. (1973). *'Cardiac Output and its Regulation.'* 2nd edn. Philadelphia; Saunders

Guyton, A. C., Polizo, D. and Armstrong, G. G. Jr. (1954). 'Mean Circulatory Filling Pressure Measured Immediately After Cessation of Heart Pumping.' *Am. J. Physiol.* **179**, 261

Guyton, A. C. and Sagawa, K. (1961). 'Compensations of Cardiac Output and Other Circulatory Functions in Areflex Dogs with Large A-V Fistulae.' *Am. J. Physiol.* **200**, 1157

Guz, A., Noble, M. I. M., Trenchard, D., Cochrane, H. L. and Makey, A. R. (1964). 'Studies on the Vagus Nerves in Man: Their Role in Respiratory and Circulatory Control.' *Clin. Sci.* **27**, 293

Hackel, D. B., Sancetta, S. M. and Kleinerman, J. (1956). 'Effect of Hypotension due to Spinal Anesthesia on Coronary Blood Flow and Myocardial Metabolism in Man.' *Circulation* **13**, 92

Häggendal, J., Hartley, L. H. and Saltin, B. (1970). 'Arterial Noradrenaline Concentration during Exercise in Relation to the Relative Work Levels.' *Scand. J. clin. Lab. Invest.* **26**, 337

Halldin, M. and Wåhlin, Å. (1959). 'Effect of Succinylcholine on the Intraspinal Fluid Pressure.' *Acta anaesth. scand.* **3**, 155

Hamilton, W. F., Woodbury, R. A. and Harper, H. T. (1936). 'Physiologic Relationships between Intrathoracic, Intraspinal and Arterial Pressures.' *J. Am. med. Ass.* **107**, 853

Hardaway, R. M. (1962). 'The Role of Intravascular Clotting in the Etiology of Shock.' *Ann. Surg.* **155**, 325

Harper, A. M. (1965). 'Discussion.' In Ledingham, I. McA., *Hyperbaric Oxygenation. Proceedings of the Second International Congress*, p. 179. Edinburgh; Livingstone

Harper, A. M., Jacobson, I. and McDowall, D. G. (1965). 'The Effect of Hyperbaric Oxygen on the Blood Flow Through the Cerebral Cortex.' In Ledingham, I. McA., *Hyperbaric Oxygenation. Proceedings of the Second International Congress*, p. 184. Edinburgh; Livingstone

Harris, P. and Heath, D. (1962). *The Human Pulmonary Circulation.* Edinburgh; Livingstone

Hartley, L. H., Grimby, G., Kilbom, A., Nilsson, W. J. ., Åstrand, I., Bjure, J., Ekblom, B. and Saltin, B. (1969). 'Physical Training in Sedentary Middle-aged and Older Men. III. Cardiac Output and Gas Exchange at Submaximal and Maximal Exercise.' *Scand. J. clin. Lab. Invest.* **24**, 335

Hauss, W. H., Kreuziner, H. and Asteroth, H. (1949). 'Über die Reizung der Pressorezeptoren im Sinus Caroticus beim Hung.' *Z. Kreislaufforsch.* **38**, 28

Henry, J. P. and Pearce, J. W. (1956). 'The Possible Role of Cardiac Stretch Receptors in the Induction of Changes in Urine Flow.' *J. Physiol.* **131**, 572

Henschel, A., Taylor, H. L. and Keys, A. (1954). 'Performance Capacity in Acute Starvation with Hard Work.' *J. appl. Physiol.* **6**, 624

Heymans, C. and Neil, E. (1958). *Reflexogenic Areas of the Cardiovascular System.* London; Churchill

Hill, D. W. (1972). *Physics Applied to Anaesthesia,* 2nd edn, p. 240. London; Butterworths

Hilton, S. M. and Lewis, G. P. (1955). 'The Cause of the Vasodilation Accompanying Activity in the Submandibular Salivary Gland.' *J. Physiol.* **128**, 235

Himmelstein, A., Harris, P., Fritts, H. W. Jr. and Cournand, A. (1958). 'Effect of Severe Unilateral Hypoxia on the Partition of Pulmonary Blood Flow in Man.' *J. thorac. Surg.* **36**, 369

Hinshaw, D. B., Peterson, M., Huse, W. M., Stafford, C. E. and Joergenson, E. J. (1961). 'Regional Blood Flow in Hemorrhagic Shock.' *Am. J. Surg.* **102**, 224

Hlastala, M. P., Wranne, B. and Lenfant, C. J. (1972). 'Single-breath Method of Measuring Cardiac Output—a Re-evaluation.' *J. appl. Physiol.* **33**, 846

Hødt-Rasmussen, K. (1965). 'Regional Cerebral Blood Flow in Man. The Intra-arterial Injection Method: Procedure and Normal Values.' In Ledingham, I. McA., *Hyperbaric Oxygenation. Proceedings of the Second International Congress,* p. 166. Edinburgh; Livingstone

Hoffman, B. F. and Cranefield, P. F. (1960). *Electrophysiology of the Heart.* New York; McGraw-Hill

Hoffman, B. F. and Cranefield, P. F. (1964). 'The Physiological Basis of Cardiac Arrhythmias.' *Am. J. Med.* **37**, 670

Hoffman, B. F., Moore, E. N., Stuckey, J. H. and Cranefield, P. F. (1963). 'Functional Properties of the Atrioventricular Conduction System.' *Circ. Res.* **13**, 308

Hollander, W., Reilly, P. and Birrows, B. A. (1956). 'Lymphatic Flow in Human Subjects as Indicated by the Disappearance of I^{131}-labelled Albumin from the Subcutaneous Tissues.' *J. clin. Invest.* **35**, 713

Hospital Technical Memorandum No. 8 (1969, revised). *Safety Code for Electro-medical Apparatus.* London; H.M.S.O.

Howitt, G. (1966). 'Therapy with Adrenergic Drugs and Their Antagonists.' *Br. J. Anaesth.* **38**, 719

Hughes, V. G. and Prys-Roberts, C. (1971). 'Intra-arterial Pressure Measurements—a Review and Analysis of Methods Relevant to Anaesthesia and Intensive Care.' *Anaesthesia* **26**, 511

Humphreys, P. W. and Lind, A. R. (1963). 'Blood Flow through Active and Inactive Muscles of the Forearm during Sustained Handgrip Contractions.' *J. Physiol.* **166**, 120

Huxley, H. E. and Hanson, J. (1954). 'Changes in the Cross-striations of Muscle during Contraction and Stretch and Their Structural Interpretation.' *Nature* **173**, 973

Insull, W. Jr., Tillotson, I. G. and Hayman, J. Jr. (1950). 'Distribution of Blood in the Rabbit's Kidney.' *Am. J. Physiol.* **163**, 676

Ivanov, S. D., Waddy, F. F. and Jennings, A. M. C. (1967). 'A Study of Carbon Dioxide Tensions during Halothane Anaesthesia using the Magill Circuit.' *Br. J. Anaesth.* **39**, 876

Janoff, A. (1964). 'Alterations in Lysosomes (Intra-cellular Enzymes) during Shock; Effects of Preconditioning (Tolerance) and Protective Drugs.' *Int. Anesth. Clin. (Boston)* **2**, 251

Johansson, B. (1962). 'Circulatory Responses to Stimulation of Somatic Afferents with Special Reference to Depressor Effects from Muscle Nerves.' *Acta physiol. scand.* **57** (Suppl. 198), 1

Johnson, P. C. (1964). 'Review of Previous Studies and Current Theories of Autoregulation.' *Circulation Res.* **14** (Suppl. 1), 2

Johnson, S. R. (1951). 'The Effect of Some Anaesthetic Agents on the Circulation in Man.' *Acta. chir. scand.* (Suppl. 158), 1

Johnstone, M. (1966). 'Propranolol in Anesthesia.' *Am. J. Cardiol.* **18**, 479

Jones, R. E., Guldmann, N., Linde, H. W., Dripps, R. D. and Price, H. L. (1960). 'Cyclopropane Anesthesia. III. Effects of Cyclopropane on Respiration and Circulation in Normal Man.' *Anesthesiology* **21**, 380

Jones, R. E., Linde, H. W., Deutsch, S., Dripps, R. D. and Price, H. L. (1962). 'Hemodynamic Actions of Diethyl Ether in Normal Man.' *Anesthesiology* **23**, 299

Kaijser, L. (1970). 'Limiting Factors for Aerobic Muscle Performance. The Influence of Varying Oxygen Pressure and Temperature.' *Acta Physiol. scand.* (Suppl. 346), 1

Kako, K. and Bing, R. J. (1958). 'Contractility of Actomyosin Bands Prepared from Normal and Failing Human Hearts.' *J. clin. Invest.* **37**, 465

Keatinge, W. R. (1972). 'Cold Immersion and Swimming.' *J. roy. Nav. med. Service* **58**, 171

Kelman, G. R. (1971). 'Interpretation of CVP Measurements.' *Anaesthesia* **26**, 209

Kelman, G. R. (1972). 'P_{CO_2} by Nitrogen Rebreathing—a Critical Theoretical Analysis.' *Resp. Physiol.* **16**, 327

Kelman, G. R. and Kennedy, B. R. (1971). 'Cardiovascular Effects of Pancuronium in Man.' *Br. J. Anaesth.* **43**, 335

Kelman, G. R. and Nunn, J. F. (1968). *Computer Produced Physiological Tables.* London; Butterworths

Kelman, G. R., Nunn, J. F., Prys-Roberts, C. and Greenbaum, R. (1967). 'The Influence of Cardiac Output on Arterial Oxygenation: a Theoretical Study.' *Br. J. Anaesth.* **39**, 450

Kelman, G. R. and Prys-Roberts, C. (1967). 'Variation of Alveolar-to-arterial Oxyge Tension Difference with Changes of $P_{a CO_2}$ in Anaesthetized Man.' *J. Physiol.* **194**, 13P

Kelman, G. R., Swapp, G. H., Smith, I., Benzie, R. J. and Gordon, N. L. M. (1972). 'Cardiac Output and Arterial Blood-gas Tensions during Laparoscopy.' *Br. J. Anaesth.* **44**, 1155

Kennedy, B. R. and Farman, J. V. (1968). 'Cardiovascular Effects of Gallamine Triethiodide in Man.' *Br. J. Anaesth.* **40**, 773

Kennedy, B. R. and Kelman, G. R. (1970). 'Cardiovascular Effects of Alcuronium in Man.' *Br. J. Anaesth.* **42**, 625

Kety, S. S. (1949). 'Measurement of Regional Circulation by the Local Clearance of Radioactive Sodium.' *Am. Heart J.* **38**, 321

Kety, S. S. and Schmidt, C. F. (1946). 'The Effects of Active and Passive Hyperventilation on Cerebral Blood Flow, Cerebral Oxygen Consumption,

Cardiac Output, and Blood Pressure of Normal Young Men.' *J. clin. Invest.* 25, 107

Kety, S. S. and Schmidt, C. F. (1948). 'The Nitrous Oxide Method for the Quantitative Determination of Cerebral Blood Flow in Man: Theory, Procedure and Normal Values.' *J. clin. Invest.* 27, 476

Kety, S. S., Shenkin, H. A. and Schmidt, C. F. (1948). 'The Effects of Increased Intracranial Pressure on Cerebral Circulatory Functions in Man.' *J. clin. Invest.* 27, 493

Keynes, R. D. and Maisel, G. W. (1954). 'The Energy Requirement for Sodium Extrusion from a Frog Muscle.' *Proc. R. Soc. B.* 142,383

Kim, T. S., Rahn, H. and Farhi, L. E. (1966). 'Estimation of True Venous and Arterial P_{CO_2} by Gas Analysis of a Single Breath.' *J. appl. Physiol.* 21, 1338

Kinsman, J. M., Moore, J. W. and Hamilton, W. F. (1929). 'Studies on the Circulation. Injection Method: Physical and Mathematical Considerations.' *Am. J. Physiol.* 89, 322

Klausen, K. (1965). 'Comparison of CO_2 Rebreathing and Acetylene Methods for Cardiac Output.' *J. appl. Physiol.* 20, 763

Kleinerman, J., Sancetta, S. M. and Hackel, D. B. (1958). 'Effects of High Spinal Anesthesia on Cerebral Circulation and Metabolism in Man.' *J. clin. Invest.* 37, 285

Klide, A. M. (1966). 'Mechanism for the Reduction in Airway Resistance Induced by Halothane.' *Fedn Proc.* 25, 229

Koehler, A. E. (1925). 'The Acidosis of Operative Anesthesia.' *J. biol. Chem.* 62, 435

Kramer, K. (1962). 'Renal Failure in Shock.' In *Shock: Ciba International Symposium*, p. 134. Heidelberg; Springer-Verlag

Kramer, K., Thurau, K. and Deetjen, P. (1960). 'Hämodynamik des Nierenmarks: Capillare Passagezeit, Blutvolumen, Durchblutung, Gewebshämatokrit and O_2-Verbauch des Nierenmarks *in situ.*' *Pflügers Arch. ges. Physiol.* 270, 251

Krasnow, N., Levine, H. J., Wagman, R. J. and Gorlin, R. (1963). 'Coronary Blood Flow Measured by I^{131} Iodo-antipyrine.' *Circulation Res.* 12, 58

Krogh, A. (1919). 'The Number and Distribution of Capillaries in Muscles with Calculations of the Oxygen Pressure Head Necessary for Supplying the Tissues.' *J. Physiol.* 52, 409

Kubota, Y., Schweiger, H. J. and Vandam, L. D. (1962). 'Hemodynamic Effects of Diethyl Ether in Man.' *Anesthesiology* 23, 306

Kukovetz, W. R., Hess, M. E., Shanfeld, J. and Haugaard, N. (1959). 'The Action of Sympathomimetic Amines on Isometric Contraction and Phosphorylase Activity of the Isolated Rat Heart.' *J. Pharmac. exp. Ther.* 127, 122

Ladefoged, J., Pedersen, F., Doutheil, U., Deetjen, P. and Selkurt, E. E. (1965). 'Renal Blood Flow Measured with Xenon[133] Wash-out Technique and with an Electromagnetic Flowmeter.' *Pflügers Arch. ges. Physiol.* 284, 195

Lamb, L. E. (1965). *Electrocardiography and Vectorcardiography.* Philadelphia; Saunders

Lambertsen, C. J., Kough, R. H., Cooper, D. Y., Emmel, A. L., Loeschicke, H. H. and Schmidt, C. F. (1953). 'Oxygen Toxicity, Effects in Man of Oxygen

Inhalation at 1 and 3.5 Atmospheres upon Blood Gas Transport, Circulation and Cerebral Metabolism.' *J. appl. Physiol.* **5**, 471

Landgren, S. (1952). 'On the Excitation Mechanism of the Carotid Baro-receptors.' *Acta physiol. scand.* **26**, 1

Landgren, S. and Neil, E. (1951). 'The Contribution of Carotid Chemoreceptor Mechanisms to the Rise of Blood Pressure Caused by Carotid Occlusion.' *Acta physiol. scand.* **23**, 152

Laragh, J. H., Angers, M., Kelly, W. G. and Lieberman, S. (1960). 'Hypotensive Agents and Pressor Substances.' *J. Am. med. Ass.* **174**, 234

Laragh, J. H., Baer, L., Brunner, H. R., Bühler, F. R., Sealey, J. E. and Darracott Vaughan, E. (1972). 'Renin, Angiotensin and Aldosterone System in Pathogenesis and Management of Hypertensive Vascular Disease.' *Am. J. Med.* **52**, 633

Lassen, N. A. (1959). 'Cerebral Blood Flow and Oxygen Consumption in Man.' *Physiol. Rev.* **39**, 183

Lassen, N. A. and Munck, O. (1955). 'The Cerebral Blood Flow in Man Determined by the Use of Radioactive Krypton.' *Acta physiol. scand.* **33**, 30

Leatham, A. (1958a). 'Systolic Murmurs.' *Circulation* **17**, 601

Leatham, A. (1958b). 'Auscultation of the Heart.' *Lancet* **ii**, 703

Ledingham, J. M. (1971). 'The Etiology of Hypertension.' *Practitioner* **207**, 5

Ledsome, J. R. and Linden, R. J. (1964). 'A Reflex Increase in Heart Rate from Distension of the Pulmonary-vein-atrial Junctions.' *J. Physiol.* **170**, 456

Lee, G. de J. and Dubois, A. B. (1955). 'Pulmonary Capillary Blood Flow in Man.' *J. clin. Invest.* **34**, 1380

Leins, T. (1927). *The Blood Vessels of the Human Skin and their Responses.* London; Shaw

Leonard, E. J. (1966). 'Excitation-contraction Coupling and Control of Cardiac Contractility.' *Circulation* **33**, 673

Lever, A. F. (1965). 'The Vasa Recta and Countercurrent Multiplication. *Acta med. scand.* **178** (Suppl. 434), 1

Levine, H. J. (1972). 'Compliance of the Left Ventricle.' *Circulation* **46**, 423

Lewis, D. H. and Mellander, S. (1962). 'Competitive Effects of Sympathetic Control and Tissue Metabolites on Resistance and Capacitance Vessels and Capillary Filtration in Skeletal Muscle.' *Acta physiol. scand.* **56**, 162

Lewis, T. and Rothschild, M. A. (1915). 'The Excitatory Process in the Dog's Heart. (Part II) (The Ventricles).' *Phil. Trans. R.Soc. B.* **206**, 181

Li, T. H. and Etsten, B. (1957). 'Effect of Cyclopropane Anesthesia on Cardiac Output and Related Hemodynamics in Man.' *Anesthesiology* **18**, 15

Light, L. H. (1969). 'Transcutaneous Observation of Blood Velocity in the Ascending Aorta in Man.' *J. Physiol.* **204**, 1P

Lillehei, R. C., Longerbeam, J. K., Bloch, J. H. and Manax, W. G. (1964a). 'The Nature of Experimental Irreversible Shock with its Implications.' *Int. Anesth. Clin.* **2**, 299

Lillehei, R. C., Longerbeam, J. K., Bloch, J. H. and Manax, W. G. (1964b). 'The Nature of Irreversible Shock: Experimental and Clinical Observations.' *Ann. Surg.* **160**, 682

Lillehei, R. C., Longerbeam, J. K. and Rosenberg, J. C. (1962). 'The Nature of Irreversible Shock: its Relationship to Intestinal Change.' In *Shock: Ciba International Symposium,* p. 106. Heidelberg; Springer-Verlag

Lind, A. R. and McNicol, G. W. (1967). 'Circulatory Responses to Sustained

Handgrip Contractions Performed during other Exercise, both Rhythmic and Static.' *J. Physiol.* **192**, 595

Linden, R. J. (1965). 'The Regulation of the Output of the Mammalian Heart.' In *The Scientific Basis of Medicine. Annual Reviews,* p. 164. London; Athens Press

Linden, R. J., Ledsome, J. R. and Norman, J. (1965). 'Simple Methods for the Determination of the Concentrations of Carbon Dioxide and Oxygen in Blood.' *Br. J. Anaesth.* **37**, 77

Linder, E. (1966). 'Measurements of Normal and Collateral Coronary Blood Flow by Close-arterial and Intramyocardial Injection of [85]Krypton and [133]Xenon.' *Acta Physiol. scand.* **68** (Suppl. 272), 1

Linzbach, A. J. (1960). 'Heart Failure from the Point of View of Quantitative Anatomy.' *Am. J. Cardiol.* **5**, 370

Lloyd, T. C. (1967). 'Influence of Po_2 and pH on Resting and Active Tensions of Pulmonary Arterial Strips.' *J. appl. Physiol.* **22**, 1101

Lorimer, A. R., Boyd, G., McCall, D., Mills, R. J. and Moran, F. (1968). 'Clinical Applications of Praecordial Counting.' In Bain, W. H. and Harper, A. M., *Blood Flow through Organs and Tissues,* p. 79. Edinburgh; Livingstone

Löwenstein, J. (1972). 'Renin Assay in Hypertensive Disease.' *Ann. Rev. Med.* **23**, 333

Luchsinger, P. C., Seipp, H. W. Jr. and Patel, D. J. (1962). 'Relationship of Pulmonary Artery-wedge Pressure to Left Atrial Pressure in Man.' *Circulation Res.* **11**, 215

Luetscher, J. A. and Johnson, B. B. (1954). 'Observations on the Sodium-retaining Corticoid (Aldosterone) in the Urine of Children and Adults in Relation to Sodium Balance and Edema.' *J. clin. Invest.* **33**, 1441

Lurie, A. A., Jones, R. E., Linde, H. W., Price, M. L., Dripps, R. D. and Price, H. L. (1958). 'Cyclopropane Anaesthesia. I. Cardiac Rate and Rhythm during Steady Levels of Cyclopropane Anaesthesia at Normal and Elevated End-expiratory Carbon Dioxide Tensions.' *Anesthesiology* **19**, 457

McBride, T. I. and Ledingham, I. McA. (1968). 'Clearance of Xenon[133] from the Myocardium as a Measure of Myocardial Blood Flow with Special Reference to the Influence on Flow of Increase of Oxygen Tension.' In Bain, W. H. and Harper, A. M., *Blood Flow through Organs and Tissues,* p. 100. Edinburgh; Livingstone

McCloskey, D. I. and Streatfield, K. A. (1975). 'Muscular Reflex Stimuli to the Cardiovascular System during Isometric Contractions of Muscle Groups of Different Mass.' *J. Physiol.* **250**, 431

MacDonald, A. G. (1969). 'The Effect of Halothane on Renal Cortical Blood Flow in Normotensive and Hypotensive Dogs.' *Br. J. Anaesth.* **41**, 644

McDonald, D. A. (1952). 'The Occurrence of Turbulent Flow in the Rabbit Aorta.' *J. Physiol.* **118**, 340

McDonald, D. A. (1960). *Blood Flow in Arteries,* 1st edn, p. 52. London; Edward Arnold

McDonald, D. A. and Taylor, M. G. (1959). 'The Hydrodynamics of the Arterial Circulation.' *Prog. Biophys. biophys. Chem.* **9**, 107

McDowall, D. G. (1966). 'Interrelationships between Blood Oxygen Tensions and Cerebral Blood Flow.' In Payne, J. P. and Hill, D. W. *Oxygen Measurements in Blood and Tissues*, p. 205. London; Churchill

McDowall, D. G. (1967). 'The Effects of Clinical Concentrations of Halothane on the Blood Flow and Oxygen Uptake of the Cerebral Cortex.' *Br. J. Anaesth.* **39**, 186

McDowall, D. G., Barker, J. and Jennett, W. B. (1966). 'Cerebro-spinal Fluid Pressure Measurements during Anaesthesia.' *Anaesthesia* **21**, 189

McGinn, F. P., Mendel, D. and Perry, P. M. (1967). 'The Effects of Alterations of CO_2 and pH on Intestinal Blood Flow in the Cat.' *J. Physiol.* **192**, 669

MacKenzie, G. J., Taylor, S. H., McDonald, A. H. and Donald, K. W. (1964). 'Haemodynamic Effects of External Cardiac Compression.' *Lancet* **i**, 1342

MacMillan, A. L. and Stott, F. D. (1968). 'Continuous Intra-arterial Blood Pressure Measurement.' *Biomed. Eng.* **3**, 20

Mahaffey, J. E., Aldinger, E. E., Sprouse, J. H., Darby, T. D. and Thrower, W. B. (1961). 'The Cardiovascular Effects of Halothane.' *Anesthesiology* **22**, 982

Mapleson, W. W. (1973). 'Circulation-time Models of the Uptake of Inhaled Anaesthetics and Data for Quantifying them.' *Br. J. Anaesth.* **45**, 319

Marsden, J. D. (1970). 'Why do Cells Pump Ions?' *New Scientist* **45**, 152

Marx, H. J., Rowell, L. B., Conn, R. D., Bruce, R. A. and Kusumi, F. (1967). 'Maintenance of Aortic Pressure and Total Peripheral Resistance during Exercise in Heat.' *J. Physiol.* **22**, 519

Mason, D. T. (1966). 'Failure and Blood Flow in the Forearm.' *Ann. int. Med.* **64**, 920

Mason, D. T. (1969). 'Usefulness and Limitations of the Rate of Rise of intraventricular Pressure (dp/dt) in the Evaluation of Myocardial Contractility in Man.' *Am. J. Cardiol.* **23**, 516

Master, A. M., Dach, S., Gresham, A., Field, L. E. and Horn, H. (1947). 'Acute Coronary Insufficiency—an Entity: Shock, Haemorrhage, and Pulmonary Embolism as Factors in its Production.' *J. Mt Sinai Hosp., N.Y.* **14**, 8

Mellander, S. (1960). 'Comparative Studies on the Adrenergic Neuro-hormonal Control of Resistance and Capacitance Blood Vessels in the Cat.' *Acta physiol. scand.* **50** (Suppl. 176), 1

Mellander, S., Johansson, B., Gray, S., Jonsson, O., Lundvall, J. and Ljung, B. (1967). 'The Effects of Hyperosmolarity on Intact and Isolated Vascular Smooth Muscle. Possible Role in Hyperaemia.' *Angiologica* **4**, 310

Mendelsohn, D. Jr. and Monheit, R. (1956). 'Electrocardiographic and Blood-pressure Changes during and after Biliary-tract Surgery.' *New Engl. J. Med.* **254**, 307

Merrill, J. P., Giorando, C. and Heetderks, D. R. (1961). 'The Role of the Kidney in Human Hypertension.' *Amer. J. Med.* **31**, 931

Merriman, J. E., Wyant, G. M., Bray, G. and McGeachy, W. (1958). 'Serial Cardiac Output Determinations in Man.' *Can. Anaesth. Soc. J.* **5**, 375

Miles, B. E. and de Wardener, H. E. (1952). 'Renal Vasoconstriction Produced by Ether and Cyclopropane Anaesthesia.' *J. Physiol.* **118**, 140

Millar, R. A. (1966). 'Post-ganglionic Sympathetic Discharge.' *Br. J. Anaesth.* **38**, 92

Millar, R. A. and Biscoe, T. J. (1965). 'Pre-ganglionic Sympathetic Activity and the Effects of Anaesthetics.' *Br. J. Anaesth.* **37**, 804

Millar, R. A., Warden, J. C., Cooperman, L. H. and Price, H. L. (1969). 'Central

Sympathetic Discharge and Mean Arterial Pressure during Halothane Anaesthesia.' *Br. J. Anaesth.* **41**, 918

Miller, G. A. H., Kirklin, J. W. and Swan, H. J. C. (1965). 'Myocardial Function and Left Ventricular Volumes in Acquired Valvular Insufficiency.' *Circulation* **31**, 374

Mills, C. J. (1968). 'A Catheter Tip Electromagnetic Velocity Probe for Use in Man.' In Bain, W. H. and Harper, A. M., *Blood Flow through Organs and Tissues*, p. 38. Edinburgh; Livingstone

Milnor, W. R. (1974). 'Regional Circulations.' In Mountcastle, V. B. *Medical Physiology*, 2nd edn, p. 1000. St Louis; C. V. Mosby

Moffitt, E. A. and Sessler, A. D. (1964). 'The Circulation in Anaesthesia.' *Can. Anaesth. Soc. J.* **11**, 173

Moran, N. C. (1966). 'Adrenergic Receptors, Drugs, and the Cardiovascular System. II. *Mod. Concepts cardiovasc. Dis.* **35**, 99

Moster, W. G., Reier, C. E., Gardier, R. W. and Hamelberg, W. (1969). 'Cardiac Output and Post-ganglionic Sympathetic Activity during Acute Respiratory Alkalosis.' *Anesthesiology* **31**, 28

Mottram, R. F. (1955). 'The Oxygen Consumption of Human Skeletal Muscle *in vivo.'* *J. Physiol.* **128**, 268

Mueller, R. P., Lynn, R. B. and Sancetta, S. M. (1952). 'Studies of Hemodynamic Changes in Humans Following Induction of Low and High Spinal Anesthesia II.' *Circulation* **6**, 894

Murray, G., Roschlan, W. and Lougheed, W. (1956). 'Homologous Aortic-valve-segment Transplants as Surgical Treatment for Aortic and Mitral Insufficiency.' *Angiology* **7**, 466

Munson, E. S., Eger, E. I. and Bowers, D. L. (1968). 'The Effects of Changes in Cardiac Output and Distribution on the Rate of Cerebral Anesthetic Equilibration Calculations Using a Mathematical Model.' *Anesthesiology* **29**, 533

Naylor, W. G. (1963). 'The Significance of Calcium Ions in Cardiac Excitation and Contraction.' *Am. Heart J.* **65**, 404

Neff, W., Stiles, J. A. and Michelson, R. (1938). 'Blood Supply Changes during Cyclopropane Anaesthesia.' *Br. J. Anaesth.* **16**, 83

Ngai, S. H., Diaz, P. M. and Ozer, S. (1969). 'The Uptake and Release of Noradrenaline.' *Anesthesiology* **31**, 45

Nickerson, M. (1962). 'Drug Therapy in Shock.' In Bock, K. D., *Shock, Pathogenesis and Therapy*, p. 356. New York; Academic Press

Niedergerke, R. (1956). 'The Potassium Chloride Contracture of the Heart and its Modification by Calcium.' *J. Physiol.* **134**, 584

Norman, J. N., Irvin, T. T. and Smith, G. (1968). 'The Effect of Inspired Oxygen Tension on Renal Blood Flow.' In Bain, W. H. and Harper, A. M., *Blood Flow through Organs and Tissues*, p. 449. Edinburgh; Livingstone

Nunn, J. F. (1969). *Applied Respiratory Physiology, with Special Reference to Anaesthesia.* London; Butterworths

Nunn, J. F. and Pouliot, J. D. (1962). 'The Measurement of Gaseous Exchange during Nitrous Oxide Anaesthesia.' *Br. J. Anaesth.* **34**, 752

Olson, R. E. (1964). 'Abnormalities of Myocardial Metabolism.' *Circulation Res.* **15** (Suppl. 2), 109

Olson, R. E. and Piatnek, D. A. (1959). 'Conservation of Energy in Cardiac Muscle.' *Ann. N.Y. Acad. Sci.* **72**, 466

Opie, L. H. (1965). 'Cardiac Metabolism. The Effect of Some Physiologic, Pharmacologic, and Pathologic Influences.' *Am. Heart J.* **69**, 401

Oriol, A., Sekelj, P. and McGregor, M. (1967). 'Limitations of Indicator-dilution Methods in Experimental Shock.' *J. appl. Physiol.* **23**, 605

Ott, H. von (1956). 'Die Errechnung des Kolloidosmotischen Serumdruckes aus dem Eiweiss-spektrum und das Mittlere Molekulargewicht der Serumeiweiss-fraktionen.' *Klin. Wschr.* **34**, 1079

Paes de Carvalho, A., de Mello, W. C. and Hoffman, B. F. (1959). 'Electrophysiological Evidence for Specialized Fiber Types in Rabbit Atrium.' *Am. J. Physiol.* **196**, 483

Palmerio, C., Zetterstrom, B., Shammash, J., Euchbaum, E., Frank, E. and Fine, J. (1963). 'Denervation of the Abdominal Viscera for the Treatment of Traumatic Shock.' *New Engl. J. Med.* **269**, 709

Pappenheimer, J. R. (1953). 'Passage of Molecules through Capillary Walls.' *Physiol. Rev.* **33**, 387

Papper, S. and Papper, E. M. (1964). 'The Effects of Preanesthetic Medication, Anesthetic and Post-operative Drugs on Renal Function.' *Clin. Pharmac. Ther.* **5**, 205

Parmley, W. W. and Sonnenblick, E. H. (1967). 'Series Elasticity in Heart Muscle. Its Relation to Contractile Element Velocity and Proposed Muscle Models.' *Circulation Res.* **20**, 112

Paterson, J. L. (1965). 'Circulation through the Brain.' In Ruch, T. C. and Patton, H. D., *Physiology and Biophysics*, p. 950. Philadelphia; Saunders

Paton, W. D. M. (1959). 'The Effects of Muscle Relaxants other than Muscular Relaxation.' *Anesthesiology* **20**, 453

Patterson, S. W., Piper, H. and Starling, E. H. (1914). 'The Regulation of the Heart Beat.' *J. Physiol.* **48**, 465

Payne, J. P., Gardiner, D. and Verner, I. R. (1959). 'Cardiac Output during Halothane Anaesthesia.' *Br. J. Anaesth.* **31**, 87

Peiss, C. N. (1964). 'Supramedullary Cardiovascular Regulation.' In Price, H. L. and Cohen, P. J., *Effects of Anesthetics on the Circulation*, p. 32. Springfield; Charles C. Thomas

Pelligrini, G. (1957). 'Einfluss der Barbiturnarkose auf die Koronardurchblutung.' *Verh. dt. Ges. Kreisl. Forsch.* **23**, 111

Pickering, G. W. (1968). *High Blood Pressure*, 2nd edn. London; Churchill

Pickering, G. W. (1974). *Hypertension: Causes, Consequences, and Management*, 2nd edn Edinburgh and London; Churchill Livingstone

Pierce, E. C. Jr., Lambertson, C. J., Deutsch, S., Chase, P. E., Linde, H. W., Dripps, R. D. and Price, H. L. (1962). 'Cerebral Circulation and Metabolism during Thiopental Anesthesia and Hyperventilation in Man.' *J. clin. Invest.* **41**, 1664

Pitts, R. F., Larrabee, M. G. and Bronk, D. W. (1941). 'An Analysis of Hypothalamic Cardiovascular Control.' *Am. J. Physiol.* **134**, 359

Pool, P. E., Covell, J. W., Levitt, M., Gibb, J. and Braunwald, E. (1967). 'Reduction of Cardiac Tyrosine Hydroxylase Activity in Experimental Congestive Heart Failure: its Role in the Depletion of Cardiac Norepinephrine Stores.' *Circulation Res.* **20**, 349

Price, H. L. (1957). 'Circulating Adrenaline and Noradrenaline during Diethyl Ether Anaesthesia in Man.' *Clin. Sci.* **16**, 377

Price, H. L. (1961). 'Circulatory Actions of General Anesthetic Agents and the Homeostatic Roles of Epinephrine and Norepinephrine in Man.' *Clin. Pharmac. Ther.* **2**, 163

Price, H. L. (1967). *Circulation during Anaesthesia and Operation.* Springfield; Charles C. Thomas

Price, H. L., Cooperman, L. H., Warden, J. C., Morris, J. J. and Smith, T. C. (1969). 'Pulmonary Hemodynamics during General Anesthesia in Man.' *Anesthesiology* **30**, 629

Price, H. L., Deutsch, S., Cooperman, L. H., Clement, A. J. and Epstein, R. M. (1965). 'Splanchnic Circulation during Cyclopropane Anesthesia in Normal Man.' *Anesthesiology* **26**, 312

Price, H. L., Deutsch, S., Davidson, I. A., Clement, A. J., Behar, M. G. and Epstein, R. M. (1966). 'Can General Anesthetics produce Splanchnic Visceral Hypoxia by Reducing Regional Blood Flow?' *Anesthesiology* **27**, 24

Price, H. L. and Helrich, M. (1955). 'The Effect of Cyclopropane, Diethyl Ether, Nitrous Oxide, Thiopental, and Hydrogen Ion Concentration on the Myocardial Function of the Dog Heart-lung Preparation.' *J. Pharmac. exp. Ther.* **115**, 206

Price, H. L., Helrich, M. and Conner, E. H. (1956). 'A Relation between Hemodynamic and Plasma Volume Alterations during General Anesthesia in Man.' *J. clin. Invest.* **35**, 125

Price, H. L., Jones, R. E., Deutsch, S. and Linde, H. W. (1962). 'Ventricular Function and Autonomic Nervous Activity during Cyclopropane Anesthesia in Man.' *J. clin. Invest.* **41**, 604

Price, H. L., Linde, H. W., Jones, R. E., Black, G. W. and Price, M. L. (1959). 'Sympatho-adrenal Responses to General Anesthesia in Man and their Relation to Hemodynamics.' *Anesthesiology* **20**, 563

Price, H. L., Jones, R. E. and Morse, H. T. (1963). 'Central Nervous Actions of Halothane Affecting the Systemic Circulation.' *Anesthesiology* **24**, 770

Price, H. L., Lurie, A. A., Black, G. W., Sechzer, P. H., Linde, H. W. and Price, M. L. (1960). 'Modification by General Anesthetics (Cyclopropane and Halothane) of Circulatory and Sympatho-adrenal Response to Respiratory Acidosis.' *Ann. Surg.* **152**, 1071

Price, H. L., Lurie, A. A., Jones, R. E., Price, M. L. and Linde, H. W. (1958). 'Cyclopropane Anesthesia. II. Epinephrine and Norepinephrine in Initiation of Ventricular Arrhythmias by Carbon Dioxide Inhalation.' *Anesthesiology* **19**, 619

Price, H. L. and Widdicombe, J. (1962). 'Actions of Cyclopropane on Carotid Sinus Baroreceptors and Carotid Body Chemoreceptors.' *J. Pharmac. exp. Ther.* **135**, 233

Price, M. L. and Price, H. L. (1962). 'Effects of General Anesthetics on Contractile Responses of Rabbit Aortic Strips.' *Anesthesiology* **23**, 16

Prime, F. J. and Gray, T. C. (1952). 'The Effect of Certain Anaesthetic and Relaxant Agents on Circulating Dynamics.' *Br. J. Anaesth.* **24**, 101

Prys-Roberts, C., Foëx, P., Biro, G. P. and Roberts, J. G. (1973). 'Studies of Anaesthesia in Relation to Hypertension. V. Adrenergic Beta-receptor Blockade.' *Br. J. Anaesth.* **45**, 671

Prys-Roberts, C., Foëx, P., Greene, L. T. and Waterhouse, T. D. (1972a).

'Studies of Anaesthesia in Relation to Hypertension. IV. The Effect of Artificial Ventilation on the Circulation and Pulmonary Gas Exchanges.' *Br. J. Anaesth.* **44**, 335

Prys-Roberts, C., Gersh, B. J., Baker, A. B. and Reuben, S. R. (1972b). 'The Effects of Halothane on the Interactions between Myocardial Contractility, Aortic Impedance, and Left Ventricular Performance. I. Theoretical Considerations and Results.' *Br. J. Anaesth.* **44**, 634

Prys-Roberts, C., Green, L. T., Meloche, R. and Foëx, P. (1971b). 'Studies of Anaesthesia in Relation to Hypertension. II. Haemodynamic Consequences of Induction and Endotracheal Intubation.' *Br. J. Anaesth.* **43**, 531

Prys-Roberts, C., Kelman, G. R., Greenbaum, R., Kain, M. L. and Bay, J. (1968). 'Hemodynamics and Alveolar-arterial P_{O_2} Differences at Varying Pa_{CO_2} in Anesthetized Man.' *J. appl. Physiol.* **25**, 80

Prys-Roberts, C., Kelman, G. R., Greenbaum, R. and Robinson, R. H. (1967). 'Circulatory Influences of Artificial Ventilation during Nitrous Oxide Anaesthesia in Man. II. Results: The Relative Influence of Mean Intrathoracic Pressure and Arterial Carbon Dioxide Tension.' *Br. J. Anaesth.* **39**, 533

Prys-Roberts, C., Kelman, G. R., Kain, C., Greenbaum, R. and Bay, J. (1967). 'Cardiac Output and Blood Carbon Dioxide Levels during Halothane Anesthesia in Man.' *Br. J. Anaesth.* **39**, 687

Prys-Roberts, C., Meloche, R. and Foëx, P. (1971a). 'Studies of Anaesthesia in Relation to Hypertension. I. Cardiovascular Responses of Treated and Untreated Patients.' *Br. J. Anaesth.* **43**, 122

Pugh, L. G. C. and Wyndham, C. L. (1950). 'The Circulatory Effects of High Spinal Anaesthesia in Hypertensive and Control Subjects.' *Clin. Sci.* **9**, 189

Raventós, J. (1961). 'The Action of Fluothane on the Autonomic Nervous System.' *Helv. chim. acta* **28**, 358

Ravin, M. B., Epstein, R. M. and Malm, J. R. (1965). 'Contribution of Thebesian Veins to the Physiologic Shunt in Anesthetized Man.' *J. appl. Physiol.* **20**, 1148

Regan, T. J., La Force, F. M., Teres, D., Block, J. and Hellems, H. K. (1965). 'Contribution of Left Ventricle and Small Bowel in Irreversible Hemorrhagic Shock.' *Am. J. Physiol.* **208**, 938

Rence, W. G., Cullen, S. C. and Hamilton, W. K. (1956). 'Observations on the Heart Sounds during Anesthesia with Cyclopropane or Ether.' *Anesthesiology* **17**, 26

Richardson, T. Q., Stallings, J. O. and Guyton, A. C. (1961). 'Pressure-volume Curves in Live, Intact Dogs.' *Am. J. Physiol.* **201**, 471

Roach, M. R. and Burton, A. C. (1957). 'The Reason for the Shape of the Distensibility Curves of Arteries.' *Can. J. Biochem. Physiol.* **35**, 681

Robertson, J. D. (1960). 'The Molecular Structure and Contact Relationships of Cell Membranes.' *Prog. Biophys. biophys. Chem.* **10**, 343

Robertson, J. D., Swan, A. A. B. and Whitteridge, D. (1956). 'Effect of Anaesthetics on Systemic Baroreceptors.' *J. Physiol.* **131**, 463

Rockoff, S. D., Ross, J. Jr., Oldham, N. N. Jr., Mason, D. T., Morrow, A. G. and Braunwald, E. (1966). 'Ventriculo-atrial Regurgitation following Prosthetic Replacement of the Mitral Valve, Angiocardiographic and Hemodynamic Findings.' *Am. J. Cardiol.* **17**, 817

Rosen, S. M., Truniger, B. P., Kriek, H. R., Murray, J. E. and Merrill, J. P. (1967). 'Intrarenal Distribution of Blood Flow in the Transplanted Dog Kidney: Effect of Denervation and Rejection.' *J. clin. Invest.* **46**, 1239

Ross, J. Jr., Mosher, P. W. and Shaw, R. F. (1961). 'Autoregulation of Coronary Blood Flow.' *Circulation* **24**, 1025

Ross, R. S., Ueda, K., Lichtlen, P. R. and Rees, J. R. (1964). 'Measurement of Myocardial Blood Flow in Animals and Man by Selective Injection of Radioactive Inert Gas into the Coronary Arteries.' *Circulation Res.* **15**, 28

Roth, F. and Wüthrich, H. (1969). 'The Clinical Importance of Hyperkalaemia following Suxamethonium Administration.' *Br. J. Anaesth.* **41**, 311

Rowe, G. G. (1959). 'The Nitrous-oxide Method for Determining Coronary Blood Flow in Man.' *Am. Heart J.* **58**, 268

Rowell, L. B. (1969). 'Circulation.' *Med. and Sci. in Sports* **1**, 15

Rowell, L. B. (1974). 'Human Cardiovascular Adjustments to Exercise and Thermal Stress.' *Phys. Rev.* **54**, 75

Rowell, L. B., Blackmon, J. R. and Bruce, R. A. (1964). 'Indocyanine Green Clearance and Estimated Hepatic Blood Flow during Mild to Maximal Exercise in Upright Man.' *J. clin. Invest.* **43**, 1677

Rowell, L. B., Taylor, H. L. and Wang, Y. (1964). 'Limitations to Prediction of Maximal Oxygen Intake.' *J. appl. Physiol.* **19**, 919

Rowlands, D. J., Howitt, G., Logan, W. F. W. E., Clarke, A. D. and Jackson, P. W. (1967). 'Haemodynamic Changes during Methohexitone Anaesthesia in Patients with Supraventricular Arrhythmias.' *Br. J. Anaesth.* **39**, 554

Rushmer, R. F. (1959). 'Constancy of Stroke Volume in Ventricular Responses to Exertion.' *Am. J. Physiol.* **196**, 745

Rushmer, R. F. (1961). *Cardiovascular Dynamics*, 2nd edn. Philadelphia; Saunders

Rushmer, R. F., Smith, O. A. Jr. and Lasker, E. P. (1960). 'Neural Mechanisms of Cardiac Control during Exertion.' *Physiol. Rev.* **40** (Suppl. 4), 27

Saidman, L. J., Eger, E. I. II., Munson, E. S., Babad, A. A. and Muallem, M. (1967). 'Minimum Alveolar Concentrations of Methoxyflurane, Halothane, Ether and Cyclopropane in Man: Correlation with Theories of Anesthesia.' *Anesthesiology* **28**, 994

Saltin, B., Blomqvist, G., Mitchell, J. H., Johnson, R. L. Jr., Wildenthal, K. and Chapman, C. B. (1968). 'Response to Submaximal and Maximal Exercise after Bed Rest and after Training.' *Circulation* **38** (Suppl. 17), 1

Saltin, B. and Stenberg, J. (1964). 'Circulatory Response to Prolonged Severe Exercise.' *J. appl. Physiol.* **19**, 833

Samet, P., Fritts, H. W., Fishman, A. P. and Cournand, A. (1957). 'The Blood Volume in Heart Disease.' *Medicine* **36**, 211

Sancetta, S. M., Lyman, R. B., Simeone, F. A. and Scott, R. W. (1952). 'Studies of Hemodynamic Changes in Humans Following Induction of Low and High Spinal Anesthesia.' *Circulation* **6**, 559

Sankawa, H. (1965). 'Cardiovascular Effects of Propanidid and Methohexital Sodium in Dogs.' *Acta Anaesth. scand.* (Suppl. 17), 55

Sarnoff, S. J. (1955). 'Myocardial Contractility as Described by Ventricular Function Curves: Observations on Starling's Law of the Heart.' *Physiol. Rev.* **35**, 107

Sarnoff, S. J. and Mitchell, J. H. (1962). 'The Control of the Function of the Heart.' In *Handbook of Physiology: Circulation Vol. 1*, p. 489. Washington; American Physiological Society

Scheinberg, P. and Jayne, H. W. (1950). 'Factors Influencing Cerebral Blood Flow and Metabolism.' *Circulation* 5, 225

Scott, D. B., Slawson, K. B. and Taylor, S. H. (1969). 'The Circulatory Effects of the Valsalva Manoeuvre during Anaesthesia and Thoracotomy.' *Cardiovasc. Res.* 3, 331

Scott, D. B., Stephen, G. W. and Davie, I. T. (1972). 'Haemodynamic Effects of a Negative (Subatmospheric) Pressure Expiratory Phase during Artifical Ventilation.' *Br. J. Anaesth.* 44,171

Scott, J. C., Bazett, H. C. and Mackie, G. C. (1940). 'Climatic Effects on Cardiac Output and the Circulation in Man.' *Am. J. Physiol.* 129, 102

Selkurt, E. E. (1946). 'The Relation of Renal Blood Flow to Effective Arterial Pressure in the Intact Kidney of the Dog.' *Am. J. Physiol.* 147, 537

Selkurt, E. E. (1963). 'The Renal Circulation.' In *Handbook of Physiology: Circulation, Vol. II*, p. 1457. Washington; American Physiological Society

Severinghaus, J. W. and Cullen, S. C. (1958). 'Depression of Myocardium and Body Oxygen Consumption with Fluothane.' *Anesthesiology* 19, 165

Shackman, R., Graber, G. I. and Melrose, B. G. (1952). 'The Haemodynamics of the Surgical Patient under General Anaesthesia.' *Br. J. Surg.* 40, 13

Shaper, A. G., Leonard, P. J., Jones, K. W. and Jones, M. (1969). Environmental Effects on the Body Build, Blood Pressure and Blood Chemistry of Nomadic Warriors serving in the Army in Kenya.' *E. Afr. Med. J.* 46, 282

Shimosato, S. and Etsten, B. E. (1969). 'The Role of the Venous System in Cardiocirculatory Dynamics during Spinal and Epidural Anesthesia in Man.' *Anesthesiology* 30, 619

Shimosato, S., Li, T. H. and Etsten, B. E. (1963). 'Ventricular Function during Halothane Anesthesia in Closed Chest Dogs.' *Circulation Res.* 12, 63

Shirer, H. W. (1962). 'Blood Pressure Measuring Methods.' *I.R.E. Trans. med. Electron.* 9, 116

Singer, R. B. and Hastings, A. B. (1948). 'An Improved Clinical Method for the Estimation of Disturbances of the Acid-base Balance of Human Blood.' *Medicine* 27, 223

Sivertsson, R. and Olander, R. (1968). 'Aspects of the Nature of the Increased Vascular Resistance and Increased "Reactivity" to Noradrenaline in Hypertensive Subjects.' *Life Sci.* 7, 1291

Sleight, P., Gribbin, B. and Pickering, T. G. (1971). 'Baroreflex Sensitivity in Normal and Hypertensive Man: the Effect of Beta-adrenergic Blockade on Reflex Sensitivity. *Postgrad. med. J.* 47 (Suppl.), 79

Smith, A. L. (1973). 'The Mechanism of Cerebral Vasodilatation by Halothane.' *Anesthesiology* 39, 581

Smith, H. W. (1951). *The Kidney: Structure and Function in Health and Disease.* New York; Oxford University Press

Smith, N. T., Eger, E. I. II., Stoelting, R. K., Whayne, T. F., Cullen, D. and Kadis, L. B. (1970). 'The Cardiovascular and Sympathomimetic Responses to the Addition of Nitrous Oxide to Halothane in Man.' *Anesthesiology* 32, 410

Smith, N. T. and Whitcher, C. E. (1967). 'Hemodynamic Effects of Gallamine and Tubocurarine Administered during Halothane Anesthesia.' *J. Am. med. Ass.* 199, 114

Smith, S. L., Webb, W. R., Fabian, L. W. and Hagaman, V. D. (1962). 'Cardiac

Excitability in Ether, Cyclopropane and Halothane Anesthesia.' *Anesthesiology* **23**, 766

Smyth, H. S., Sleight, P. and Pickering, G. W. (1969). 'Reflex Regulation of Arterial Pressure during Sleep in Man: a Quantitative Method of Assessing Baroreflex Sensitivity.' *Circulation Res.* **24**, 109

Sonnenblick, E. H. (1962). 'Force-velocity Relations in Mammalian Heart Muscle.' *Am. J. Physiol.* **202**, 931

Sonnenblick, E. H., Parmley, W. W., Urschel, C. W. and Boutsaert, D. L. (1970). 'Ventricular Function: Evaluation of Myocardial Contractility in Health and Disease.' *Prog. in cardiovasc. Dis.* **12**, 449

Spence, A. A. and Ellis, F. R. (1970). 'A Critical Evaluation of a Nitrogen Rebreathing Method for the Estimation of $P\bar{v}o_2$.' *Respir. Physiol.* **10**, 313

Spencer, M. P. and Greiss, F. C. (1962). 'Dynamics of Ventricular Ejection. *Circulation Res.* **10**, 274

Starling, E. H. (1896). 'On the Absorption of Fluid from the Connective Tissue Spaces.' *J. Physiol.* **19**, 312

Starling, E. H. (1918). *The Linacre Lecture on the Law of the Heart. (Cambridge, 1915.)* London; Longmans Green and Co

Starling, E. H. (1920). 'On the Circulatory Changes Associated with Exercise.' *J. roy. Army med. Corps* **34**, 258

Starr, A. (1960). 'Total Mitral Valve Replacement: Fixation and Thrombosis.' *Surg. Forum* **11**, 258

Starr, I. (1967). 'The Place of the Ballistocardiogram in a Newtonian Cardiology, and the New Light it Sheds on Certain Old Clinical Problems.' *Proc. R. Soc. Med.* **60**, 1297

Stead, E. A., Warren, J. V. and Brannon, E. S. (1948). 'Cardiac Output in Congestive Heart Failure.' *Am. Heart J.* **35**, 529

Stevens, W. C., Cromwell, T. H., Halsey, M. J., Eger, E. I., Shakespeare, T. F. and Bahlman, S. H. (1971). The Cardiovascular Effects of a New Inhalational Anaesthetic, Forane, in Human Volunteers at Constant Arterial Carbon Dioxide Tension.' *Anesthesiology* **35**, 8

Stone, J. E., Wells, J., Draper, W. B. and Whitehead, R. W. (1958). 'Changes in Renal Blood Flow in Dogs during the Inhalation of 30 per cent Carbon Dioxide.' *Am. J. Physiol.* **194**, 115

Sutton, J. R., Cole, A., Gunning, J., Hickie, J. B. and Seldon, W. A. (1967). 'Control of Heart-rate in Healthy Young Men.' *Lancet* ii, 1398

Swan, H. J. C., Ganz, W., Forrester, J., Marsuc, H., Diamond, G. and Chonette, D. (1970). 'Catheterisation of the Heart in Man with Use of a Flow Directed Balloon-tipped Catheter.' *N. Engl. J. Med.* **283**, 447

Sykes, M. K. (1963). 'Venous Pressure as a Clinical Indication of Adequacy of Transfusion.' *Ann. R. Coll. Surg. Eng.* **33**, 185

Sykes, M. K. (1967). 'Resuscitation of the Apparently Dead.' In Hewer, C. D., *Recent Advances in Anaesthesia and Analgesia*, p. 278. London; Churchill

Sykes, M. K., Davies, D. M., Chahrabarti, M. K. and Loh, L. (1973). 'The Effects of Halothane, Trichlorethylene and Ether on Pulmonary Vascular Resistance in the Isolated Perfused Cat Lung.' *Br. J. Anaesth.* **45**, 655

Taylor, H. L., Buskirk, E. and Henschel, A. (1955). 'Maximal Oxygen Intake as an Objective Measure of Cardio-respiratory Performance.' *J. appl. Physiol.* **8**, 73

Tenney, S. M. (1960). 'The Effect of Carbon Dioxide on Neurohumoral and Endocrine Mechanisms.' *Anesthesiology* **21**, 674

Thompson, S. P. (1946). *Calculus Made Easy*. London; Macmillan

Thomson, W. J. (1967). 'The Effect of Induction of Anaesthesia on Peripheral Haemodynamics.' *Br. J. Anaesth.* **39**, 210

Tobian, L. (1960). 'Interrelationship of Electrolytes, Juxtaglomerular Cells and Hypertension.' *Physiol. Rev.* **40**, 280

Trautwein, W. and Kasselbaum, D. G. (1961). 'On the Mechanism of Spontaneous Impulse Generation in the Pacemaker of the Heart.' *J. gen. Physiol.* **45**, 317

Trueta, J., Barclay, A. E., Daniel, P. M., Franklin, K. J. and Pritchard, M. M. L. (1947). *Studies of the Renal Circulation*. Oxford; Blackwell

Udhoji, V. N. and Weil, M. H. (1965). 'Hemodynamics and Metabolic Studies on Shock Associated with Bacteremia: Observations on Sixteen Patients.' *Ann. int. Med.* **62**, 966

Uvnäs, B. (1960). 'Sympathetic Vasodilator System and Blood Flow.' *Physiol. Rev.* **40** (Suppl. 4), 69

Vance, J. P., McBride, T. I. and Ledingham, I. McA. (1967). 'Effects of Alteration of Arterial Carbon Dioxide Tension on Myocardial Blood Flow.' *Br. J. Anaesth.* **39**, 688

Veall, N. (1968). 'Diagnostic Uses of Radioisotopes. 8. Blood Flow.' *Hosp. Med.* **2**, 460

Veragut, V. P. and Krayenbühl, H. P. (1965). 'Estimation and Quantification of Myocardial Contractility in the Closed-chest Dog.' *Cardiologia* **57**, 96

Vick, R. L. (1966). 'Effects of Altered Heart Rate on Chloroform-epinephrine Cardiac Arrhythmia.' *Circulation Res.* **18**, 316

Vickers, M. D. (1966). 'Adrenergic Drugs and Their Antagonists in Anaesthesia.' *Br. J. Anaesth.* **38**, 728

Viles, P. H. and Shepherd, J. T. (1968). 'Evidence for a Dilator Action of Carbon Dioxide on the Pulmonary Vessels of the Cat.' *Circulation Res.* **22**, 325

Wade, O. L. and Bishop, J. M. (1962). *Cardiac Output and Regional Blood Flow*. Oxford; Blackwell

Waldhausen, J. A., Kilman, J. W., Abel, F. L. (1965). 'Effects of Catecholamines on the Heart.' *Archs Surg.* **91**, 86

Wall, P. D. and Davis, G. D. (1951). 'Three Cerebral Cortical Systems Affecting Autonomic Function.' *J. Neurophysiol.* **14**, 507

Wallace, A. G. and Daggett, W. M. (1964). 'Re-excitation of the Atrium, "the Echo Phenomenon".' *Am. Heart J.* **68**, 681

Wang, S. C. (1964). 'Bulbar Regulatory Mechanisms.' In Price, H. L. and Cohen, P. J., *Effects of Anesthetics on the Circulation*, p. 16. Springfield; Charles C. Thomas

Warner, H. R., Swan, J. H. C., Connolly, D. C., Tompkins, R. G. and Wood, E. H. (1953). 'Quantitation of Beat-to-beat Changes in Stroke Volume from the Aortic Pulse Contour in Man.' *J. appl. Physiol.* **5**, 495

Warren, J. V., Brannon, E. S., Weens, H. S. and Stead, E. A. Jr. (1948). 'Effect of Increasing the Blood Volume and Right Atrial Pressure on the Circulation of Normal Subjects by Intravenous Infusion.' *Am. J. Med.* **4**, 193

Watson, W. E., Seelye, E. and Smith, A. C. L. (1962). 'The Action of Thiopentone on the Vascular Distensibility of the Hand.' *Br. J. Anaesth.* **34**, 19

Weideman, M. P. (1963). 'Dimensions of Blood Vessels from Distributing Artery to Collecting Vein.' *Circulation Res.* **12**, 375

Weideman, M. P. (1967). 'Architecture of the Terminal Vascular Bed.' In Reeve, E. B. and Guyton, A. C., *Physical Bases of Circulatory Transport*, p. 307. Philadelphia; Saunders

Weiderhielm, C. A. (1967). 'Analysis of Small Vessel Function.' In Reeve, E. G. and Guyton, A. C., *Physical Bases of Circulatory Transport*, p. 313. Philadelphia; Saunders

Webster, M. E. and Pierce, J. V. (1963). 'The Nature of the Kallidins Released from Human Plasma by Kallikreins and other Enzymes.' *Ann. N.Y. Acad. Sci.* **104**, 91

Weissler, A. M., Harris, W. S. and Schoenfeld, C. D. (1969). 'Bedside Technics for the Evaluation of Ventricular Function in Man.' *Am. J. Cardiol.* **23**, 577

Weissler, A. M., Peeler, R. G. and Roehill, W. H. (1961). 'Relationships between Left Ventricular Ejection Time, Stroke Volume and Heart Rate in Normal Individuals and Patients with Cardiovascular Disease. *Am. Heart. J.* **62**, 367

West, J. B. (1966). 'Regional Differences in Blood Flow and Ventilation in the Lung.' In Caro, C. G. (Ed.), *Advances in Respiratory Physiology*, p. 198. London; Edward Arnold

West, J. B. and Dollery, C. T. (1965). 'Distribution of Blood Flow and the Pressure-flow Relations of the Whole Lung.' *J. appl. Physiol.* **20**, 175

Westgate, H. D., Gordon, J. R. and Bergen, F. H. van (1962). 'Changes in Airway Resistance Following Intravenously Administered d-Tubocurarine.' *Anesthesiology* **23**, 65

White, C. de B. and Udwadia, B. P. (1975). 'β-Adrenoceptors in the Human Dorsal Hand Vein, and the Effects of Propranolol and Practolol on Venous Sensitivity to Noradrenaline.' *Br. J. clin. Pharmac.* **2**, 99

Whitney, R. J. (1953). 'The Measurement of Volume Changes in Human Limbs.' *J. Physiol.* **121**, 1

Whittaker, S. R. F. and Winton, F. R. (1933). 'The Apparent Viscosity of Blood Flowing in the Isolated Hind Limb of the Dog, and its Variation with Corpuscular Concentration.' *J. Physiol.* **78**, 339

Whitteridge, D. (1960). 'Cardiovascular Reflexes Initiated from Afferent Sites other than the Cardiovascular System Itself.' *Physiol. Rev.* **40** (Suppl. 4), 198

Whittingham, H. E. (1938). 'Preventive Medicine in Relation to Aviation.' *Proc. roy. Soc. Med.* **32**, 455

Wiggers, C. J. and Werle, J. M. (1942). 'Cardiac and Peripheral Resistance Factors as Determinants of Circulatory Failure in Hemorrhagic Shock.' *Am. J. Physiol.* **136**, 421

Wildenthal, K., Mierzwiak, D. S., Myers, R. W. and Mitchell, J. H. (1968). 'Effects of Acute Lactic Acidosis on Left Ventricular Performance.' *Am. J. Physiol.* **214**, 1352

Winsor, T. and Burch, G. E. (1945). 'Phlebostatic Axis and Phlebostatic Level, Reference Levels for Venous Pressure Measurements in Man.' *Proc. Soc. exp. Biol. Med. N.Y.* **58**, 165

Wollman, H., Smith, T. C., Stephen, G. W., Colton, E. T., Gleaton, H. E. and

Alexander, S. C. (1968). 'Effects of Extremes of Respiratory and Metabolic Alkalosis on Cerebral Blood Flow in Man.' *J. appl. Physiol.* **24**, 60

Womersley, J. R. (1955). 'Method for the Calculation of Velocity, Rate of Flow and Viscous Drag in Arteries when the Pressure Gradient is Known.' *J. Physiol.* **127**, 553

Wong, K. C., Martin, W. E., Hornbein, T. F., Freund, F. G. and Everett, J. (1973). 'The Cardiovascular Effects of Morphine Sulfate with Oxygen and with Nitrous Oxide in Man.' *Anesthesiology* **38**, 542

Wood, E. H., Bowers, D., Shepherd, J. T. and Fox, I. J. (1955). 'O_2 Content of "Mixed" Venous Blood in Man during various Phases of the Respiratory and Cardiac Cycles in Relation to Possible Errors in Measurement of Cardiac Output by Conventional Application of the Fick Method.' *J. appl. Physiol.* **7**, 621

Wood, J. E. (1968). 'The Venous System.' *Sci. Am.* **218**, 86

Wood, J. E., Litter, J. and Wilkins, R. W. (1956). 'Peripheral Venoconstriction in Human Congestive Heart Failure.' *Circulation* **13**, 524

Woodbury, J. W. (1962). 'Cellular Electrophysiology of the Heart.' In *Handbook of Physiology, Circulation, Vol. 1*, p. 237. Washington; American Physiological Society

Woodbury, J. W. (1965). 'The Cell Membrane: Ionic and Potential Gradients and Active Transport.' In Ruch, T. C. and Patton, H. D., *Physiology and Biophysics*, p. 1. Philadelphia; Saunders

Woodbury, J. W. and Crill, W. E. (1961). In Florey, E., *Nervous Inhibition*, p. 124. New York; Pergamon

Wright, J. T. M. (1972). 'The Heart, its Valves and their Replacement.' *Biomed. Eng.* **7**, 26

Wyant, C. M., Merriman, J. E., Kilduff, C. J. and Thomas, E. T. (1958). 'The Cardiovascular Effects of Halothane.' *Can. Anaesth. Soc. J.* **5**, 384

Zahony, I., Winnie, A. P., Rosello, L. and Collins, V. J. (1964). 'The CPZ Test. A Bedside Method of Estimating Blood Volume.' AMA 113th Annual Convention. San Francisco

Zierler, K. L. (1962). 'Theoretical Basis of Indicator-dilution Methods for Measuring Flow and Volume.' *Circulation Res.* **10**, 393

Zweifach, B. W. (1959). 'The Microcirculation of the Blood.' *Sci. Am.* **200**, 54

Zweifach, B. W. (1974). 'Mechanisms of Blood Flow and Fluid Exchange in Microvessels.' *Anesthesiology* **41**, 157

Index

311